U0233532

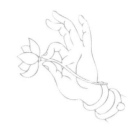

中国针灸

（中英双语版）

主编 张卫东 王丕敏

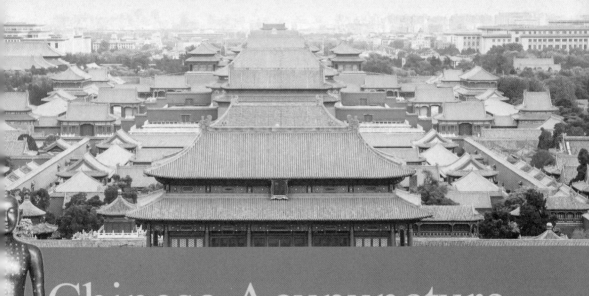

Chinese Acupuncture and Moxibustion

山西出版传媒集团　　山西科学技术出版社

编委会名单

主　编：张卫东　王丕敏

副主编：王麒琰　杜宇征

编　委：乔　丽　陈雪玲　巴　特　田　雨

　　　　杨　凯　刘文晶

编者的话

张卫东，女，54岁，教授，主任医师，硕士生导师，中国工程院院士石学敏弟子，山西针灸学会理事，中国医疗保健国际交流促进会中医药质量优化分会常务委员。自1989年以优异成绩从天津中医学院（现为天津中医药大学）针灸推拿专业毕业后，一直忙碌在针灸推拿领域的教育教学和临床工作的第一线，辛勤育人，扎实临床。从教31年来，培育了一大批中医药事业的优秀接班人，同时在中医针灸的对外交流工作中表现突出。

1998年至今，我一直受邀担任山西省卫计委（原山西省卫生厅）国际交流中心承办的国家商务部援外针灸推拿培训项目的任课教师，并一步步从助教、主讲教师成长为课程负责人。至今，已圆满完成了36期的培训任务，共培训针灸推拿技术人员和中医爱好者1095名，学员来自亚、非、欧、美、大洋洲以及加勒比海的100多个发展中国家和地区，授课语言涉及英语、法语和葡萄牙语，其中英语针灸推拿培训班，我全程用英文授课。授课内容涵盖了中医基础理论、经络腧穴、刺法灸法、针灸治疗学、临床示教等各种中医培训课程，获得了外国学员的一致好评和省卫计委相关领导的高度赞誉，每年被学员评为最优秀授课教师。

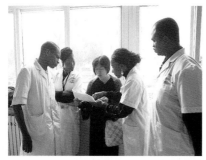
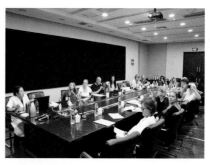
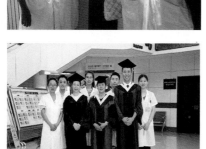
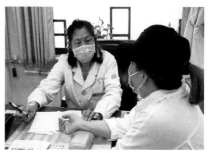
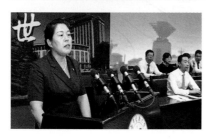

　　从教31年，中医针灸双语教学和对外交流成为我职业生涯的重要组成部分。在与前来学习的外国友人交谈的过程中，我了解到选择来华学习中医针灸的大多是没有中医学背景的临床技师，甚至是没有医学背景的中医爱好者。他们被中医针灸简、便、廉、验的特点所吸引，渴望把针灸推拿技术带回本国运用于临床。这些学员都面临一个共同的问题：中医基础知识薄弱，培训时间不足。学员们希望能够在有限的时间内获得最有价值的知识，掌握最实用的技能。他们多次向我提出希望有一本综合实用的教材供他们学习以及回国后随时查阅。经过三年多的筹备，这本综合了中医基础理论、中医诊断学、针灸学、经络腧穴学、针灸处方学等多方面内容的综合双

语教材终于完成。希望仅以此书给来华学习针灸推拿技术的外国友人以及肩负针灸推拿对外交流任务的各位同仁提供参考。

张卫东

2020 年 6 月

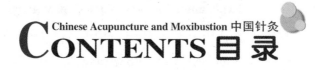

CONTENTS 目录

Chinese Acupuncture and Moxibustion 中国针灸

Chinese Acupuncture

中国针灸

Chinese Acupuncture and Moxibustion

Part 1

Important Knowledge Points of Basic Theory of Traditional Chinese Medicine (TCM)

To master the basic theory of TCM and the basic knowledge of TCM diagnostics

❖ 1. Basic characteristics of theoretical system of Traditional Chinese Medicine

❖ 2. *Yin-yang* Theory

❖ 3. Five-element Theory

❖ 4. The Theory of visceral manifestation (*Zang-xiang* Theory)

❖ 5. *Qi* and Blood Theory

❖ 6. Causes of Disease (Etiology Theory)

❖ 7. The four diagnostic methods

❖ 8. Syndrome Differentiation Principles

Knowledge point 1   Basic characteristics of theoretical system of Traditional Chinese Medicine

The theoretical system of Traditional Chinese Medicine (TCM) has evolved in the long course of clinical practice under the guidance of classic Chinese materialism and dialectics. It originates from practice and, in turn, guides the practice. This unique theoretical system is essentially characterized by the concept of holism and treatment based on syndrome differentiation.

1. The Concept of holism

The holism means that the human body is an organic whole and that human beings are interrelated with nature.

1. 1 The unity within the body

TCM believes that the human body is composed of various tissues and organs. These different tissues and organs are united into an organic whole. They are closely related to each other in structure, physiology, pathology, diagnosis and treatment.

1. 1. 1 The unity of the structure

The component parts of the body are inseparable from each other. The unity of the structure is realized through the five-*zang* organs, with the assistance of the six-*fu* organs and the communications of the meridian system. (Table 1-1-1)

1. 1. 2 The unity of physiological functions

Each of the visceral organs has its own functions. Each of the visceral organs is related, subsided and conditioned by the others. The heart controls all the physiological functions.

1. 1. 3 The unity of pathology

The disease transmits among the visceral organs. The disease transmits from visceral organs to other structures.

1. 1. 4 The unity of the diagnosis

The four diagnosis methods include inspection, auscultation and olfaction, inquiry as well as pulse-taking and palpation. The human body is an organic whole. Local pathological changes may affect the viscera and the whole body and can be detected from the manifestations of the sensory organs, limbs and surface of body.

1. 1. 5 The unity of the treatment

Since the human body is an organic whole, treatment of a local disease has to take the whole body into consideration.

Table 1 – 1 – 1 The unity of the structure

system	five-*zang*	six-*fu*	five constituents	five sensory organs	meridians and collaterals
Heart system	Heart	Small-intestine	Vessel	Tongue	Heart meridian of hand *shaoyin* Small intestine meridian of hand-*shaoyang*
Liver system	Liver	Gllbladder	Tendon	Eyes	Liver meridian of foot-*jueyin* Gallbladder meridian of foot-*shaoyang*
Spleen system	Spleen	Spleen	Muscle	Mouse	Spleen meridian of foot-*taiyin* Stomach meridian of foot-*yangming*

Continued

Lung system	Lung	Large intestine	Skin	Nose	Lung meridian of hand-*taiyin* Large intestine meridian of hand-*yangming*
system	five-*zang*	six-*fu*	five con-stituents	five sens-ory organs	meridians and collaterals
Kidney system	Kidney	Bladder	Bone	Ears and the external genitals and the anus	Kidney meridian of foot-*shaoyin* Bladder meridian of foot-*taiyang*

1. 2 The unity within the nature

Human beings live in nature and nature provides them with various necessities, such as sunlight, air and water. On the other hand, various changes taking place in nature may directly or indirectly affect the human body and bring on corresponding physiological or pathological responses. Geographical conditions, similar to the seasonal variations, also affect the physiological activity and pathological state of the body.

2. Treatment based upon syndrome differentiation

Treatment based upon syndrome differentiation is the distinguishing feature of TCM and represents the application of TCM theories in clinical practice. It can be divided into two stages. The first one is syndrome differentiation and the second is treatment. Syndrome differentiation means that the clinical data collected by the four diagnostic techniques and the patient's symptoms and signs detected are analyzed and summarized in order to identify the location, cause, property and the relationship of the evils and body resistance, thus establishing a diagnosis. Treatment means that a proper therapeutic program is drown up according to the diagnosis made.

Knowledge point 2 *Yin-yang* Theory

1. Conception of *Yin-yang*

Yin-yang is the generalization for the two aspects of some things or phenomena which are interrelated in the natural world. *Yin* and *yang* represent not only two inter-opposite things or forces, but also the two inter-opposite aspects existing within one object.

The properties of things signified by *yin* and *yang* are quite abstract. In order to make the meaning of *yin* and *yang* explicit, people in ancient China used specific things, namely water and fire, as metaphors to analogize. (Table 1 – 2 – 1)

Table 1 – 2 – 1 The categorization of things according to *Yin-yang*

yang	invigorate	warm	excited	function
yin	accumulate	moist	depressed	material

yang	active	external	upward	hot	bright	functional	hyper-functional
yin	static	internal	downward	cold	dark	substantial	hypo-functional

2. Interactions between *Yin* and *Yang*

The *yin* and *yang* aspects within an object or phenomena are not simply arbitrary divisions. In fact they are in constant and complicated interactions. The interactions between *yin* and *yang* are various in manifestations. The following is a brief description of the major ones.

2. 1 Opposition of *Yin* and *Yang*

Yin-yang theory holds that everything in nature has two opposite aspects, namely *yin* and *yang*, which are mainly manifested in their mutual strugle and restriction. The opposition of *yin* and *yang* leads to the restriction. The restriction keeps the dynamic equilibrium. Dynamic equilibrium keeps the unities exist.

2. 2 Interdependence between *Yin* and *Yang*

Yin and *yang* not only oppose but also contain each other. Any aspect of them can not exist singly without the other one, and each must take the other as the prerequisite for its existence. This relationship is known as the interdependence of *yin* and *yang*.

2. 3 Wane and wax between *Yin* and *Yang*

Wane and wax between *yin* and *yang* implies that, in the interaction between *yin* and *yang*, one side is developing while the other side is declining and vice verse. Normally, alternation and repetition of wane and wax maintain a dynamic balance between *yin* and *yang*. If the state of wane and wax between *yin* and *yang* exceeds the normal level, relative predominance or relative decline of either *yin* or *yang* will arise, consequently damaging the dynamic balance between *yin* and *yang* and leading to imbalance of *yin* and *yang*.

2. 4 Mutual transformation between *Yin* and *Yang*

If *yin* or *yang* wanes or waxes to the extreme point, it will turn to the opposite. That means *yin* will change into *yang* and *yang* into *yin*. The key element involved in such a mutual transformation is the degree of wane and wax. The degree that leads to transformation is termed "extreme point" or "excess" in TCM.

3. Application of the theory of *Yin* and *Yang* in TCM

3.1 Explain the histological structure of human body

TCM believe that the human body is an organic whole. The histological structure is organically connected, and can be divided into opposite *Yin-yang* parts according to their location and functional characteristics.

3.1.1 According to anatomical locality

Table 1 −2 −2 Explain the *Yin* and *Yang* attributes of histological structure according to anatomical locality

yang	the upper part of the body	exterior	lateral aspects of limbs
yin	the lower part of the body	interior	medial aspects of limbs

3.1.2 According to viscera function

The five-*zang* organs pertain to *yin* because they store essence, but never discharge it. The six-*fu* organs pertain to *yang* because they transport and transform food, but never store it. Among the five-*zang* organs, the heart and lung are located in the chest, so they pertain to *yang*. But the live, the spleen and the kidney are located in the abdomen, so they pertain to *yin*. Each organ itself can be further divided into *yin* and *yang* aspects, such as heart-*yin* and heart-*yang*, kidney-*yin* and kidney-*yang*, etc.

Table 1 – 2 – 3 Explain the *Yin* and *Yang* attributes of histological structure according to viscera function

yang	six-*fu*	small intestine, large intestine, stomach, gallbladder and bladder			each *zang* organs, *fu* organs can be further divided into *yin* and *yang* parts, like *kidney-yang* and *kidney-yin*
yin	five-*zang*	in the chest (*yang*)	heart	*yang* within *yang*	
			lung	*yin* within *yang*	
		in the abdomen (*yin*)	liver	*yang* within *yin*	
			spleen	*zhi-yin* within *yin*	
			kidney	*yin* within *yin*	

3. 1. 3 Divide meridians

Table 1 – 2 – 4 *Yin* and *Yang* attributes of meridians

meridians	*yang* meridians	travel in the lateral aspects of limbs and back
	yin meridians	travel in the medial aspects of limbs and abdomen

3. 1. 4 Divide *qi*-blood-body fluid

The theory of *yin* and *yang* holds that the normal activities of life result from the balance between *yin* and *yang* and that the close relationship between histological structure and physiological functions signifies the opposition and the unity between *yin* and *yang*. The histological structure of the body pertains to *yin* because they are all substantial. However, their functions all pertain to *yang*.

Table 1 – 2 – 5 *Yin* and *Yang* attributes of *qi*-blood-body fluid

yang	*qi*	representing the physiological function of the body
yin	blood and body fluid	representing the material basis of human body

3. 2 Explanation of the physiological function of human body

The physiological functions of the human body are based on the storage of the essence and the movement of *qi* within the meridians and *zang-fu* organs. Essence is stored in the *zang-fu* organs and belongs to *yin*. *Qi* transformed by essence is circulating around the whole body continually and belongs to *yang*. The mutual reinforcement and promotion of essence and *qi* maintain the stable and orderly function of the viscera, orifices and meridians. The normal physiological function of the human body is the result of the dynamic balance of *yin* and *yang* in the body.

3. 3 Explanation of pathogenesis

When the balance between *yin* and *yang* in the body is damaged, it leads to various diseases known as "imbalance between *yin* and *yang*". Complicated pathological changes generally fall into two categories: relative predominance of *yin* or *yang* and relative decline of *yin* or *yang*, according to the analysis of pathogenesis with the theory of *yin* and *yang*.

3. 3. 1 Relative predominance of *yin* or *yang*

Relative predominance of *yin* and *yang*, refers to *yin* exuberant or *yang* exuberant, belongs to the disease that *yin* or *yang* is excess beyond normal level.

(1) Relative predominance of *yang*.

Relative predominance of *yang*, usually caused by invasion of pathogenic factors of *yang* nature, is a manifestation of excess-heat syndrome known as "predominance of *yang* leading to heat" in *Inner Canon of Yellow Emperor*.

(2) Relative predominance of *yin*.

Relative predominance of *yin* is usually caused by invasion of pathogenic factors of *yin* nature, leading to exuberance of *yin*-cold and bringing on excess cold syndrome known as "predominance of *yin* leading to cold "in *Inner Canon of Yellow Emperor*.

3. 3. 2 Relative decline of *yin* or *yang*

Relative decline of *yin* or *yang* refers to *yin* deficiency or *yang* deficiency, belongs to the disease that *yin* or *yang* is insufficient beyond normal level.

(1) Relative decline of *yang*.

Refers to deficiency-cold syndrome due to insufficiency of *yang-qi* that fails to restrain *yin*-cold and warm the visceral organs.

(2) Relative decline of *yin*.

Relative decline of *yin* refers to deficiency-heat syndrome due to insufficiency of *yin*-fluid that fails to restrain *yang*-heat and nourish the visceral organs.

3. 4 Application to clinical diagnosis and syndrome differentiation

The occurrence, development and changes of the diseases, according to the theory of *yin* and *yang*, lie in the imbalance between *yin* and *yang*. Generally all kinds of diseases, including pathological changes of complexion, voice and pulse condition as well as the nature of diseases, can be generalized and analyzed with the theory of *yin* and *yang*.

Diagnostically, the theory of *yin* and *yang* can be used to analyze the data collected with the four diagnostic methods and differentiate the nature of disease.

3. 5 Guiding clinical treatment and herb application

3. 5. 1 Making the therapeutic principles

(1) Therapeutic principles for relative predominance of *yin* and *yang*: "excess should be reduced".

(2) Therapeutic principles for relative decline of *yin* and *yang*: "deficiency should be supplemented".

3. 5. 2 Generalization of the properties of drugs

TCM believes that all drugs possess four properties, five flavors and act-ing tendencies (namely ascending, descending, sinking and floating) which are generalized according to the theory of *yin* and *yang*.

Knowledge point 3   Five-element Theory

1. The interpretation of the five-element theory

In Chinese, "*Wu*" refers to five categories of things in the nature world, namely wood, fire, earth, metal and water. "*Xing*" means movement and transformation. So the five elements refer to the movement and transformation of these five elements as well as their interrelationship.

2. The Conception of the five-element theory

The five-element theory is to summarize the attributes of things and phenomena according to the functional properties of five kinds of matter: wood, fire, earth, gold and water. The mutual promotion and mutual restraint among these five elements is used to explain and deduct the relationship between things and the complex laws of movement among them. The five-element theory, an ancient Chinese philosophical thought, has been introduced into the theory of traditional Chinese medicine to analyz the functional activities and internal connection of *zang-fu* organs, meridians, body structure, orifice and mental emotions. The five-element theory is widely used to guidance Diagnosis and prevention of diseases.

"Wood" stands for germinating, stretching, and smoothing. "Fire" for warming, flaming upward, and burning. "Earth" for growing, bearing, and supplying. "Metal" for solidity, purging, and changing. "Water" for moistening, cooling, and flowing downward. These characteristics were used to illustrate and correlate different types of matter.

3. Categorization of things according to the properties of the five-element

The five-element theory holds that all objects and phenomena of nature and man can be classified into five categories according to the characteristics of the five-element mentioned above. (Table 1 −3 −1, Table 1 −3 −2)

Table 1 −3 −1 Five-element Attribute Classification of Things

nature						five-element
five musical notes	five flavors	five colors	five trans-formation	five kinds of *qi*	five seasons	
jue	sour	cyan (blue)	germina-tion	wind	spring	wood
zhi	bitter	red	growth	heat (summer heat)	summer	fire
gong	sweet	yellow	trans-formation	dampness	late summer	earth
shang	pungent	white	reaping	dryness	autumn	metal
yu	salty	black	storing	cold	winter	water

Table 1 −3 −2 Five-element Attribute Classification of Human Body

human body							
five element	five-*zang* organ	five-*fu* organs	five sensories	five emotions	five con-stituents	five kinds of liquids	five tastes of pulse
wood	liver	gall-bladder	eye	anger	tendon	tear	taut
fire	heart	small intestine	tongue	joy	vessel	sweating	bounding
earth	spleen	stomach	mouth	contem-plation	muscle	saliva	moderate

Continued

human body							
metal	lung	large intestine	nose	grief	skin & hair	snivel	superficial
water	kidney	urinary bladder	ear	fear	bone	spittle	deep

4. Interactions among the five-element

Five-element possess specific properties respectively. They are related to each other and act on each other. The interactions among the five-element are either normal or abnormal. The former includes inter-promotion and inter-restraint and the latter includes over-restraint and reverse restraint which are actually the abnormal manifestations of inter-restraint.

4.1 Inter-promotion and inter-restraint among the five-element

4. 1. 1 Inter-promotion

Inter-promotion means that one thing can promote, produce and assistant another one in the five-element. The order of inter-promotion among the five-element follows certain rules and forms a circle, i. e, wood promoting fire, fire promoting earth, earth promoting metal, metal promoting water, and water promoting wood.

4. 1. 2 Inter-restraint

Inter-restraint means that one thing can restrict, conquer and suppress another one in the five-element. The order of inter-restraint among the five-element follows certain rules and forms a circle, i. e, wood restraining earth, earth restraining water, water restraining fire, fire restraining metal, metal restraining wood.

4. 1. 3 The relationship between inter-promotion and inter-restraint

Both inter-promotion and inter-restraint among the five-element are indispensable relationships by which living things exist and move normally. Without inter-promotion there would be no birth and development. Without inter-restraint, there will be no way to prevent harm caused by excessive development of things. Only when restraint exists in promotion and promotion in restraint can the normal development and harmonious balance of thing be maintained.

4. 2 Over-restraint and reverse restraint

4. 2. 1 Over-restraint

Over-restraint refers to an abnormal state in which one element among the five-element excessively restrains another element. The order of inter-restraint among the five elements is the same as that of inter-restraint.

4. 2. 2 Reverse-restraint

Reverse-restraint refers to an abnormal state in which one element among the Five-element reversely restrains and bullies another element. The order of reverse-restraint is just the opposite of that of inter-restraint.

4. 3 Application of the five-element theory in TCM

4. 3. 1 Explaining the physiological functions of the five-*zang* organs and the relationships among them

The theory of the five-element explains the physiological characteristics and functions of the five-*zang* organs according to the attributes of the five-element, pairing each of the five-*zang* organs with the corresponding one of the five-element.

Some of the intrinsic relationships among the functional activities of the five-*zang* organs also reflect the relationship of inter-promotion and inter-restraint among the five-element. So they can be explained with the theory of inter-promotion and inter-restraint among the five-element.

4. 3. 2 Explaining pathogenesis transmission among the five-*zang* organs

The *zang-fu* organs are related to each other and act on each other. When one organ is disorder, other organs will be affected. Such pathological interaction is called pathogenesis transmission. The law of pathogenesis transmission can be described with the inter-promotion and inter-restraint among the five-element.

(1) Pathogenesis transmission according to inter-promotion.

Mutual involvement or affection of the mother-organs and the child-organs reflects pathological transmission due to abnormal change of inter-promotion relationship.

Disorder of the mother-organs involving or affecting the child-organs means that the disease is transmitted from the mother-organs into the child-organs.

Disorder of the child-organs involving or affecting the mother-organs indicates that disease is transmitted from the child-organs to the mother-organs. Such a transmission is also known as " the child-organs consuming*qi*of the mother-organs".

(2) Pathogenesis transmission according to over-restraint and reverse-restraint.

Over-restraint and reverse-restraint are pathological transmissions due to abnormal change of inter-restraint relationship. Over-restraint refers to transmission of disease due to excessive restraint. Reverse-restraint refers to transmission of disease due to opposite restraint.

4. 3. 3 Guiding the diagnosis and treatment

(1) Guiding the clinical diagnosis.

Since the five-*zang* organs pair with the five-element, the five colors, the five flavors and the five pulses respectively, and because the disorders of the internal organs can manifest on the surface of the body, clinically the theory of the five-element can be used to analyze the changes of complexion, taste and pulse in order to decide which viscus and meridian are involved.

(2) Guiding the treatment of disease.

In the treatment of disease, the theory of five-element is mainly used to control the disease transmission and decide therapeutic principles.

Knowledge point 4   The Theory of visceral manifestation (*Zang-xiang* Theory)

The term "*zang*" refers to viscera which are seated in the interior of the body, and "*xiang*" refers to the physiological and pathological activities of the viscera which appear exteriorly. *Zang-fu* organs are classified into three categories according to their functional features, which are the five-*zang* organs, the six-*fu* organs, and the extraordinary *fu* organs.

The five-*zang* organs include the heart, the lung, the liver, the spleen and the kidney. The five-*zang* organs produce and store vital essence, *qi*, and mind. The six-*fu* organs in TCM include the gall bladder, stomach, large intestine, small intestine, bladder and triple energizer. Their common physiological function is to transport and digest food stuff, and excrete the waste. The extraordinary *fu* organs are similar to the *fu* organs in morphology but store vital essence like and subordinate to the five-*zang* organs. The extra ordinary *fu* organs include the brain, marrow, bone, blood vessels, gallbladder and uterus. In morphology, most of these organs are hollow and are similar to the six-*fu* viscera. however, they function in storing the essential *qi*, and this is similar to the five-*zang* viscera.

◆Five-*zang* System

1. Heart

The heart occupies the first place among the five-*zang* organs and governs the life activities of the whole body. That is why it is said that the heart is "an organ of monarch" in Inner Canon of Yellow Emperor.

1. 1 Physiological functions of the heart

1. 1. 1 Governing the blood and vessels

It means that heart-*qi* keeps the heart beating normally and propelling the blood flow through the vessels to nourish and moist all the components of the body.

1. 1. 2 Controlling the mind (storing the spirit)

It means that the heart can produce and dominate human body, spirit, consciousness and thinking. It also can regulate the other viscera to keep harmony.

1. 2 The relationships between the heart and the body, the sensory organs and the orifices, and emotions

1. 2. 1 The heart governs the vessels

In structure, the heart is directly connected with the vessels. In function, the heart propels blood to flow inside the vessels by beating. In fact normal blood circulation is maintained by the heart and vessels working together. Pulse shape can reflect the functional state of the heart governing the blood.

1. 2. 2 External manifestation on the face

Since the condition of heart-*qi*, heart-blood, heart-*yin* and heart-*yang* mainly display on the face, observation of facial color and expressions can reflect the functional state of the heart.

1. 2. 3 The heart opens into the tongue

The idea that the heart opens into the tongue indicates that there is a special relationship between the heart and the tongue. The state of the tongue can reflect the physiological functions and pathological changes of the heart because a branch of the heart meridian runs into the tongue.

1. 2. 4 The heart is responsible for joy

Normal joy promotes the harmony of *qi* and blood of body, benefits the heart functions. Excess joy hurts the heart and leads to the heart *qi* slack, the patient cannot concentrate on anything, even crazy.

2. Pericardium

The concept is closely related to the heart, and its stipulated main function is to protect the heart from attacks by Exterior Pathogenic Factors. Like the heart, the Pericardium governs blood and stores the mind. The Pericardium's corresponding *yang* meridian is assigned to the *Sanjiao* (triple energizer). The Pericardium is not distinguished from the heart. It is also the first line of defense against the heart from external pathogenic influences.

3. Lung

The lung's location is highest among the internal organs. It is compared to a "canopy". The lung is delicate, intolerable to cold and heat, and is easy to be attacked by pathogenic factors. That is why it is called "delicate organ".

3. 1 Physiological functions of the lung

3. 1. 1 Domination of *qi*

It implies that the *qi* of the whole body is dominated and controlled by the lung. It includes two aspects: dominating the *qi* of respiration, and dominating the *qi* of the whole body.

(1) The lung dominates the *qi* of respiration.

It means that the inhalation and exhalation all depend on the function of the lung. The lung is a place of exchanging *qi* between interior and exterior of the body.

(2) The lung dominates the *qi* of whole body.

It implies that the lung controls and regulates the *qi* of visceral organs and meridians. It includes three aspects: the formation of *qi*, regulation of *qi* activity and assisting the heart to promote blood circulation.

3. 1. 2 Dominating of dispersing and depurative descending function

Dominating dispersing function here means that the lung has physiological functions characterized by upward dispersion and distribution. This function of the lung depends on the exhaling function of the lung.

Dominating depurative descending function means cleaning and descending, and "cleaning" also contains elimination in meaning, clearing away poison-evil and getting rid of foreign bodies. The descending of lung-*qi* can ensure deep, even and smooth breath. This function depends on the inhaling function of lung.

3. 1. 3 Regulation of water passage

The lung governing the regulation of water passage refers to the function of the lung in propelling, adjusting and discharging water.

After taken into the body, water is absorbed by means of transportation and transformation of spleen, and then transmitted upwards to the lung. On the one hand, lung-*qi*, by means of dispersing to the upper and external, transmits water to the surface of the body and transforms it into sweat to be discharged. At the same time, part of the water is excreted through respiration. On the other hand, lung-*qi*, by means of descending to the lower and internal, transmits water to the viscera and then to the kidney where it is transformed into urine to be excreted out of body. Besides, the descending function of the lung assists the large intestine in transmission, through which part of the water is discharged in defecation.

3. 2 The relationships between the lung and the body, the sensory organs and the orifices, and emotions

3. 2. 1 The lung governing the skin

The relationship between the lung and skin can be understood from the following two aspects. One is that the lung can disperse and transport the *wei-qi*(defensive-*qi*) and body fluid to the skin to warm, nourish and moisten the skin so as to maintain the normal function of the skin. The other is that the normal opening and closing activities of the sweat pores on the skin can excrete sweat, adjust body temperature, assist the lung to respire and discharge the turbid *qi*.

3. 2. 2 External manifestation on the body hair

Since the lung dominates the skin, the defensive *qi* and body fluid dispersed by the lung nourish the skin and the body hair. With proper nourishment of the defensive *qi* and body fluid, the body hair appears lustrous and is not easy to lose. Thus the condition of the body hair reflects the functional states of the lung.

3. 2. 3 The lung opening into the nose

The nose is a route for air to be breathed in and out of the body. Since the lung controls respiration and dominates *qi* in the whole body, so the nose is called "the outward orifice of lung".

3. 2. 4 The lung being responsible for grief

The lung's function has the relationship with the emotional activities of grief.

4. Spleen

The spleen governs digestion and absorption. As the source of *qi*, blood and body fluid, the spleen plays a vital role in maintaining life activity. Such a function of the spleen only comes into play after birth. So TCM regards the spleen as "the acquired base of life" and "the source of qi, blood and body fluid".

4. 1 Physiological functions of the spleen

4. 1. 1 Governing transportation and transformation

The function of the spleen to govern transportation and transformation means that the spleen can digest food, absorb nutrients of food and drink, and then transport them to the heart and lung. The function of the spleen to govern transportation and transformation are usually divided into two parts: transporting and transforming food nutrients, transporting and transforming drink.

4. 1. 2 In charge of "elevation"

It means that the spleen function is characterized by leading up and ascending. It includes two aspects: the first one is to send the essence of food and drink upward (the spleen governs the activity of elevating the lucid). The second one means to lift and fixate so as to keep the internal organs in their fixed positions.

4. 1. 3 Commanding blood

It means that the spleen functions in controlling the blood circulation inside the vessels and prevent it from flowing out of the vessels.

4. 2 The relationships between the spleen and the body, the sensory organs and the orifices, and emotions

4. 2. 1 The spleen governing the muscles and the extremities

The spleen-qi distributes the essence of food and drink to the muscles and limbs to nourish them.

4. 2. 2 The spleen opens to the mouth

The mouth is the starting point of the digestive canal. Since digestion is governed by the spleen, the mouth is the orifice into which the spleen opens. The state of diets and appetite are related to the physiological function of the spleen.

4. 2. 3 The external manifestation on the lips

The functional state of the spleen can be reflected on the lips. The lips are nourished by the essence of food and drink and the spleen is the source of essence of food and drink.

4. 2. 4 The spleen being responsible for contemplation

Excessive contemplation affects the function of spleen, leads to stagnation of spleen-*qi*.

5. Liver

The physiological characteristics of the liver are that "pertains to *yin* in entity and *yang* in function". As one of the five-*zang* organs, the liver pertain to *yin* because it stores *yin*-blood. However, in function the liver pertains to *yang* because *yang-qi* in the liver is very active and resolute, tending to disperse. That is why the liver is described as "general-organs".

5. 1 Physiological functions of the liver

5. 1. 1 To dredge and regulate

It means the liver dredges the routes and regulates the *qi* activity so as to ensure smooth flow of *qi* in the body. The function of the liver to regulate *qi* activity is demonstrated in the following aspects.

(1)To promote circulation of blood and metabolism of body fluid.

Blood circulation and body fluid metabolism all depend on the propelling function of the visceral qi, the normal flow of which relies on the regulating and dredging function of the liver which are prerequisite to constant blood circulation and normal metabolism of body fluid.

(2)To assist the spleen and the stomach to digest food.

The liver regulates the activity of spleen-qi and stomach-qi with its dredging and regulating functions, ensuring a harmonious balance between the function of spleen-qi to elevate the lucid and the function of the stomach-qi to descend the turbid so as to guarantee a normal process of digestion. Besides, the bile accumulation of surplus liver-qi, comes from the liver and excretes into small intestine to assist digestion. The normal secretion and excretion of the bile are closely related to the dredging and regulating functions of the liver.

(3)To regulate mental activity.

Mental activity, part of spiritual activity, is dominated by the heart and closely related to the dredging and regulating functions of the liver. The normal mental activity depends on sufficiency of blood and smooth activity of qi which can be promoted by the liver.

(4)To regulate menstruation.

The physiological characteristics of women, such as menstruation, pregnancy and delivery, are closely related to blood. The liver regulates the activity of qi to enable blood to flow downward into the uterus to meet the need for menstruation, pregnancy and delivery.

5. 1. 2 To store blood

The liver storing blood means that the liver is capable of storing blood, regulating its volume in circulation and preventing from hemorrhage. If the function of the liver to store blood is in disorder, it may lead to two kinds of pathological changes. One is insufficiency of liver-blood. In this case the body cannot get enough nourishment, leading to dizziness, vertigo, weakness of limbs, scanty and light-colored menses or menorrhea. The other is failure of the liver to store blood which may lead to abnormal flow of blood, causing various symptoms such as hematemesis, epistaxis, and profuse menorrhea.

5. 2 The relationship between the liver and the body, the sensory organs and the orifices

5. 2. 1 The liver governing the tendons

The liver governing the tendons means that the physiological functions of the tendons depend on liver-blood to nourish and liver-*yin* to moisten.

5. 2. 2 The external manifestation of the liver on the nails

Nails include the fingernails and toenails. They are nourished by the liver-blood. So their formation and quality can reflect the functional state of liver-blood.

5. 2. 3 The liver opening into the eyes

The liver and the eyes are connected closely in physiology and pathology. The liver meridian runs upward into the eyes. The eyes are nourished by liver-*yin* and liver-blood. Besides, the liver can regulate the activities of the eyes with its dredging and regulating functions. Thus eyesight is closely related to the liver. The conditions of liver can be observed from the manifestations of eyes.

6. Kidney

The kidney is the source of genuine *yin* and genuine *yang*, so the kidney is closely related with the essence, *qi*, blood, *yin* and *yang*. Since the kidney-essence comes from parents and is the primary substance for constituting human body and conceiving new life. TCM regards the kidney as "the prenatal base of life".

6. 1 Physiological functions of the kidney

6. 1. 1 Kidney storing essence

The kidney stores essence. Essence has two meanings: In the narrow sense, it refers to the reproductive essence stored in the kidney, including the one inherited from the parents and the one proved by the spleen and the stomach. In the broad sense, it refers to all the essential materials of the body, including essence, marrow, *qi*, blood and body fluid, etc. The essence transforms *qi* and produces blood.

The main functions of the essence storage in the kidney are to promote growth and development, to govern reproduction and to participate in blood production.

(1)Governing growth and development.

The kidney stores essence, *qi*, *yin* and *yang*. The growth and development of the body mainly depend on the kidney-essence, kidney-*yin* and kidney-*yang*. After birth, the kidney-essence gradually becomes abundant with the development of the body. At different stages of life process, the body and its physiological functions vary with the changes of the essence in the kidney. That is to say that the essence, *qi*, *yin* and *yang* in the kidney decide the growth and development of the body.

(2)Governing reproduction.

The reproduction function includes the development of sex organs, maturity and maintenance of sex as well as fertility which are all closely related with the kidney-essence, kidney-*yin* and kidney-*yang*. When the body develops to the period of youth, the essence in the kidney enriches to a certain degree and produces a kind of reproductive substance known as *Tiangui* which can promote the development of sex organs and maintain normal sex function. Consequently man has sperm and experiences seminal emission, and woman has menarche. Man and woman maintain such a sex function and genitality after their middle age. At the period of old age, the kidney-essence gradually declines. Subsequently *Tiangui* becomes exhausted and, accordingly, genitality declines and disappears in the end.

(3) Participating in blood production.

The kidney stores essence and the essence stored in the kidney can produce marrow. The narrow produced by kidney can transform to blood. The marrow includes cerebral marrow, spinal cord and bone marrow.

6. 1. 2 Governing water

It implies that kidney manages and regulates the water metabolism of the human body. The metabolism of water is related to many organs like the lung that regulates water passage, the spleen that transports and transforms water, the liver that promotes the metabolism of water and the triple energizer that serves as the passage of water. However, the function of the kidney to govern water is key to the water metabolism. The kidney regulates the whole process of transporting and excreting water. The function of the kidney to govern water is accomplished with its function of *qi-hua* (*qi* transformation). With its function of *qi*-transformation, the kidney separates the lucid part of from the water and elevates it again to the lung to keep certain amount of water inside the body on the one hand, and transforms the rest part into urine to be transported to the bladder and excreted out of the body on the other.

6. 1. 3 Governing the reception of *qi*

Governing the reception of *qi* implies that the kidney has a physiological function in receiving fresh *qi* inhaled by the lung, and regulating respiration in order to prevent shallow breath and to maintain a normal exchange of gases outside and inside the body.

6. 1. 4 To nourish and warm the viscera

Kidney-*yin*, also known as primordial *yin* or genuine *yin*, can nourish *yin* in all the viscera, serving as the source of *yin*-fluid in the body. Kidney-*yang*, also known as primordial *yang* or genuine *yang*, can warm *yang* in all the viscera, serving as the source of *yang-qi* in the whole body.

6.2 The relationship between the kidney and the body, the sensory organs and the orifices

6.2.1 The kidney governing the bones

The kidney governing the bones means that the development and the function of the bones depend on the kidney-essence. The kidney stores essence and the essence can transform into bone marrow to nourish the bones, promote the growth and repair of the skeleton and strengthen the skeleton. The teeth are the extensions of the bones. Both bones and teeth need kidney-essence to nourish.

6.2.2 External manifestation on the hair

The hair is called "the extension of blood". It is nourished by the essence and blood. Kidney essence transforms into blood, both of them nourish the hair.

6.2.3 Opening into the ears, the external genitals and the anus

(1)Opening into the ears.

Kidney-essence produces marrow and the ears are connected with the cerebral marrow.

(2)Opening into the external genitals and anus.

It implies that the functions of discharging urine and reproduction of the external genitals and the functions of discharging stool of anus depend on the kidney. The relationship between the kidney and external genitals can be understood from the functions of the kidney to govern water and reproduction. The relationship between the kidney and anus refers to the fact that the kidney influences the functions of the spleen, the large intestine and the anus to control defecation though kidney-*yin* and kidney-*yang*.

◆Six-*fu* System

1. Gallbladder

The gallbladder is connected with the liver and contains bile. The bile comes from the liver and is the accumulation of the surplus part of liver-*qi*.

1. 1 Physiological functions of the gallbladder

1. 1. 1 Storing and excreting the bile and aiding digestion

The gallbladder itself is empty. After produced by the liver, the bile is stored in the gallbladder and directed by the dredging and dispersing functions of the liver, excreted into the small intestine to participate in the process of digestion and absorption of food and promote the small intestine to separate the lucid from the turbid.

1. 1. 2 Dominating decision-making and relating with emotions

It means that the gallbladder has the ability to judge and make decision in the mental activities.

2. Stomach

The stomach is connected with the esophagus in the upper and the small intestine in the lower, usually divided into three parts, namely Shangwan (CV 13, the upper part of the stomach and cardia), Zhongwan (CV 12, the middle part of the stomach) and Xiawan(CV 10, the lower part of the stomach and pylorus).

2. 1 Physiological functions of the stomach

2. 1. 1 Receiving and digesting of food and water

It implies that the stomach can receive and digest the food and water. The chime transformed in the stomach is then transmitted to the small intestine. Since the stomach is big and can contain large amount of food, it is called "the sea of food and water".

2. 1. 2 Dominating descending for maintenance of health

After the digesting of food and water, the stomach sends the chyme into small intestine, large intestine, and helps the stool being discharged from the anus.

3. Large intestine

The large intestine is connected with the small intestine in the upper and the anus in the lower.

The physiological function of the large intestine is mainly to receive the waste of food transmitted down from the small intestine. After absorbing part of the water in it, the large intestine transmits the waste downward and transforms it into feces to be excreted feces from the anus. Transmits means: absorbs the water of the waste again, and transforms it into feces.

4. Small intestine

The small intestine is located in the abdomen, connected with the stomach at the pylorus in the upper and the large intestine at ileocecal junction in the lower.

4. 1 Physiological functions of the small intestine

4. 1. 1 Receiving and absorbing the food and drink

Receiving means: Receives the chyme transported from the stomach and the chyme must stay in the small intestine for a period of time. Absorbing means: Digests the chyme coatingther, transforms the chyme into essence and waste, and absorbs the essence.

4. 1. 2 Separating the lucid from the turbid

The lucid refers to nutrients of food and the turbid refers to the residues of food. After coating the digestion and absorption of the nutrients and part of the water, the small intestine transmits the waste to the large intestine.

5. *Sanjiao* (The triple energizer)

It is a special *fu* organs, serving to divide the internal organs in the chest and abdomen and generalize certain functional systems of the body. It is composed of three parts, i. e. the upper energizer, the middle energizer and the lower energizer.

5. 1 Physiological functions of triple energizer

5. 1. 1 The passage for primordial *qi*

It means that triple energizer is the passage for the ascending, descending, and going-out and entering of the primordial *qi*, it is also the place for life activities of visceral organs. The primordial *qi* originates from the kidney, but it needs the triple energizer as its pathway for distribution in order to stimulate and promote the functional activities of the *zang* organs, *fu* organs and tissues of the whole body.

5. 1. 2 The passage for water fluid

The triple energizer is the passage for ascending and descending of water fluid.

5. 2 Functional characteristics of the triple energizer

5. 2. 1 The upper energizer functions as a sprayer

The upper energizer refers to the part above the diaphragm, mainly including heart and lungs. Its main physiological function is to disperse and distribute the defensive *qi*, food nutrient, and body fluid so as to nourish the whole body. So it is said in *Lingshu Jing*, *Miraculuos Pivot* that "The upper energizer functions as a sprayer".

5. 2. 2 The middle energizer described as a fermentor

The middle energizer refers to the part between the diaphragm and umbilicus, mainly including the spleen and stomach. Its main physiological function is to digest the foodstuff and to absorb and distribute its essence that is coatingther transformed into *qi* and blood. Such a function in *Lingshu Jing*, *Miraculuos Pivot* is"The middle energizer described as a fermentor".

5. 2. 3 The lower energizer described as a drainer

The lower energizer refers to the part below the umbilicus, mainly including the small intestine, large intestine, kidney and bladder. Its main physiological function is to discharge food residues and urine. So the function of the lower energizer in *Miraculous Pivot* is "The lower energizer described as a drainer".

6. The bladder

The bladder is located in the middle of the lower abdomen. There is an exterior and interior relation between kidney and bladder.

6. 1 Physiological functions of the bladder

Storing and discharging urine: the water and turbid *qi* produced in the process of metabolism are changed into urine through *qi*-transforming function of the kidney and transmitted to the bladder. When certain amount of urine is accumulated in the bladder, it is excreted naturally out of the body through the action of *qi*-transformation.

◆ Extraordinary-*fu* organs System

1. Brain

The brain is located in the skull and is composed of marrow and connects with the spinal cord. That is why the brain is called "the sea of marrow" in *Inner Canon of Yellow Emperor*.

1. 1 Physiological functions of the brain

1. 1. 1 The center of life activities

The brain plays a very important role in life activities. It governs the five-*zang* organs and six-*fu* organs and regulates life activities. Impairment of the brain will threaten life.

1. 1. 2 Governing the mental activities

The brain is the organ related to the spirit, consciousness and thinking. In the *Ming* Dynasty, Li Shizhen pointed out that "the brain is the house of original spirit". In the *Qing* Dynasty, Wang Qingren pointed out that "the intelligence and memory come from the brain but not from the heart" and that "thinking, memory, vision, hearing, smelling and speaking are all controlled by the brain". However, traditionally Chinese medicine ascribes the functions of the brain to the heart and the five-*zang* organs respectively. That is why it is said that "the heart stores the spirit".

2. The uterus

The uterus is located in the lower abdomen. The physiological function of the uterus is to produce menses and conceive fetus.

3. The gallbladder

In morphology, gallbladder is a hollow organ. In function, it takes part in the digestive process, so it belongs to six-*fu* organs. But it also stores essence juice, and relates with emotions, it is different from ordinary six-*fu* organs, so it belongs to extraordinary-*fu* organs.

4. Marrow

"Marrow" the common matrix of bone-marrow and brain, is produced by the kidney-essence, it fills the brain and spinal cord and forms bone marrow.

The Chinese medicine concept of "marrow" should not be confused with bone-marrow as defined by western medicine. In Chinese medicine, the function of marrow is to nourish the brain and spinal cord and to form bone-marrow. Marrow is closely related to the kidneys, as the kidney-essence is the origin of marrow. If the kidney is deficient, marrow cannot be abundant.

5. The bones

The bones, like all the other extraordinary organs, are also related to the kidney. They are considered one of the extraordinary organs because they store bone-marrow. If kidney-essence and marrow are deficient, the bones lose nourishment, cannot sustain the body and there will be inability to walk or stand.

In clinical practice, the relationship between kidneys and bones can be exploited, by treating the kidney to speed up the healing of bone fractures.

6. The blood vessels

Blood vessels are considered one of the extraordinary organs because they contain blood. They are also indirectly related to the kidneys because kidney-essence produces marrow which contributes to producing blood, and the original *qi* of the kidney also contributes to the transformation of the food-*qi* into blood.

Knowledge point 5   *Qi* and Blood Theory

Qi and blood are the basic substances of the human body, and are the basis of all its physiologic activities. *Qi* is a kind of energy, flowing around the whole body to maintain its life activities, while blood is the nourishing and moistening substances, circulating in every corner of our body. It is really important to note that *qi* belongs to *yang* while blood belongs to *yin*.

1. *Qi*

1.1 The basic concept of *qi*

Qi is the fundamental substance to make up the human body and to maintain the life activities. It has two aspects. One refers to the vital substances comprising the human body and maintaining its life activities, the other refers to the physiological functions of viscera, meridians and collaterals.

1.2 The production of *qi*

Qi exists right after the formation of individual life. This kind of *qi* is inherited from the parents, stored in the kidney. So it is called "congenital *qi*".

After birth, the human body keeps absorbing nutrients from the external world to nourish the congenital *qi*. This is acquired *qi*. Acquired *qi* comes from food nutrients and fresh air inhaled into the body.

1.3 Classification of *qi*

1.3.1 Primordial *qi*

It is also called primary *qi* or genuine *qi*, which is the most essential *qi* stored in the kidney and nourished and enriched by the nutrients provided by the spleen and stomach.

1. 3. 2 Pectoral *qi*

It is a kind of acquired *qi*, and produced by combing the fresh air inhaled by the lung with the essential *qi* transformed by stomach and spleen from the essence of drink and food.

1. 3. 3 *Ying-qi* (nutritive *qi*)

It comes from the pectoral *qi*, and belongs to "the most essential part" of the food nutrients, existing in the blood vessels.

1. 3. 4 *Wei-qi*(defensive *qi*)

It comes from the pectoral *qi* too, and belongs to "the most active and powerful part" of the food nutrients, flowing outside the vessels.

1. 4 The physiological functions of *qi*

Qi is the essential substance that makes up the body and maintains various physiological activities. *Qi* in different viscera and organs functions differently. Generally speaking, there are five physiological functions of *qi*.

1. 4. 1 Propelling function

Qi is the motivation of the physiological functions of all the viscera and organs in the body. The propelling function of *qi* can stimulate and maintain the physiological functions of viscera and other organs. *Qi* in different viscera and organs functions differently. For example, kidney-*qi* promotes the development of the body and reproduction, transformation of water and receive lung-*qi*.

1. 4. 2 Warming function

Qi warms the body and is the source of heat energy in the body. It is important in maintaining normal body temperature and ensuring the physiological functions of all the viscera and organs. Since *qi* can warm the body, it is similar to *yang* in nature. So the kind of *qi* that warms the body is called *yang-qi*.

1. 4. 3 Protecting function

The protection function of *qi* is shown in two aspects. One is to protect the surface of the skin against the invasion of pathogenic factors. The other is to fight against the pathogenic factors to ward it off.

1. 4. 4 Fixating function

Fixation of *qi* means that *qi* can astringe and control liquid substances, such as blood, body fluid and sperm, to prevent them from losing. Besides defecation and location of the viscera are under the influence of the fixating function of *qi*.

1. 4. 5 *Qi*-transforming function

Qi-transformation means changes caused by the movement of *qi*, which is the essential cause of the conception, development, growth and decline of life. This action refers to the metabolism and mutual transformation of essence, *qi*, blood, and body fluid. Firstly, through food and respiration the body absorbs nutrients from the external world and transforms into essence, *qi*, blood, and body fluid essential to the body. Secondly, waste substance and turbid *qi* are excreted out of the body in the process of life. Thirdly, inter-promotion among the essence, *qi*, blood, and body fluid, are the process of automatic regulation, improvement and balance of life.

2. Blood

Blood is a kind of red fluid substance flowing within the blood vessels. It is a basic material of body composition and for the life activities with function of nourishing and moistening.

2. 1 The basic concept of blood

Blood, mainly composed of the nutrient *qi* and body fluid, circulates inside the vessels. It is red in color and sticky in texture.

2. 2 The production of blood

The basic substance for producing blood is essence, including the congenital essence (kidney-essence) and the acquired essence (food nutrients). The transformation of essence into blood is in fact a process of *qi*-transformation.

2. 3 The physiological functions of blood

2. 3. 1 Nourishing and moistening the body

Since blood contains nutrient *qi*, through the meridians, it can transport nutrient substances to all parts of the body to nourish the five-*zang* organs, six-*fu* organs, the five constituents, the five sensory organs and the nine orifices.

2. 3. 2 The blood is the substantial basis for the mental activities

Blood is also the material basis of mental activities. Sound mental activity results from normal circulation and a sufficient supply of blood. So any blood trouble, whatever the causes maybe, will bring about symptoms of mental activities in degrees. Deficiency of blood will cause mental disorder. For example, heart-blood or liver-blood deficiency will lead to such symptoms as palpitation, insomnia and dreaminess.

2. 4 The circulation of blood

2. 4. 1 The direction of blood circulation

Blood circulates within the vessels, by which it is carried to the *zang-fu* organs internally and to the skin, muscles, tendons and bones externally. It circulates ceaselessly like a ring without end to nourish and moisten all the organs and tissues. Normal physiological activities are maintained based on the continually circulation of blood.

2. 4. 2 The mechanism of blood circulation

Normal blood circulation comes of the joint action of the heart, the lung, the spleen and the liver. The heart-*qi* is the fundamental motive power to propel blood circulation. The lungs control the respiration and regulates the *qi* movement of the whole body, so it help the heart to promote the circulation of the blood in the vessels. The spleen may keep blood flowing within the vessels and prevent it from extravasating. And the liver, besides its function of storing blood, adjusts the volume of blood flow and maintain the normal flow of *qi* and blood. In case any one of the above organs fails to work properly, abnormal blood circulation is certain to occur. The heart-*qi* deficiency, for instance, may lead to heart-blood stagnation. The spleen-*qi* deficiency fails to control blood, leading to bleeding, The disturbance of *qi* flow of the liver and blood circulation may bring about such pathological changes as blood stasis or swelling, abnormal menstruation, dysmenorrhea or amenorrhea in women.

3. The relationship between *qi* and blood

Qi and blood are closely related. *Qi* is the "commander" of blood, and blood is the "mother" of *qi*.

3. 1 *Qi* is the "commander" of blood

Qi is the "commander" of blood, and blood is the "mother" of *qi*. As the commander of blood, for one thing, *qi* is the motive power for blood formation, or rather, it produces blood. Blood is formed from mutritive *qi* and body fluid, both of which come from food and water. All these cannot be separated from the functions of *qi*. Blood circulation depends on the propelling function of heart-*qi*. For another, *qi* controls blood and keep it flowing in the blood vessels without extravasation. This function of *qi* is performed by spleen-*qi*. When *qi* is deficient, it fails to control blood, thus leading to hemorrhage.

3. 2 Blood is the "mother" of *qi*

Blood is referred to as the mother of *qi*. On the one hand, blood is the carrier of *qi*. On the other hand, blood provides adequate nutrients for *qi*. Blood is the material basis of *qi*. Without blood, *qi* will no longer exist.

Knowledge point 6　Causes of Disease(Ettiology Theory)

The causes of disease refer to the factors that lead to imbalance between *yin* and *yang* in the body, impairment of the *zang-fu* organs and abnormality in their physiological functions and result in disease.

The TCM summarized the causes into four categories, namely internal causes including seven emotions, improper diet and overstrain, etc. External causes include six climatic factors and pestilence. Secondary pathogenic factors are phlegm, retention of fluid and blood stasis. Besides, other pathogenic factors include various traumatic injuries, injuries due to physical and chemical factors and injuries caused by insects and animal.

1. The six climatic factors

The six climatic factors are pathogenic wind, pathogenic cold, pathogenic summer-heat, pathogenic dampness, pathogenic dryness and pathogenic heat (fire).

General pathogenic characteristics of the six climatic factors are as follow. (1) The diseases caused by six climatic factors are mostly related with seasonal changes and living or working conditions. (2) The six climatic factors may singly or collectively attack people. (3) After the six climatic factors cause disease, they affect each other in the process of disease development, and some pathological properties, under certain conditions, can be transformed into other pathological factors. (4) The six climatic factors usually get into the body and cause diseases through the skin and muscle, or the mouth and nose, or through both ways, so they are also termed "the six exogenous pathogenic factors".

1. 1 Wind

Wind is the main climatic factor in spring. Although the diseases caused by wind-evil are mostly in spring, they can also occur in other seasons. Diseases caused by wind-evil have the following characteristics.

1. 1. 1 Lightness and pertaining to the *yang*

Wind is a pathogenic factor of *yang* nature, characterized by floating and dispersion because of lightness. That is why wind attacks the upper part and skin first when it invades the body.

1. 1. 2 Movable and changeable

Wind is mobile and the disease caused by it is also migration. Besides, wind tends to change. So the disease caused by wind is often characterized by sudden onset, immediate transmission and change as well as fast healing.

1. 1. 3 Wind tends to be complicated by other pathogenic factors

It is because that wind is easier to attacked body, other factors in the six exogenous pathogenic factors often attach themselves to wind when they invade the body. So TCM regards wind as "the leading one among the six exogenous pathogenic factors".

1. 2 Cold

Cold is the dominant climatic factor in winter, so diseases caused by cold-evil are usually seen in winter. Diseases caused by cold-evil have the following characteristics.

1. 2. 1 Tending to impair *yang-qi*

Cold pertains to *yin* and tends to impair *yang*. When cold attacks the surface of the body, it will impair *yang* in the superficies. When it attacks the internal of the body, it will impair the visceral *yang*.

1. 2. 2 Tending to coagulate

Qi, blood and body fluid in the body flow continuously inside the body because they are constantly warmed and propelled by *yang-qi*. If the pathogenic cold obstructs *yang-qi*, then *qi*, blood and body fluid cannot flow freely and will coagulate in the vessels, bringing on pain. If cold attacks the viscera, the visceral *qi* and blood will be stagnated, causing abdominal pain. If cold attacks the muscles and joints, *qi* and blood in the muscles and joints will coagulate, resulting in pain in the muscles and joints.

1. 2. 3 Tending to contract

Cold pertains to *yin* and tends to restrain the activity of *qi*, leading to contracture of muscles, tendons and vessels.

1. 3 Summer-heat

Summer-heat is transformed from heat and fire in summer. Summer-heat pertains to *yang* and usually appears after summer solstice and before autumn solstice. The attack by summer-heat is either due to hot weather or due to low adaptability of the body to the environment. Diseases caused by summer-heat-evil have the following characteristics.

1. 3. 1 Summer-heat is hot

Summer-heat pertains to *yang* and is hot in nature. So the disease caused by summer-heat is usually marked by a series of *yang* symptoms such as fever, dysphoria, reddish complexion, etc.

1. 3. 2 Tending to ascend and disperse

Summer-heat pertains to *yang* and tends to disperse and ascend. Summer-heat disturbs the mind when it ascends. Summer-heat induces sweating and consumes *qi* and impairs body fluid when it disperses.

1. 3. 3 Summer-heat is often complicated by dampness

In the hot season, heat fumigates dampness. That's why dampness is exuberant in summer and often mixes up with heat to attack people.

1. 4 Dampness

Dampness is predominant in late summer but also can be encountered in other seasons. Since it is hot in late summer, dampness permeates everywhere due to fumigation and frequently causes disease. Diseases caused by dampness-evil have the following characteristics.

1. 4. 1 Dampness is heavy and turbid

Dampness pertains to *yin*, so it is heavy. Dampness is similar to water and it often mixes up with water. That's why it is turbid. Invasion of dampness into the body often brings on the symptoms of turbid secreta and excreta, dirty complexion, etc.

1. 4. 2 Dampness tends to block *qi*

Dampness moves slowly because it is heavy. So it tends to retain in the viscera and meridians, inhibits the flow of *qi* and blood and disturbs the activity of *qi*, frequently leading to chest oppression and fullness, scanty urine and unsmooth defecation. On the other hand, dampness pertains to *yin* and tends to impair *yang-qi*.

Since dampness pertains to earth in the five elements and is related to the spleen, it tends to impair the spleen, bringing on encumbrance of the spleen by the dampness and stagnation of *qi* in the middle energizer.

1. 4. 3 Dampness is sticky and stagnant

These characteristics of dampness usually affect people in two ways. One is that the disease caused by dampness is not brisk. The second is that the disease caused by dampness is obstinate and recurring with long duration.

1. 4. 4 Dampness tends to move downward

Dampness is similar to water, so it tends to move downward. Firstly, it impairs the lower part when it attacks the body. Secondly, the disease caused by dampness usually involves the lower part of the body. For example, edema often mostly involves the lower limbs. Thirdly, the disease caused by dampness usually transmitted from the upper to the lower.

1. 5 Dryness

Dryness is predominant in autumn. So disease caused by dryness mostly appears in autumn. Diseases caused by dryness-evil have the following characteristics:

1. 5. 1 Dryness is xerotic and unsmooth

Dryness is usually caused by insufficiency of body fluid. So the attack by dryness tends to consume body fluid and lead to dryness of the mouth and nose, dry throat, dry skin or even rhagas, scanty urine and retention of dry feces.

1. 5. 2 Dryness tends to impair the lung

Dryness is prevailing in autumn and is associated with the lung. Lung is the important respiratory organ which is directly connected with the external environment by mouth and nose. Dryness-evil mostly attack the human body through mouth and nose, so dryness-evil tends to impair the lung when it invades the body.

1. 6 Heat (Fire)

Heat is the predominant climatic factor in summer, so disease due to pathogenic heat usually occurs in summer. Diseases caused by heat(fire)-evil have the following characteristics.

1. 6. 1 Heat (Fire) tends to flame up

Heat (Fire) pertains to *yang* and tends to flame up. So the disease caused by the pathogenic heat is marked by high fever, aversion to heat, extreme thirst, sweating and full pulse. Since the pathogenic heat is responsible for irritability and rapid movement, the disease caused by it is characterized by acute onset and rapid transmission.

1. 6. 2 Heat (Fire) tends to consume *qi* and impairs the body fluid

Heat pertains to *yang* and tends to consume *yin*-fluid. If there is superabundant heat, it will drive body fluid out of the body in the form of sweat. The pathogenic heat is strong fire, so it consumes the healthy *qi*.

1. 6. 3 Heat (Fire) tends to produce wind and disturb blood

When heat (Fire) invades the body, it usually scorches the liver meridians, consumes body fluid and deprives the tendons of moisture and nourishment, leading to occurrence of liver-wind with the manifestations of high fever, delirium, coma, convulsion of four limbs, etc. Blood coagulates with cold and moves fast with heat. But if the heat is excessive, it will drive blood to flow very fast or scorch the vessels or even compel blood to flow out of the vessels, leading to various hemorrhages.

1. 6. 4 Heat (Fire) tends to cause swelling and ulceration

When heat invades blood phase and accumulates in local area, it will putrefy blood and muscles. It easily lead to swelling and ulcer on the body surface.

1. 6. 5 Heat(Fire) easily disturbs the mind

When the pathogenic heat (Fire) attacks the body, it may disturb the mind, leading to dysphoria, insomnia, etc.

2. Seven emotions

2. 1 The concept of seven emotions

The seven emotions are seven sentimental changes, which include joy, anger, anxiety, contemplation, grief, fear and fright, and reflect the mental state of human beings.

The seven emotions are the physiological responses of visceral *qi*, blood, *yin* and *yang*. Different visceral *qi*, blood, *yin* and *yang* differ from each other in moving styles, leading to different emotional responses.

Normally the seven emotions will not cause disease. But those sudden, violent or prolonged emotional stimuli which is beyond the range of physiological activities, will cause disorder of *qi* activity and disharmony of visceral *yin*, *yang*, *qi* and blood which consequently lead to disease.

2. 2 The pathogenic feature of the seven emotions

2. 2. 1 Directly impairing the internal visceral organs

Since the seven emotions are endogenous, they can directly impair the internal organs. The disorder of the seven emotions usually directly affects the relevant viscera because of the close relationship between the viscera and emotions. For example, excessive joy impairs the heart, excessive anger impairs the liver, excessive contemplation impairs the spleen, excessive grief impairs the lung, excessive fear impairs the kidney, etc.

2. 2. 2 Disordering the activity of visceral *qi*

When the seven emotions impair the internal organs, they mainly affect the activity of visceral *qi*, leading to disorder of the activity of *qi*, in turn, bringing on the disorder of blood circulation. For example, "excessive anger drives *qi* to flow upward", "excessive joy makes *qi* sluggish ", "excessive grief consumes *qi* ", "excessive anxiety inhibits *qi*", "excessive fear drives *qi* to flow downward", "excessive fright disorders *qi*" and "excessive contemplation stagnates *qi*".

2. 2. 3 Causing or aggravating certain diseases

Emotional factors are certain diseases. For example, people with frequent superabundance of liver-*yang* tend to flare into violent rage which brings on violent hyperactivity of liver-*yang*, leading to sudden dizziness and syncope or unconsciousness, paralysis and distorted face. Besides, other diseases may become aggravated or worsened because of abnormal change of emotions.

3. Improper diet

Diet is indispensable to human existence and is the main route for human being to obtain nutrient substances from the natural world. However, improper diet or imbalanced diet frequently leads to diseases. Because it affect the physiological functions of the spleen and stomach, eventually resulting in the accumulation of dampness, production of phlegm, transformation of heat or other pathological changes.

4. Phlegm and retained fluid

Phlegm retention is a pathological substance caused by disturbance of body fluid. Generally speaking, the thick part is called phlegm while the thin part is called retained fluid.

"Phlegm" not only refers to sputum expectorated from the throat, but also includes scrofula, nodules and the thick liquid substance retained or stagnated in the viscera and meridians. Phlegm usually results in asthmatic cough with expectoration if it is retained in the lung. Phlegm stagnated in the heart will causes chest distress and palpitation. When the phlegm blocks the *qi* movement of the head and brain, unconsciousness and dementia will appear. Vomiting and stomach fullness could be caused by phlegm retained in the stomach. If the phlegm retains in the meridians, tendons and bones, scrofula, numbness of limbs or paralysis will come out. Vertigo is one of the symptoms after the phlegm attacks the head.

Retained fluid includes four categories according to their location, namely phlegmatic rheum in the abdomen, suspending rheum in the chest and diaphragm, sustaining rheum in the rib-sides and overflowing rheum in the skin and muscles.

5. Blood stasis

Blood stasis is a kind of pathological substance caused by disturbance of blood circulation.

5. 1 The formation of blood stasis

The formation of blood stasis can be caused by internal and external factors. All the factors which can cause poor blood circulation even blood stagnate or blood stasis due to flowing outside meridians. It can be divided into blood stasis due to bleeding, *qi* stagnation and blood stasis, blood stasis due to deficiency, blood stasis due to cold and blood stasis caused by blood heat.

5. 2 The characteristics of blood stasis in causing diseases

Static blood cause pain marked by stabbing, fixed and un-pressure pain that turns worse at night. Protracted blood stasis gradually develops into lumps which appears hard and fixed. Blood stasis retained in the vessels tends to bring on repeated hemorrhage. The patient with blood stasis is characterized by cyanotic complexion, lips and nails. For those patients, their tongue is cyanotic or has ecchymosis and petechia. Their pulse is thin, unsmooth, deep and taut, or knotted or even has slow regular intermittent.

Knowledge point 7   The four diagnostic methods

Diagnostic methods are the methods used to collect data related to pathological conditions, including inspection, auscultation and olfaction, inquiry as well as pulse-taking. The four diagnostic methods are used to examine disease from different angles and they cannot replace each other in diagnosis. So in clinical practice, they are usually used in combination for systematic understanding of diseases.

1. Inspection of tongue

Inspection means that the doctor purposefully observes the whole body or local regions and excreta of the patient in order to understand the pathological conditions. Here we will focus on tongue inspection. Inspection of the tongue mainly includes the examination of tongue proper and the tongue coating.

1. 1 The relation between tongue and viscera

The body of the tongue is composed of muscles and vessels. In the ancient time some people believes that the surface of the tongue corresponded to the viscera. That is to say the tip of the tongue reflects the pathological changes of the heart and lung, the center of the tongue reflects the changes of spleen and stomach, the root of the tongue reflects the changes of the kidney and the margins of the tongue reflect the changes of liver and the gallbladder. (Fig. 1 –7 –1)

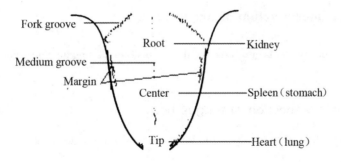

Fig. 1 – 7 – 1

1. 2 Instruction for inspection of tongue

The patient is asked to sit down or lie in supination, exposed to the natural light source. The tongue is protruded naturally and the tip of the tongue is kept slightly downwards. The mouth is opened wide to make the tongue exposed fully.

The sequence of inspection of the tongue begins from the tip from the tongue, then the middle and margin of the tongue, and finally the root of the tongue. The inspection begins with the tongue body first and then moves to the tongue coating.

1. 3 Normal state of the tongue

Normal states of the tongue marketed by suitable size, softness, flexibility, light-red color, luster and moisture, even and whitish thin coating neither dry or greasy and slippery, closely attached to the surface of the tongue, distributed more on the center and root and less on margins and tip. The normal conditions of the tongue is usually described as "light-reddish tongue with thin and whitish coating", suggesting normal functions of the viscera, sufficiency of qi, blood and body fluid as well as superabundance of gastric qi.

1. 4 Interpretation of tongue image

Tongue image is analysis by the inspection of tongue body and tongue coating.

1. 4. 1 Inspection of tongue body

Inspection of the body of the tongue includes the color, shape and movement of the tongue.

(1) Color of the tongue.

Light-reddish tongue: it is usually seen among healthy people. Sometimes it is also seen in mild cases.

Light-whitish tongue: such a condition suggests deficiency of qi and blood or deficiency of $yang$-qi.

Red and deep-red tongue: red and deep-red tongue both indicates heat syndrome.

Cyanotic and purplish tongue: such a condition indicates inhibited circulation of qi and blood. Besides, it is also seen in case of congenital heart disease or intoxication by drugs of food.

(2) Shape of tongue.

Rough tongue and tender tongue: rough tongue usually indicates excess syndrome and heat syndrome. Tender tongue signifies deficiency and cold syndrome.

Bulgy tongue: it usually indicates the internal retention of dampness and phlegm.

Swollen tongue: swollen tongue usually suggesting excess syndrome.

Thin and emaciated tongue: The tongue is thinner than usual, indicating deficiency of qi and blood or consumption of yin fluid.

Fissured tongue: it indicates deficiency of fluid or essence and blood. However, fissured tongue may be seen in some healthy people, known as congenital fissured tongue. Such a tongue is marked by fine fissures and covered with tongue coating.

Prickly tongue: the tongue is covered with reddish prickles, suggesting superabundance of pathogenic heat.

Tooth-marked tongue: it indicates *qi* deficiency or *yang* deficiency and internal retention of dampness. Tooth-marked tongue is also seen among some healthy people, characterized by constant existence of slight tooth marks and no bulging manifestation.

(3) Movement of the tongue.

Stiff tongue: such a change of tongue is usually seen in exogenous disease due to exuberant heat consuming body fluid, or due to invasion of heat into the pericardium, or due to phlegm or turbid substance confusing the heart.

Shivering tongue: the tongue is involuntarily trembling, indicating endogenous liver wind.

Deviated tongue: the tongue is deviated to one side, suggesting wind stroke or premonitory sign of wind stroke.

Flaccid tongue: the tongue is too weak to protrude and withdraw, suggesting extreme consumption of *yin* fluid, or by decline of *qi* and blood.

Shrunk tongue: the tongue is contracted and cannot protrude, or cannot even reach the teeth, usually indicating critical condition. However, congenital short sublingual frenum also prevents the tongue from protruding.

Protruding and wagging tongue: Both protruding and wagging tongue suggest heat in the heart and the spleen.

1. 4. 2 Inspection of tongue coating

(1) Nature of tongue coating.

Thickness and thin of tongue coating: the thickness and thin of the tongue coating reflects the degree and severity of the pathogenic factors as well as the development of disease.

Moistening and dryness of tongue coating: the moistening and dryness of the tongue coating reflect the conditions and the distribution of body fluid.

Greasy and putrid tongue coating: the greasiness and putridity of the tongue coating reflect the decline and development of *yang-qi* and turbid dampness.

Exfoliating tongue coating: exfoliation of the tongue coating can tell whether the gastric *qi* and *yin* still exist or not and how the prognosis of a disease will be.

The tongue coating with or without root: Inspecting whether the tongue coating is with or without coating is helpful for understanding whether gastric *qi* still exist or not and whether the pathogenic factors are exuberating or declining.

(2) The colors of tongue coating.

White tongue coating: apart from normal tongue coating, white tongue coating is usually seen in external syndrome and cold syndrome.

Yellow tongue coating: yellow tongue coating usually indicates internal syndrome and heat syndrome.

Grayish black tongue coating: grayish and black tongue coating suggests severity of internal heat syndrome or internal cold syndrome.

2. Auscultation and olfaction

2. 1 Auscultation

Auscultation is a diagnostic method whereby the doctor listens to the patient's speech, respiration, cough, and special sounds like vomit, hiccough etc. In general if the sound is rough and sonorous and its form is strong, then it is an excess type. If the sound is low and weak and the breath is timorous then it is a deficiency type.

2. 2 Olfaction

The smelling examination includes abnormal odors emitted from the patient's body, excretions and secretions. Foul or rotten odor usually indicates heat syndromes of excess (*shi*) type while fishy odor indicates cold syndromes of deficiency (*xu*) type. Foul breath indicates heat in the stomach or food retention.

3. Inquiry

Inquiry means investigating into the occurrence, development and treatment of the disease as well as the present manifestations and other related problems by means of inquiry the patient or other people accompanying the patient.

Inquiry includes general information, chief complaint, present disease history, present symptoms, past medical history and family history.

4. Pulse-taking and palpation

4. 1 Pulse-taking

Pulsing-taking means that doctor uses his or her hand to press certain part of the patient's pulse to examine the conditions of the pulse and diagnose disease.

4. 1. 1 Regions for taking pulse

Cunkou is the usual region selected to take pulse. *Cunkou* refers to pulsation of radial artery on the wrist. Pulse over *Cunkou* can be divided into three portions, *Cun*, *Guan*, and *Chi*. The part slightly below the styloid process of radius is *Guan* pulse, the part anterior the *Guan* pulse is *Cun* pulse, and the part posterior the *Guan* pulse is the *Chi* pulse. (Fig. 1 −7 −2)

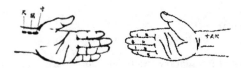

Fig. 1 −7 −2

Clinically the correspondence of *Cunkou* pulse and viscera is decided according to the description in *Neijing* (Table 1 − 7 − 1), that is the upper pulse (*Cun* pulse) corresponds to the upper part of the body and the lower pulse (*Chi* pulse) corresponds to the lower part of the body.

Table 1 −7 −1 The relationships between pulse and viscera

pulses	left corresponding viscera	right corresponding viscera
cun	heart	lung
guan	liver	spleen(stomach)
chi	kidney-*yin*	kidney-*yang*

4. 1. 2 The methods for taking pulse

(1) Time.

Early morning is the ideal time for taking pulse. However, this requirement is difficult to fill in clinical practice. To ensure accurate pulse taking, the patient should rest for a while to tranquilize the heart and breathe before taking pulse. The pulse should be taken at least for one minute each time in order to correctly exam the condition of pulse.

(2) Normal and calm breath.

Normal and calm breath means that the doctor keeps his or her own breath quiet to exam the pulse of the patient and calculate the beat of pulse according to his or her own cycle of exhalation and inhalation, about 60 ~ 90 beats per time.

(3) Posture.

The patient sits erect or lies in supination and the forearms stretches out naturally to the level of heart. The wrist is put straight, the palm turns over and the fingers are relaxed to extend the *Cunkou* region and enable *qi* and blood to flow freely.

(4) Arrangement of fingers.

The three fingers of the doctor are put at the same level and slightly arched to press the pulse with the belly of fingers. The middle finger presses on the *Guan* pulse, the index finger presses on the region anterior the *Guan* pulse, the ring finger on the *Chi* pulse posterior to the *Guan* pulse. In diagnosing disease in children, "one finger is used to press just *Guan* pulse". It is unnecessary to divide the pulse into three parts in the case.

4. 1. 3 Normal pulse

Normal pulse refers to the pulse conditions of the healthy people. The normal pulse is marked by gastric-*qi*, spirit and root. Gastric-*qi* means that the pulse is located in the middle, neither floating or sunken, regular in beating, moderate in size, gentle in sensation and floating. Spiritual means that pulse is soft, powerful and rhythmic. Root means that the *Chi* pulse is powerful and constantly beating under heavy pressure.

4. 1. 4 Morbid pulse

The pulse in a morbid condition is called morbid pulse, in which the manifestations of pulse conditions are either the changes of position of the pulse, or the difference in rhythm, or variation in morphology, or changes in strength. Sometimes morbid pulse may show difference in various aspects, such as the position, rhythm and strength of the pulse.

(1) Floating pulse.

Floating pulse is marked by superficial beating. Floating pulse indicates external syndrome, floating and powerful pulse signifying external excess syndrome while floating and weak pulse manifesting external deficiency syndrome.

(2) Sunken pulse.

Sunken pulse is marked by sensibility only under heavy pressure, indicating internal syndrome. Sunken and powerful pulse signifies excess internal syndrome, while sunken and weak pulse shows internal deficiency internal syndrome.

(3) Slow pulse.

Slow pulse means no more than 4 beats in a cycle of breath (< 60/ min), indicating cold syndrome. Slow and powerful pulse signifies excess cold syndrome, while slow and weak pulse shows deficiency cold syndrome.

(4) Moderate pulse.

The pulse is moderate and powerful. Beating 4 times in a cycle of breath, or moderate and sluggish, beating 4 times in a cycle of breath (60 ~ 70/ min), indicating damp disease and weakness of stomach and spleen.

(5) Fast pulse.

The pulse beats 5 ~ 6 times in a cycle of breath (90 ~ 110/min), indicating heat syndrome. Fast and powerful pulse signifies excess heat syndrome, while fast and weak pulse shows deficiency heat syndrome.

(6) Swift pulse.

The pulse beats over 7 times in a cycle of breath($\geqslant$ 140/min), indicating loss of control of hyperactive *yang*, declination of kidney *yin* and near depletion of primordial *qi*.

(7) Weak pulse.

Weak pulse is marked by weak beating of the pulse at all the *Cun*, *guan* and *Chi* regions, indicating deficiency syndrome, usually seen in deficiency of both *qi* and blood, especially in *qi* deficiency.

(8) Powerful pulse.

Powerful pulse is marked by powerful sensation of pulse beating at *Cun*, guan and chi regions under superficial, moderate and heavy pressure, indicating excess syndrome.

(9)Slippery pulse.

The pulse is beating freely and smoothly like the movement of beads of an abacus, indicating retention of phlegm and fluid, dyspepsia and excess heat.

(10)Unsmooth pulse.

The pulse is beating in an inhibited way like scraping a piece of bamboo, unsmooth powerful pulse indicates *qi* stagnation and blood stasis. unsmooth and weak pulse signifies lack of essence and insufficiency of blood.

(11)Full pulse.

Full pulse is marked by wide size and full content, beating like roaring waves and sensibility under light pressure and surges as well as sudden flowing and ebbing, indicating exuberant internal heat.

(12)Thin pulse.

The pulse is as thin as a thread, weak and quite sensible under pressure, indicating deficiency of both *qi* and blood, various overstrain and disease due to pathogenic dampness.

(13)Soft pulse.

Soft pulse is superficial and thin as well as sensible and weak under light pressure, indicating insufficiency of *qi* and blood, and dampness syndrome.

(14)Taut pulse.

Taut pulse appears straight, energetic and hard like the feeling of pressing the string of violin, indicating disorders of liver and gallbladder, pain syndrome and retention of phlegm and fluid.

(15)Tense pulse.

Tense pulse feels like the pulling of a rope and licks the finger when pressed, indicating cold syndrome, pain syndrome and retention of food.

(16)Rapid and intermittent pulse.

Rapid and intermittent pulse beats fast with occasional and irregular intermittence.

Fast and powerful pulse indicates hyperactive of *yang* heat, *qi* stagnation and blood stasis and retention of phlegm and food. Fast and weak pulse signifies weakness of visceral *qi* and insufficiency of blood.

(17) Slow and intermittent pulse.

The pulse beats slowly with occasional and irregular intermittence. Slow intermittent and powerful pulse indicates predominates of *yin*, *qi* stagnation, retention of phlegm and blood stasis. While slow, intermittent and weak pulse signifies declination of *qi* and blood.

(18) Slow-intermittent-regular pulse.

The pulse beats slow with regular and longer intermittent, indicating declination of visceral *qi* and deficiency of primordial *qi*.

(19) Long pulse.

The pulse surpasses the range of *Cun*, *guan* and *Chi* regions, indicating *yang* syndrome, heat syndrome and excess syndrome.

(20) Short pulse.

The pulse appears shorter content of *Cun*, *guan* and *Chi*, indicating *qi* disorders. Short and powerful pulse indicates *qi* stagnation, while short and weak pulse indicates deficiency of *qi*.

4. 2 Palpation

Palpation means to use fingers or palms to feel or press certain regions of the patient's body to understand whether the local regions are cold or warm, dry or moist and soft or hard as well as whether there are tenderness, lump or other abnormal changes.

Knowledge point 8   Syndrome Differentiation Principles

1. Concept of syndrome differentiation

Differentiation of syndromes (Bian-zheng) in TCM is a method to analyse and recognize the syndrome of disease. In other words, it is also a process in which the location, nature, occurrence and development of a disease as well as the condition of vital *qi* and pathogenic factors are identified according to the clinical data obtained from the four diagnostic methods. From the above it becomes obvious that differentiation of syndromes is the premise and foundation of treatment. Correct differentiation and appropriate treatment are the prerequisite for achieving the hoped-for results.

There are a number of methods to differentiate syndromes in TCM, such as differentiation of syndromes according to the eight principles, differentiation of syndromes according to the theory of *qi*, blood and body fluid, differentiation of syndromes according to the *zang-fu* theory, and differentiation of syndromes according to the theory of *wei*, *qi*, *ying* and *xue*. Each method, while having its own features and laying stress, they should be applied flexibly and accurately so as to understand a disease comprehensively, thereby providing the basis for treatment.

2. Syndrome differentiation principles

2.1 Syndrome differentiation with eight-principles

Syndrome differentiation with eight-principles means differentiating syndromes according to the principles of *yin* and *yang*, internal and external aspects, cold and heat, as well as deficiency and excess. Complicated as the clinical manifestations of diseases may be, they are classified under the eight principles. For example, diseases can be classified into *yin* or *yang* syndrome in terms of the categorization, internal or external syndrome in terms of the location of disease, cold or heat syndrome in terms of the nature as well as deficiency or excess syndrome in terms of the states of the pathogenic factors and healthy *qi*.

The eight-principles concentrate on specific syndromes respectively. However, they are inseparable and not static. Among the eight-principles, *yin* and *yang* are the general principles which can be used to generalize the other six principles. In diagnosis, all diseases can be generalized into either *yin* or *yang* according to the clinical manifestations. Generally speaking, any syndromes that correspond to *yin* in nature are termed *yin* syndromes, such as internal syndrome, cold syndrome and deficiency syndrome. While any syndrome that correspond to *yang* in nature are termed *yang* syndromes, such as external syndrome, heat syndrome and excess syndrome. *Yin* syndrome is characterized by deficiency of *yang-qi* and excess of *yin* in the body. *Yang* syndrome is characterized by the hyperactivity of *yang-qi* and hyperfunctions of the *zang-fu* organs, resulting from excess of *yang*-heat in the body.

Although this differentiating method classifies various syndromes into eight categories, they are interrelated and inseparable from each other. For instance, the exterior syndrome and interior syndrome are related to the cold, heat, deficiency and excess syndromes. The cold syndrome and heat syndrome are related to the exterior, interior deficiency and excess syndromes. The deficiency syndrome and excess syndrome are related to cold, heat, exterior and interior syndromes. These pathologic changes do not occur singly, the exterior and interior, cold and heat, deficiency and excess syndromes are usually found simultaneously. For instance, the disease with both the exterior and interior syndromes. The deficiency syndrome mingling with excess syndromes, intertwinement of the cold and heat syndromes. Under certain conditions these syndromes are often transformed into one another. For example, the exogenous pathogens may invade the interior and vice versa the cold syndrome may be transformed into heat syndrome and vice versa. The deficiency syndrome may be transformed into the excess syndrome and vice versa. With the progress of disease, some false appearances contrary to its nature may appear. For example, cold syndrome with pseudo-heat symptoms and vice versa, deficiency syndrome with pseudo-excess symptoms and vice versa. Thus, when applying differentiation of syndrome according to the eight-principles, physicians are required not only to have a masterly command of the characteristics of each syndrome, but also to pay attention to their coexisting, interlacing, transforming, and true or false conditions, so and so only can the disease be understood in an all-round way. Thereby, providing reliable basis for treatment.

Yin and *yang* are a pair of principles used to summarize the other three pairs of principles and are also the key principles in the eight-principles. So the other three pairs of principles are classified under either *yin* or *yang*. Exterior, heat and excess syndromes are classified into the category of *yang*, while interior, cold and deficiency syndromes fall into the category of *yin*. *Yin* syndrome is characterized by deficiency of *yang-qi* and excess of *yin* in the body. *Yang* syndrome in characterized by the hyperactivity of *yang-qi* and hyperfunctions of the *zang-fu* organs, resulting from excess of *yang*-heat in the body. *Yin* and *yang* are also used to explain the pathological changes of the *zang-fu* organs, eg. *yin* depletion, *yang* depletion, *yin* deficiency and *yang* deficiency, etc.

2.2 Differentiation of syndromes according to the theory of *qi*, blood and body fluid

Differentiation of syndromes according to the theory of *qi*, blood and body fluid is a differentiating method to analyse and identify the pathological changes of *qi*, blood and body fluid according to the theory of *qi*, blood and body fluid. *Qi*, blood, and body fluid, are the material basis for the functional activities of the *zang-fu* organs, their formation and circulation depend upon the normal functions of the *zang-fu* organs. Therefore the pathological changes of *qi*, blood and body fluid may bring about the dysfunction of the *zang-fu* organs, and the dysfunction of the *zang-fu* organs will be bound to cause the pathological changes of *qi*, blood and body fluid. Hence, both of them should closely coordinate and complement each other.

Qi has many syndromes, which are usually classified into four classes: *qi* deficiency, *qi* sinking, *qi* stagnation and reversed flow of *qi*. As concerns blood syndromes, TCM tends to group them under four heads: blood deficiency, blood stasis, heat in blood and cold in blood. Physiologically, they complement each other and, pathologically, affect each other. Thereby, forming differentiation of syndromes of the same disease of *qi* and blood. Clinically, there is *qi* stagnation and blood stasis, *qi* deficiency and blood loss, deficiency of both *qi* and blood, *qi* deficiency and blood stasis, and *qi* prostration resulting from hemorrhage. Syndromes of body fluid may be classified into two categories: insufficiency of body fluid and water retention. Insufficiency of body fluid may cause the clinical manifestations: dryness of the mouth and throat, dry lips and tongue, subsidence of eyes, dry skin, scanty urine, constipation, a red tongue with scanty saliva and thready, rapid pulse. Whereas, retention of water may form such pathological substances as water, dampness and phlegm retention. Usually seen in edema, tympanites and phlegm-retention.

2.3 Differentiation of syndromes according to the theory of *Wei-qi-ying-xue*

Differentiation of syndromes according to the theory of *wei* (defensive), *qi* (vital-*qi*), *ying* (nutrient) and *xue* (blood) is a differentiating method applied to analyse and differentiate exogenous febrile diseases. It was developed and created by Ye Tianshi in the Qing Dynasty. It supplements the differentiation of syndromes by the theory of the six meridians and enriches the differentiation of syndromes and treatment for exogenous febrile diseases in TCM. This theory is the basis used to classify syndromes, to identify transformation and determine treatment. The theory of *wei-qi-ying-xue* is of great practical value because, for one thing, it generalizes the pathological changes of febrile diseases as the four kinds of syndromes: *weifen*, *qifen*, *yingfen* and *xuefen*; for another, it represents the four different stages: superficial or deep and mild or serious in the development of exogenous febrile diseases. It is also believed as a law of the development and changes of exogenous febrile diseases. Diseases of the *wei* and *qi* stages are mild and superficial, whereas those of the *ying* and *xue* stages are deep and serious.

2. 4 Differentiation of syndromes according to the *zang-fu* theory

Differentiation of syndromes, according to the *zang-fu* theory, a differential method by which symptoms and signs are analyzed to clarity the cause, the location and nature of disease as well as the conditions between vital *qi* and pathogens in light of the theories viscera figure (manifestation), *yin-yang* and five elements. It is the basis of various kinds of differentiation of syndromes and the basic diagnostic method of all clinical branches of TCM, and an important component part of all differential system in TCM. Differentiation of syndromes according to the theory of the *zang-fu* organs includes differentiating syndromes of *zang* organs diseases, *fu* organs diseases and complicated diseases of both *zang* organs with *fu* organs.

As a whole, conditions of differentiating syndromes are complex. What has been discussed in this unit is only those common and typical syndrome differentiation principles, they should be applied flexibly so as to decide the therapeutic principle on the basis of correct syndrome differentiation.

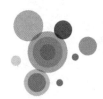

Part 2

Important Knowledge Points of Science of Acupuncture and Moxibustion

Study Objective

Master the basic theory of meridians and acupoints, needling and moxibustion methods as well as acup-moxibustion therapeutics for common diseases.

List of knowledge points

❖1. Basic Theory of Meridians and Collaterals

❖2. Basic Theory of Acupoints

❖3. Methods for locating acupoints

❖4. Meridians and their acupoints

❖5. Acupuncture and Moxibustion techniques

❖6. Acupuncture and Moxibustion treatment

Essential Knowledge

Knowledge point 1　Basic Theory of
Meridians and Collaterals

1. Conception

The meridians and collaterals refer to the pathways for *qi* and blood to circulate in the whole body. They pertain to the *zang-fu* organs interiorly and extend over the body exteriorly, link the upper part of the body with the lower part and associate the interior portions with the exterior, forming a network and linking the tissues and organs into an organic whole. They are collectively termed *Jingluo* (meridians and collaterals) in TCM.

2. Compositions

This system of meridians and collaterals includes the twelve main meridians, eight extra meridians, fifteen collaterals, twelve divergent meridians (the twelve meridian branches), muscles along twelve meridians (twelve meridian tendons) and twelve cutaneous regions (twelve skin areas). (Table 2 – 1 – 1)

Table 2 – 1 – 1 The composition of the meridian and collateral systems

meridians	twelve regular meridians	three *yin* meridians of hand
		three *yang* meridians of hand
		three *yang* meridians of foot
		three *yin* meridians of foot
		twelve divergent meridians (twelve meridian branches)
		muscles along twelve meridians (twelve meridian tendons)
		twelve cutaneous regions (twelve skin areas)
	eight extraor- dinary meridians	the *du* meridian
		the *ren* meridian
		the *chong* meridian
		the *dai* meridian
		the *yinwei* meridian
		the *yangwei* meridian
		the *yinqiao* meridian
		the *yangqiao* meridian
collaterals	fifteen collaterals	
	minute collaterals	
	superficial collaterals	

3. Brief introduction of the meridians and collaterals system

3. 1 The twelve meridians

The twelve meridians are the main parts of the meridian system which are also known as "the twelve regular meridians" including three *yin* meridians of the hand, three *yang* meridians of the hand, three *yin* meridians of the foot, and three *yang* meridians of the foot.

3. 1. 1 Distribution on the surface of the body

The twelve meridians distribute in symmetry on the face, head, trunk and limbs.

Four limbs: the *yin* meridians distribute along the inner side of the four limbs, *yang* meridians on the lateral side of the four limbs. According to *yin* and *yang*, *taiyin* and *yangming* meridians distribute along the anterior side, *shaoyin* and *taiyang* along the posterior side and *jueyin* and *shaoyang* along the middle side.

Among these meridians, only *jueyin* meridian of the foot turns and converges with others in distribution. It runs anterior to the *taiyin* meridian of the foot 8 *cun* down to the medial malleolus, from the region 8 *cun* above the medial malleolus, it converges with *Taiyin* meridian and runs between the *Taiyin* and *Shaoyin* meridians.

Trunk: the six meridians of the foot distribute in the way mentioned above. The only difference is that they pertain to either *yin* or *yang* according to the inner side and lateral side of the trunk. The three *yang* meridians of the foot distribute the surface of the trunk, *yangming* on the front, *taiyang* on the back and *shaoyang* on the lateral side. While the three *yin* meridians of the foot run in the interior part corresponding to the *yang* meridians that they are internally and externally related to. Among the six meridians of the hand, the three *yang* meridians all run over the shoulder to the neck while the three *yin* meridians all come out of the chest from the armpit.

Head and face: the six *yang* meridians of the hand and foot all reach the head and face to connect with the five sense organs. That is why it is said the head is the convergence of all *yang* meridians. All the six *yin* meridians run deep in the head and neck to connect with the throat, tongue and eyes.

3. 1. 2 Association of the twelve meridians with the viscera

As to its rule, the association of the twelve meridians with the viscera is mainly demonstrated as "pertaining and connection". *Yin* meridians pertain to the *zang* organs and connect with the *fu* organs, while *yang* meridians pertain to the *fu* organs and connect with the *zang* organs. Besides the regular "pertaining and connection", the *taiyang* meridians of the hand and the foot in the six *yang* meridians also associate with the stomach and the brain. The six *yin* meridians usually associate with the other *zang* and *fu* organs. The following table is a thorough demonstration of such relations among the meridians. (Table 2 – 1 – 2)

Table 2 – 1 – 2 Association of the twelve meridians with the viscera

meridians	pertaining viscera	connecting viscera
lung meridian of hand-*taiyin*	lung	large intestine
large intestine meridian of hand-*yangming*	large intestine	lung
stomach meridian of foot-*yangming*	stomach	spleen
spleen meridian of foot-*taiyin*	spleen	stomach
heart meridian of hand-*shaoyin*	heart	small intestine
small intestine meridian of hand-*taiyang*	small intestine	heart
bladder meridian of foot-*taiyang*	bladder	kidney
kidney meridian of foot-*shaoyin*	kidney	bladder
pericardium meridian of hand-*jueyin*	pericardium	*san Jiao*
triple energizer meridian of hand-*shaoyang*	*san Jiao*	pericardium
gallbladder meridian of foot-*shaoyang*	gallbladder	liver
liver meridian of foot-*jueyin*	liver	gallbladder

3. 1. 3 Running direction, circulation and convergent principle of the twelve meridians

(1) Running direction.

The three *yin* meridians of the hand run from the chest to the hand, the three *yang* meridians run from the hand to the heads, the three *yang* meridians of the foot run from the head to the foot, the three *yin* meridians run from the foot to the abdomen.

(2) Circulation.

The twelve meridians form a cycle of *qi* and blood circulatory system with their regular and adverse circulatory directions. (Fig. 2 – 1 – 1)

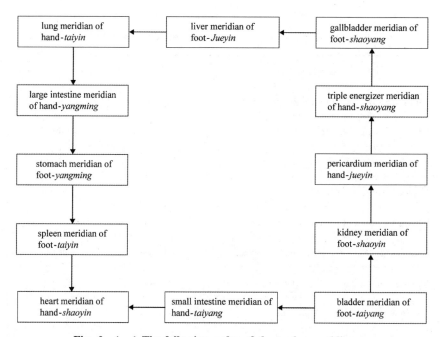

Fig. 2 – 1 – 1 **The following order of the twelve meridians**

(3) Convergent principle.

The *yin* and *yang* meridians in external and internal relationship converge over the end of the four limbs. The *yang* meridians with the same name converge over the head and face. The *yin* meridians and *yang* meridians (in a cycle-like connection) converge over the chest.

The running direction, circulation and convergence are interrelated and reflect the circulatory order of *qi* and blood in the twelve meridians from different perspectives.

3. 2 The twelve divergent meridians (The meridian branches of the twelve meridians)

The twelve divergent meridians stem from the twelve meridians, run deep into the trunk, associate with the viscera and join the meridians in external and internal relation.

3. 2. 1 Distribution characteristics

The running of the twelve divergent meridians is marked by "stemming, entering, outthrusting (leaving) and combination".

"Stemming" means that the twelve divergent meridians stem from the areas below or up the knees and elbows, usually the meridian branches run parallel to or together with the meridians in external and internal relation.

"Entering" means that the divergent meridians enter the body and usually associate with the viscera in external and internal relation, the branches of three *yang* meridians of the foot also associate with the heart.

"Outthrusting (leaving)" means that the divergent meridians come out to run in the superficial areas over the head and neck.

"Combination" means that the *yin* divergent meridians combine with the *yang* meridians that they are in external and internal relation with, while the *yang* divergent meridians combine with the meridians that they stem from.

3. 2. 2 Function

The twelve divergent meridians strengthen the meridians in external and internal relation, especially the association of the meridians with the viscera in external and internal relation. With such activities, the divergent meridians also widen the distribution of the meridians, reinforce the association of the twelve meridians with the whole body, and enlarge the indication of the acupoints.

3. 3 Muscles along twelve meridians (The tendons of the twelve meridians)

Muscles along twelve meridians refer to the areas where *qi* from the twelve meridians accumulates and are the regions where the twelve meridians are connected with the musculature and joints.

3. 3. 1 The distribution rule

The same like the projection of the meridians that they are connected with on the body surface, especially on the four limbs.

3. 3. 2 Function

Nourish and govern the musculature and joints to maintain the normal activities of the body and strengthen the relation of the twelve meridians with the three *yin* and three *yang* meridians on the same side.

3. 4 Twelve cutaneous regions (The twelve skin areas)

Twelve cutaneous regions refers to the regions where the twelve meridians distribute on the skin, are the regions where the *qi* of the collateral spreads, and the functional activities of the twelve meridians reflected on the body surface.

3. 4. 1 The distribution rule

The same distribution of the twelve meridians on the body surface.

3. 4. 2 Function

Twelve cutaneous regions are regarded as the defensive screen of the body. Under pathological conditions, skin areas may act as the routes to transmit pathogenic factors inside and reflect the pathological conditions of the viscera and meridians.

3. 5 The eight extraordinary meridians

The eight extraordinary meridians is a collective term for the governor vessel (*Du* meridian), conception vessel (*Ren* meridian), thoroughfare vessel
(*Chong* meridian) ,belt vessel(*Dai* meridian) ,*yin* link vessel(*Yinwei* meridian) , *yang* link vessel(*Yangwei* meridian) ,*yin* heel vessel(*Yinqiao* meridian)
and *Yang* heel vessel(*Yangqiao* meridian).

3. 5. 1 The differences between twelve meridians and the eight extraordinary meridians (Table 2 – 1 – 4)

Table 2 – 1 – 4 Difference between twelve meridians

and the eight extraordinary meridians

visceral association	close relation with extraordinary *fu* organs
external and internal relation	no
distribution	no their own distributing routes and just run around among the twelve meridians except the governor and conception vessels
acupoints	no their own specific acupoints except the governor and conception vessels
function	they do not transport *qi* and blood like that of the twelve meridians just accumulate and regulate *qi* and blood in the twelve regular meridians

3. 5. 2 The functions of the eight extraordinary meridians

The functions of the eight extraordinary meridians are reflected in two aspects.

One is to associate the twelve meridians to command *qi* and blood in certain meridians as well as to regulate *yin* and *yang*. The governor vessel meets
all the *yang* meridians ,thus it is called "the sea of *yang* meridians" , its func-

tion is to govern the *qi* of all the *yang* meridians of the body. The conception vessel meets all the *yin* meridians, thus it is called "the sea of *yin* meridians", its function is to govern the *qi* of all the *yin* meridians of the body. The thoroughfare vessel meets the governor vessel, the conception vessel, the stomach meridian, the kidney meridian, so it is termed as "the sea of the twelve regular meridians", or "the sea of blood".

The other is accumulate, effuse and regulate *qi* and blood in the twelve meridians, when the *qi* and blood of *zang-fu* organs are vigorous, the eight extraordinary meridians can store them; while the body needs them for its activity, they can be supplied by the eight extraordinary meridians.

3. 6 The fifteen collaterals

The fifteen collaterals is a collective term for the collaterals of twelve meridians, the govern and conception vessels as well as the major collateral of the spleen meridian. They are named respectively after the name of the points from where they start.

3. 6. 1 Regularity of distribution of the fifteen collaterals

①The collaterals of the twelve meridians stem from the ' *luo*-connecting" acupoints of twelve meridians located below the knees and elbows, run to their internal and external relation meridians. ②The collateral of the conception vessel comes out from Jiuwei(CV 15) and spreads over the abdomen. ③The collateral of governor vessel arises from Changqiang(GV 1) and spreads over the head. It goes along the Bladder meridian on the right and left. ④The major collateral of the spleen meridian starts from Dabao (SP 21) and spreads through the chest and hypochondriac region. ⑤"The superficial collaterals" are those which are distributed on the superficies of the body, and the smallest branches of the collaterals are called "Minute collaterals".

3. 6. 2 Functions of the fifteen collaterals

The collaterals of the twelve meridians strengthen the relations of the *yin*-

yang and the internal-external meridians. The collaterals of the conception vessel communicate with the *qi* of the abdomen. The collaterals of governor vessel communicate with the *qi* of the back. The major collaterals of spleen meridian communicate with the *qi* of meridian in the lateral side of the chest.

4. Functions of the meridian system and clinical application of the theory of meridians

4. 1 The functions of meridians system

4. 1. 1 Connecting the external with the internal as well as connecting the viscera with other organs

The body is organic whole. It is the meridians and collaterals that connect the viscera, the body, the five sensory organs and the nine orifices together.

4. 1. 2 Transporting *qi* and blood and regulating *yin* and *yang*

All the viscera and other parts of the body depend on *qi*, blood, *yin* and *yang* to nourish and maintain their physiological functions. It is meridians that transport *qi*, blood, *yin* and *yang* to the whole body. In fact, the meridians and collaterals are passages of *qi*, blood *yin* and *yang*.

4. 1. 3 Resisting pathogens and defending the body

Because the meridians can transport the *qi* and blood, regulate *yin* and *yang*, the nutrient *qi* circulate the meridians interiorly, the defensive *qi* along the meridians exteriorly. This makes the nutrient *qi* and defensive *qi* spread over the whole body and strengthen the body resistance against the diseases.

4. 1. 4 Transmitting needling sensation and regulating deficiency and excess conditions

Acupuncture and moxibustion can prevent and treat diseases depend on the functions of meridians of transmitting needling sensation and regulating deficiency and excess conditions. The meridians can regulate deficiency and excess conditions based on the functions of meridians of regulating *yin* and *yang*.

4. 2 Clinical application of the theory of meridians

4. 2. 1 To explain the pathological transmission

Physiologically, the meridians serve as the pathways for *qi* and blood to circulate in the body. Pathologically, the meridians transmit pathogenic factors into the body. When the meridian *qi* becomes weak or fails to protect the body due to certain factors, exogenous factors may invade the body and the pathogenic factors will be transmitted to the viscera through meridians. Similarly, when the pathological changes have taken place in the viscera, they may be transmitted to the surface of the body through the system of meridians. Due to the association of the viscera by meridians, the pathogenic factors are transmitted from one viscera to another.

4. 2. 2 To explain the functions of treatment

The treatment of diseases with acupuncture and moxibustion is accomplished by the transmitting activities of the meridians in regulating meridian *qi* to restore the normal functions of the viscera and meridians. Such a function of the meridians lies in their physiological activities in transporting *qi* and blood as well as in harmonizing *yin* and *yang*.

4. 2. 3 To guide the diagnosis of disease

Since the meridians run along certain routes and pertain to certain viscera, there is a special relationship between different parts of the body and the internal organs. Clinically the relationship between the pathological location or disease and the meridians can be used to decide which meridian and viscera are involved so as to make an accurate diagnosis. Besides, doctors can diagnose diseases according to the special reactive changes along the course of the meridians such as sensitive tenderness, tubercles and cord-like things.

4. 2. 4 To guide the treatment of disease

The theory of the meridians and collaterals is extensively used in clinical treatment, especially in acupuncture and moxibustion, massage and drug treatment.

The treatment of disease by acupuncture, moxibustion and massage is usually done by needling or massaging the acupoints proximal or distal to the affected part on the meridians to regulate the functional activities of the meridian *qi* and blood. The selection of points along the course of meridians is the basic principle. Besides, in view of the close relation of the skin areas to the meridians and collaterals and *zang-fu* organs, diseases of the meridians and collaterals and *zang-fu* organs can be treated by using plum-blossom needle to stimulate the skin or embedding an intradermal needle and needling collaterals to let blood out. The pathological changes of tendons are characterized by muscle pain, spasm, rigidity or convulsion, sluggish, etc. The treatment for the pathological changes of tendons are to chose local *Ashi* points.

Drug treatment also has to be done according to the theory of meridians and collaterals because the meridians and collaterals can transport the effect of the drugs to the affected part. In the long course of clinical practice, TCM has developed the theory of "meridian tropism of drugs" which holds that each drug can enter one or more meridians. With the guidance of the theory, clinically drugs are selected, based on syndrome differentiation, according to their state of "meridian tropism " to treat disease so as to improve the therapeutic effect.

Knowledge point 2   Basic Theory of Acupoints

1. Conception

Acupoints are the regions where qi and blood from the viscera and meridians effuse and infuse beneath the body surface, usually located in the interstices of the thick muscles or between tendons and bones.

The viscera, meridians and acupoints in the interior and exterior form an organic whole with close relation and harmonious unity. The meridians are connected with the viscera in the interior and with the acupoints in the exterior. Under pathological conditions, disorders of the viscera can reflected on certain acupoints through the meridians. Stimulation the acupoints may regulate the functional activities of the corresponding viscera.

2. Classifications

Acupoints can usually be classified into meridian acupoints, extraordinary acupoints and *Ashi* points according to the characteristics of acupoints. (Table 2 – 2 – 1)

Meridian acupoints, also known as acupoints of the fourteen meridians, refer to the acupoints located on the twelve meridians as well as the governor and conception vessels. Meridian acupoints, the main part of the acupoints and frequently selected for acupuncture treatment, pertain to definite meridians with fixed names and location.

Extraordinary acupoints refer to the acupoints excluding the ones located on the fourteen meridians. These acupoints have definite locations and name and are effective in treating certain diseases. But they usually do not pertain to any meridians. However, the extraordinary acupoints and meridian acupoints are closely related to each other. Some extraordinary acupoints include certain meridian acupoints.

Ashi acupoints actually refer to tenderness spots. Such acupoints are characterized by absence of fixed locations, definite names and pertaining meridians.

Table 2 – 2 – 1 Classifications of acupoints

	name	location	number	meridian
meridian acupoints	regular names	regular locations	361	pertaining to definite meridians
extraordinary acupoints	regular locations	regular locations	no	no pertaining meridians
ashi points	no specific names	no definite locations	no	no pertaining meridians

3. Therapeutic effects of acupoints

The functions of acupoints are marked by proximal therapeutical effect, distal therapeutical effect and special therapeutical effect.

3. 1 Proximal therapeutic effect

Proximal curative effect is the common feature of all acupoints. That means that all acupoints can be punctured to treat disorders to the regions, tissues and organs around them, especially the acupoints located on the head, face and trunk. That is "where acupoints, indication lies".

3. 2 Distal therapeutic effect

Distal curative effect is the feature of the acupoints of the fourteen meridians, especially the acupoints of the twelve meridians located below the knees and elbows which not only can be needled to treat disorders of the regional tissues, but also can be applied to treat the disorders of the viscera, tissues and organs associated with the meridians in their distribution. Some of the meridian acupoints even can be needled to treat the disorders of the whole body. That is "the indication extends to where the meridian reaches".

3. 3 Special therapeutic effect

Special therapeutical effect of acupoints includes *bi*-directional and relative specific effect.

3. 3. 1 *Bi*-directional effect

Bi-directional effect, also known as favourable *bi*-directional regulating effect, refers to the needling of the same acupoints with different manipulating techniques to stimulate meridian *qi* to regulate different functional activities of the body *bi*-directionally. That means to balance the functions of the body when they become hyperactive with the inhibiting effect and to restore the normal functions of the body when they become hypoactive with the exciting effect.

3. 3. 2 Relative specific effect

Relative specific effect means that some of the acupoints bear special or specific therapeutical effect on certain diseases.

4. Special acupoints

Special acupoints refer to the acupoints on the fourteen meridians with special therapeutical effect. A majority of the acupoints bears special effect and are commonly used in clinical treatment.

There are ten types of special acupoints, including five-*shu* acupoints below the knees and elbows, *yuan*-source acupoints, *luo*-connecting acupoints, lower *he*-sea acupoints, *xi-cleft* acupoints and eight convergent acupoints.

back-shu acupoints and front-*mu* acupoints located on the trunk, as well as eight confluent acupoints and crossing acupoints located on the whole body.

4. 1 Five-*shu* acupoints

Five-*shu* acupoints refer to *jing*-well, *ying*-spring, *shu*-stream, *jing*-river and *he*-sea which are five acupoints located on the twelve meridians below the knees and elbows. They are situated in the above mentioned order from the distal extremities to the elbows or knees. From these five acupoints, we can see reflect the indication of the acupoints below the knees and elbows.

4. 2 *Yuan*-source acupoints

Yuan-source acupoints, as the regions where the primary *qi* of the viscera flows through and retains, are usually located around the wrists and ankles, reflecting the pathological changes of the viscera. They are clinically used to diagnose and treat the disorders of the related viscera.

4. 3 *Luo*-connecting acupoints

Luo-connecting acupoints refer to the points where the fifteen collaterals stem from the twelve meridians, the governor and conception vessels as well as the major collateral of the spleen. All the *luo*-connecting acupoints of the twelve meridians are located below the elbows and knees. These acupoints are used to treat the disorders of the regions that the meridians and collaterals run through as well as the disorders to the meridians in external and internal relation.

4. 4 *Xi*-cleft acupoints

Xi-cleft acupoints are the sites where *qi* and blood from the meridians are deeply converged. Each of the twelve meridians and the four extraordinary vessels (*yin* heel vessel, *yang* heel vessel, *yin* link vessel and *yang* link vessel) has a *xi*-cleft acupoint on the limbs, amounting to sixteen in all.

Clinically *xi*-cleft acupoints are used to treat severe acute disorders of the meridians. The *xi*-cleft acupoints on the *yin* meridians are usually used to treat various blood syndromes and the *xi*-cleft acupoints on the *yang* meridians are often used to treat various pain syndromes.

4. 5 The eight convergent acupoints

The eight convergent acupoints refer to the eight acupoints on the twelve meridians that are connected with the eight extraordinary vessels. These eight acupoints are all located below the knees and elbows and are used to treat disorders involving the face, head and trunk related to the eight extraordinary vessels.

4. 6 The lower *He*-sea acupoints

The lower *he*-sea acupoints refer to six acupoints on the three *yang* meridians of the foot where *qi* from the six-*fu* organs converge and are the key acupoints for the treatment for the disorders of the six-*fu* organs.

4. 7 Back-*shu* acupoints

Back-*shu* acupoints are located on the back and waist along the first lateral line of the bladder meridian(1. 5 *cun* lateral to the back middle line) and are the regions where *qi* of the viscera is infused. The distributing order of back-*shu* acupoints is similar to that of the location of the viscera.

Clinically these acupoints are used to treat the disorders of the related viscera, tissues and organs.

4. 8 Front-*mu* acupoints

Front-*mu* acupoints are those located on the chest and abdomen where *qi* of the viscera is infused and converged. The location of the front-*mu* acupoints is similar to that of the related viscera. Among these acupoints, six on the conception vessel are unilateral acupoints and the rest are bilateral ones.

Front-*mu* acupoints can be used to treat disorders of the related viscera, especially the disorders of the six-*fu* organs. These acupoints are usually needled with the combination of back-*shu* acupoints.

4. 9 Eight confluent acupoints

Eight confluent acupoints, located on the trunk and four limbs below the knees and elbows, are the regions where the essence of *qi*, blood, tendons, vessels, bones, marrow, *zang* organs and *fu* organs converge.

Apart from treating diseases of the meridian proper, these acupoints are frequently used to treat diseases of the corresponding tissues and organs.

4. 10 Crossing acupoints

Crossing acupoints are those at the intersections of two or more meridians. Most of them are located on the head. Face and trunk, except a few which are located on the lower limbs. Crossing acupoints are clinically used to treat diseases related to the meridian proper and the meridians crossed with the meridian proper.

Knowledge point 3　Methods for locating acupoints

Location of acupoints, whether accurate or not, will affect the therapeutic results. However, accurate location of acupoints depends on proper selection of locating acupoints. At present, commonly used in clinics are four methods of acupuncture point location, i. e. , proportional measurement, anatomical landmarks, finger measurement and simple measurement.

1. Proportional Measurements (Bone-length measurement)

The width or lengths of various portions of the human body are divided respectively into definite numbers of equal units as the standards for the proportional measurement. These standards are applicable on any patient of different sexes, ages and body sizes. (Fig. 2 – 3 – 1, Fig. 2 – 3 – 2 and Table 2 – 3 – 1)

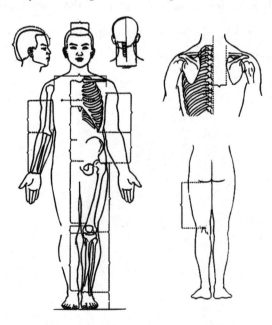

Fig. 2 – 3 – 1 Front of the body　Fig. 2 – 3 – 2 Back of the body

Table 2 – 3 – 1 Proportional Measurements（Bone-length measurement）

body part	distance	bone-length	indications	notes
head	anterior hairline → posterior hairline	12	vertical *cun* for the vertex	*cun* measurement from *yin-tang*（GV 14）to dazhui（GV 14）can be used if hairline is not clear
	between the two mastoid prcesses	9	transverse *cun* for back head	
chest and abdomen	sternocostal angle → umbilicus centre	8	vertical *cun* for the upper abdomen	sternocostal symphysis is usually parllel to the fifth costal space
	umbilicus center → upper margin of pubic symphysis	5	vertical *cun* for the lower abdomen	
	between two nipples	8	transverse *cun* for chest and abdomen	usually used for women
back	the medial border of the scapula → the posterior midline	3		
lateral side of the chest	anterior axillary fold	12		
upper extremities	anterior axillary fold	9	vertical *cun* for the upper arm	
	cubital transverse crease → wrist transverse crease	12	vertical *cun* for the forearm	

Continued

body part	distance	bone-length	indications	notes
lower extremities	upper border of pubic symphysis →medial epicondyle of malleolus	18	vertical *cun* for lateral side of the thigh	bone measurement of the medial side of the lower limbs is applicable to the location of acupoints on the three *yin* meridians of foot
	lower margin of the medial condyle → tip of medial malleous	13	vertical *cun* for the medial side of the shank	
	great trochanter of femur→ middle of patella	19	vertical *cun* for the lateral side of thigh	applicable to the location of acupints on the three *yang* meridians o f foot. the horizontal line in the knee is parallel anteriorly to the lower margin of the patella, posteriorly to the popliteal transverse crease and to the *Dubi* (ST 35) when the knee is bent
	buttock crease → popliteal crease	14	vertical *cun* for theback of thigh	
	basis patellae → apex patellae	2		
	middle of patella → tip of lateral malleolus	16	vertical *cun* for the lateral side of shank	
	from the tip of the lateral malleolus to the heel	3	vertical *cun* for the lateral side of foot	

2. Anatomical landmarks

Various anatomical landmarks on the body surface are the basis for locating points. Those landmarks fall into two categories.

2. 1 Fixed landmarks

Fixed landmarks are those that would not change with body movement. They include the five sense organs, hair, nails, nipple, umbilicus, and prominence and depression of the bone.

2. 2 Moving landmarks

Moving landmarks refer to those that will appear only when a body part keeps in a specific position.

3. Finger measurement

The length and width of the patient's finger(s) are taken as a standard for point location. The following three methods are commonly used in clinic.

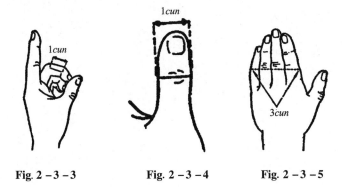

Fig. 2 – 3 – 3   Fig. 2 – 3 – 4   Fig. 2 – 3 – 5

3. 1 Middle finger measurement (Fig. 2 – 3 – 3)

When the patient's middle finger is flexed, the distance between the two medial ends of the creases of the interphalangeal joints is taken as 1 *cun*.

This method is employed for measuring the vertical distance to locate the limb points of the *yang* meridians, or measuring the horizontal distance to locate the points on the back.

3. 2 Thumb measurement (Fig. 2 – 3 – 4)

The width of the interphalangeal joint of the patient's thumb is taken as 1 *cun*. The method is also employed for measuring the vertical distance to locate the points on the limbs.

3. 3 Four-finger measurement（Fig. 2 − 3 − 5）

The width of the four fingers（index, middle, ring and little）close together at the level of the dorsal skin crease of the proximal interphalangeal joint of the middle finger is taken as 3 *cun*. It is used to locate the points on the limb and in the abdominal region.

Knowledge point 4   Meridians and their acupoints

1. The Lung Meridian of Hand-*taiyin*

1.1 The course of the Lung Meridian of Hand-*taiyin* (Fig. 2 −4 −1)

The lung meridian of hand-*taiyin* originates from the middle energizer, running downward to connect with the large intestine. Winding back, it goes along the upper orifice of the stomach, passes through the diaphragm, and enters the lung, its pertaining organ. From the lung system, which refers to the portion of the lung communicating with the throat, it comes out transversely. Descending along the radial border of the medial aspect of the upper arm, it reaches the cubital fossa,

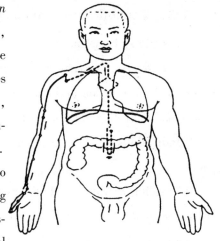

Fig. 2-4-1 The course of the
lung meridian of hand-*taiyin*

then goes continuously downward along the anterior border of the radial side in the medial aspect of the forearm. and enters *Cunkou*. Passing the thenar eminence, and going along its radial border, it ends at the medial side of the tip of the thumb.

The branch proximal to the wrist emerges and runs directly to the radial side of the tip of the index finger and ends at the medial side of the tip of the index finger where it links with the large intestine meridian.

[**Associated viscera**]Lung, large intestine, stomach and middle energizer.

[**Associated organs**] Trachea and throat.

1. 2 Indications

Disorders of the chest, lung, throat and regions the meridian running by.

1. 3 Commonly used acupoints of the Lung Meridian of Hand-*taiyin*

The acupoints of the Lung Meridian of Hand-*taiyin* starts from LU 1, ends at Shaoshang(LU 11), bilateral each consisting of 11 acupoints.

1. 3. 1 Zhongfu (front-*mu* acupoint)

[**Location**] Laterosuperior to the sternum at the lateral side of the first intercostals space, 1 *cun* below *Yunmen*(LU 2), parallel to the first costal interstice and 6 *cun* lateral to the median line. The patient sit straight or lies in supination for locating this point. (Fig. 2-4-2)

[**Indications**] (1) Cough, asthma, chest pain. (2) Shoulder and back pain.

[**Needling Method**] Oblique insertion towards the lateral aspect of the chest or subcutaneous insertion 0. 5 ~0. 8 *cun*. Deep perpendicular insertion or towards the medial aspect is prohibited in order to avoid puncturing the lungs, causing pneumatothorax.

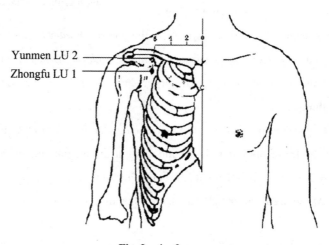

Yunmen LU 2
Zhongfu LU 1

Fig. 2 −4 −2

1. 3. 2 Chize（LU 5, *he*-sea acupoint of the lung meridian of hand-*taiyin*）

[**Location**] When the palm is turned upward and slightly bent, this point is located on the cubital crease and on the radial side of the tendon of the m. biceps brachii. （Fig. 2 − 4 − 3）

[**Indications**] (1)Cough, asthma, hemoptysis, and sore throat. (2)Sun stroke. (3)Acute abdominal pain with vomiting and diarrhea. (4)Infantile convulsion. (5)Spasmodic pain of the elbow and arm.

[**Needling Method**] Perpendicular insertion 0. 8 ~ 1. 2 *cun*. When treating acute abdominal pain with vomiting and diarrhea, prick the cephalic vein on this point to make bleeding.

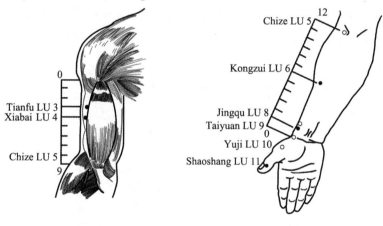

Fig. 2 − 4 − 3　　　　　　Fig. 2 − 4 − 4

1. 3. 3 Kongzui（Lub, *xi*-cleft acupoint of the lung meridian of hand-*taiyin*）

[**Location**] The elbow is bent slightly and the palms turn to face each other. Or when the forearm is stretched and the palm turn over. This point is located on the palmar aspect of the forearm on the line joining Taiyuan （LU 9）and Chize（LU 5）and 7 *cun* above the transverse crease of the wrist. （Fig. 2 − 4 − 4）

[**Indications**] (1) Cough, hemoptysis, epistaxis and sore throat. (2)Febrile diseases without sweating. (3)Spasmodic pain of the elbow and arm.

[**Needling Method**] Perpendicular insertion 0. 5 ~ 1 *cun*.

1. 3. 4 Lieque (LU 7, *luo*-connecting point of the lung meridian of hand-*taiyin* and one of the eight convergent points associating with the conception vessel)

[**Location**] The elbow is bent slightly and the palm turns to face each other. This point is superior to the styloid process of the radius, 1. 5 *cun* above the transverse crease of the wrist.

When the index finger of one hand placed on the styloid process of the radius of the other, the depression right under the tip of the index finger is the acupoint. (Fig. 2 – 4 – 5)

Lieque LU 7

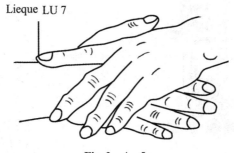

Fig. 2 – 4 – 5

[**Indications**] (1)Cough, asthma, and sore throat. (2)Headache, stiff neck, facial paralysis, and toothache. (3)Pain in the penis and hematuria. (4)Weakness and pain of the wrist.

[**Needling method**] Insert obliquely upwards 0. 3 ~0. 5 *cun*.

1. 3. 5 Taiyuan (LU 9, *shu*-stream and *yuan*-source point of lung meridian of the hand-*taiyin* and one of the eight confluent acupoints-the vessel-confluent point)

[**Location**] The arm is stretched and the palm is turned over, the point is located at the radial end of the transverse crease of the wrist and in the depression on the radial side of the radial artery. (Fig. 2 – 4 – 6)

Taiyuan LU 9

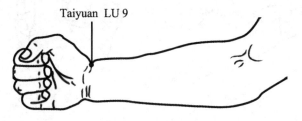

Fig. 2 – 4 – 6

[**Indications**] (1) Cough with large amount of phlegm and asthma. (2) Headache, hemiplegia, cold. (3) Wrist pain.

[**Needling method**] Keep clear of artery. Perpendicular insertion 0. 3 ~ 0. 5 *cun*.

1. 3. 6 Yuji (LU 10, *xing*-spring acuptiont)

[**Location**] This point is located at the radical side of the midpoint of the first metacarpal bone and the junction of the red and white skin, in the depression proximal to the first metacarpophalangeal joint. (Fig. 2 – 4 – 7)

[**Indications**] (1) Febrile disease, sore throat, aphonia, cough, asthma. (2) Feverish sensation in the palms.

[**Needling method**] Puncture perpendicularly 0. 5 ~ 0. 8 *cun*. Moxibustion is applicable.

1. 3. 7 Shaoshang (LU 11, *jing*-well acupoint)

[**Location**] Thumb is stretched, the point is located on the radial side of the thumb, about 0. 1 *cun* lateroposterior to the corner of the nail. (Fig. 2 – 4 – 8)

[**Indications**] (1) Sore throat, cough, epistaxis. (2) Fever, coma, manic depression.

[**Needling method**] Insert obliquely 0. 1 *cun* towards upper direction, or prick the point to cause bleeding.

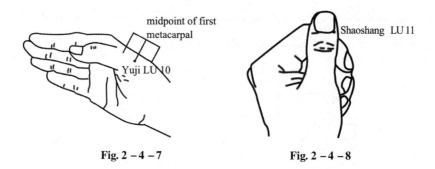

Fig. 2 – 4 – 7   Fig. 2 – 4 – 8

2. The Large Intestine Meridian of Hand-*yangming*

2. 1 The course of the Large Intestine Meridian of Hand-*yangming* (Fig. 2 – 4 – 9)

The large intestine meridian starts from the tip of the index finger (*Shangyang* , LI 1). It runs upward along the radial side of the index finger and passes through the interspace of the first and second metacarpal bones (Hegu, LI 4), in enters into the depression between the tendons of m. extensor pollices longus and brevis. Following the lateral anterior aspect of the forearm, it reaches the lateral side of the elbow where it ascends along the lateral anterior aspect of the upper arm to the highest point of the shoulder (Jianyu, LI 15). Along the anterior border of the acromion, it goes up to the seventh cervical vertebral (the confluence of the three *yang* meridians of the hand and foot) and descends to the supraclavicular fossa to connect with its corresponding *zang-fu*—the lung. It then passes through the diaphragm and enters the large intestine, its pertaining organ. The branch from the supraclavicular fossa runs upward to the neck, passes through the cheek and enters the lower gums. Then it turns back to the upper lip and crosses the opposite meridian at philtrum From there, the left meridian goes to the right and the right meridian to the left, to the contralateral sides of the nose (Yingxiang, LI 20) , where the large intestine meridian connects with the stomach meridian.

[**Associated viscera**] Large intestine and lung.

[**Associated organs**] Mouth, lower teeth and nose.

2. 2 Indications

Disorders of the mouth, teeth, nose and throat as well as diseases involving the lateral border of the upper limbs, anterior part of the shoulder and neck.

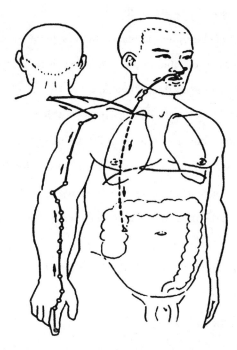

Fig. 2 – 4 – 9 The coures of the large intestine meridian of hand-*yangming*

2. 3 Commonly used acupoints of the Large Intestine Meridian of Hand-*yangming*

The acupoints of the large intestine meridian of hand-*yangming* starts from Shangyang(LI 1) ,ends at yingxiang(LI 20). Bilateral each consisting of 20 acupoints.

2. 3. 1 Hegu(LI 4 , *yuan*-source acupoint)

[**Location**] The point is located on the dorsum of the hand, between the first and second metacarpal bones, approximately in the middle of the second metacarpal bone on the radial side. (Fig. 2 – 4 – 10)

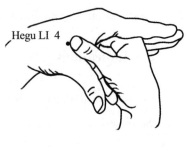

Fig. 2 – 4 – 10

When the transverse crease of the interphalangeal joint of the thumb is placed in coincident position with the margin of the web between the thumb and the index finger of the other hand, the point is where the tip of the thumb touches.

[**Indications**] (1) Headache, dizziness, swelling and pain of the eye, toothache, epistaxis, facial paralysis. (2) Aversion to cold, fever, febrile disease, anhidrosis, hidrosis. (3) Abdominal pain, diarrhea, constipation, dysentery. (4) Dysmenorrheal, amenorrhea, dystocia. (5) Infantile convulsion, trismus. (6) Urticaria, acne. (7) Hemiplegia, finger spasm, pain in the arm.

[**Needling method**] Perpendicular insertion 0. 5 ~ 1 *cun*. This point is prohibited in pregnancy.

2. 3. 2 Shousanli(LI 10)

[**Location**] It is located on the line joining Yangxi (LI 5) and Quchi (LI 11), 2 *cun* below the cubital transverse crease. (Fig. 2 – 4 – 11)

[**Indications**] (1) Abdominal pain, diarrhea. (2) Paralysis of the upper extremities, stop aching and distention sensation caused by incorrect needling technique.

[**Needling method**] Perpendicular insertion 0. 8 ~ 1. 2 *cun*.

2. 3. 3 Quchi(LI 11, *he*-sea acupoint)

[**Location**] When the elbow is flexed 90°, the acupoint is located on the middle point on the line joining Chize (LU 5) and the external epicondyle of the humerous. (Fig. 2 – 4 – 12)

[**Indications**] (1) Febrile diseases, sore throat, headache, dizziness, redness, swelling, swelling and pain of the eye, toothache. (2) Paralysis of the upper limbs, spasmodic pain of the elbow and arm. (3) Abdominal pain, vomiting, diarrhea. (4) Eczema, urticaria, acne. (5) Hypertension, manic depression.

[**Needling method**] Perpendicular insertion 1 ~ 1.5 *cun*.

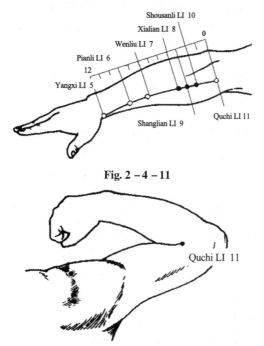

Fig. 2 – 4 – 11

Fig. 2 – 4 – 12

2.3.4 Jianyu(LI 15)

[**Location**] The acupoint is located anterior-inferior to the acromion, on the upper portion of m. deltoideus and between the acromion and greater tuberosity of humerus. When the arm is in full abduction, the acupoint is in the depression at the anterior border of the acromioclavicular joint. (Fig. 2 – 4 – 13)

[**Indication**] Paralysis of the upper extremities, pain and motor impairment of the shoulder.

[**Needling method**] Perpendicularly or obliquely downward insertion

0. 8 ~ 1. 5 *cun*.

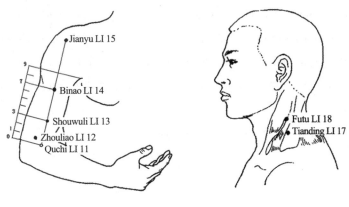

Fig. 2 − 4 − 13   Fig. 2 − 4 − 14

2. 3. 5 Futu(LI 18)

[**Location**] The acupoint is located on the lateral side of the laryngeal protuberance and between the sternal head and clavicular head of m. sternocleidomastoideus. (Fig. 2 − 4 − 14)

[**Indication**] (1) Sore throat, scrofula, goiter. (2) Paralysis of the upper extremity, pain and limitation of the shoulder.

[**Needling method**] Perpendicularly insertion 0. 5 ~ 0. 8 *cun*.

2. 3. 6 Yingxiang(LI 20)

[**Location**] The acupoint is located in the nasolabial groove and at the level of the midpoint of the lateral border of the nose. (Fig. 2 − 4 − 15)

[**Indications**] (1) Nasal obstruction, epistaxis, nasosinusitis, facial paralysis. (2) Biliary ascariasis.

[**Needling method**] Oblique or subcutaneous insertion 0. 3 ~ 0. 5 *cun*.

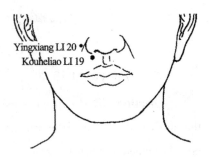

Fig. 2 − 4 − 15

3. The Stomach Meridian of Foot-*yangming*

3. 1 The course of the Stomach Meridian of Foot-*yangming* (Fig. 2 –4 –16)

The stomach meridian of foot-*yangming* starts from the lateral side of nose (Yangxing, LI 20), ascending to the bridge of the nose, turning downward along the lateral side of the nose, entering the upper gums, reemerging, curving around the lips, descending to meet the *Ren* meridian at the mentolabial groove, running posterolaterally across the lower portion of the cheek at Daying (ST 7), winding along the angle of the mandible (Jiache, ST 6), ascending in front of the ear and traverse Shangguan (GB 3), following the anterior hairline, reaching the forehead (Shenting, GV 24).

Facial branch meridian: running downward Daying (ST 9), then going along the throat, entering the supraclavicular fossa, descending and passing through the diaphragm.

The straight portion of the meridian arising from the supraclavicular fossa, running downward, passing through the nipple, descending by the umbilicus and entering Qichong (ST 30) on the lateral side of the lower abdomen.

The branch from the lower orifice of the stomach: descending inside the abdomen and joining the previous portion of the meridian at Qichong (ST 30). Running downward, traversing Biguan (ST 31), and further through Futu (ST 32), reaching the knee, continuing downward along the anterior border of the lateral aspect of the tibia, passing through the dorsum of the foot, reaching the lateral side of the tip of the 2nd toe.

The tibial branch: emerging from 3 *cun* below the knee (Zusanli, ST 36), entering the lateral side of the middle toe.

The branch from the dorsum of foot arising from Chongyang (ST 42), terminating at the medial side of the tip of the great toe (Yinbai, SP 1), where linking with the spleen meridian of foot-*taiyin*.

[**Associated Viscera**] Stomach and spleen.

[**Associated organs**] Eyes, nose, lower teeth, ears, mouth, larynx and breast.

3. 2 Indications

Diseases involving stomach, intestine, head, face, nose, mouth and tooth as well as mental problems and disorders involving the regions through which the meridian runs.

3. 3 Commonly used acupoints of the Stomach Meridian of Foot-*yangming*

This meridian starts at Chengqi(ST 1) and ends at Lidui(ST 45), biliterally each consisting of 45 acupoints.

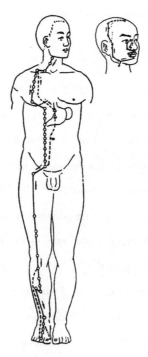

Fig. 2 – 4 – 16 The coures of the stomach meridian of foot-*yangming*

3. 3. 1 Sibai(ST 2)

[**Location**] This point is located on the face, directly below the pupil and in the depression at the infraorbital foramen when the eyes look straight forward. (Fig. 2 – 4 – 17)

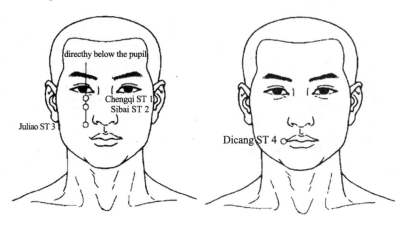

Fig. 2 – 4 – 17   Fig. 2 – 4 – 18

[**Indication**] (1) Redness, pain and itching of eyes, cataract, twitching of eyelids, myopia. (2) Facial paralysis, headache, trigeminal neuralgia.

[**Needling method**] Puncture perpendicular or obliquely 0. 3 ~ 0. 5 *cun*. Usually do not use moxa.

3. 3. 2 Dicang(ST 4)

[**Location**] This point is located lateral to the corner of the mouth and directly below the pupil. (Fig. 2 – 4 – 18)

[**Indications**] Facial paralysis, salivation (drooling), twitching of the corner of the mouth.

[**Needling method**] Oblique or subcutaneous insertion 0. 5 ~ 0. 8 *cun* or puncture towards to Jiache(ST 6).

3. 3. 3 Jiache(ST 6)

[**Location**] This point is one finger-breadth (middle finger) anterior and superior to the lower angle of the mandible where m. masseter attaches at the prominence of the muscle when the teeth are clenched. (Fig. 2 – 4 – 19)

[**Indications**] Swelling of the cheek, facial paralysis, toothache, trismus, difficulty in opening the mouth.

[**Needling method**] Perpendicular insertion 0. 3 ~ 0. 5 *cun* or subcutaneous towards Dicang(ST 4).

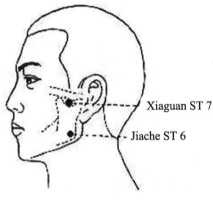

Fig. 2 – 4 – 19   Fig. 2 – 4 – 20

3. 3. 4 Xiaguan(ST 7)

[**Location**] This point is located before the ear and in the depression anterior to the condyloid process of the mandible. This point is located with the mouth opened. (Fig. 2 – 4 – 19)

[**Indications**] (1) Toothache, trigeminal neuralgia, facial paralysis, difficulty in opening the mouth. (2) Deafness, tinnitus, otopyorrhea.

[**Needling method**] Perpendicular insertion 0. 5 ~ 1 *cun*.

3. 3. 5 Touwei(ST 8)

[**Location**] This point is located on the lateral side of the head, 0. 5 *cun* within the anterior hairline at the corner of the head, 4. 5 *cun* laterals to the midline of the head. (Fig. 2 – 4 – 20)

[**Indications**] Headache, vertigo, blurred vision, twitching of eyelids.

[**Needing method**] Subcutaneous insertion 0. 5-1 *cun*.

3. 3. 6 Rugen(ST 18)

[**Location**] This acupoint is located directly below the nipple, on the root of breast, in the fifth intercostal space and 4 *cun* lateral to the anterior midline. (Fig. 2 – 4 – 21)

[**Indications**] Cough, asthma, chest pain, mastitis, insufficiency of lactation.

[**Needling method**] Obliquely or subcutaneous insertion 0. 5 ~ 0. 8 *cun*.

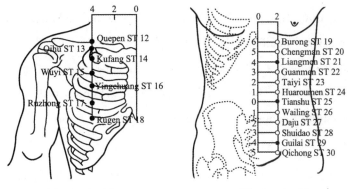

Fig. 2 – 4 – 21   Fig. 2 – 4 – 22

3. 3. 7 Liangmen(ST 21)

[**Location**] This point is located 4 *cun* above the umbilicus and 2 *cun* laterals to anterior midline. (Fig. 2 – 4 – 22)

[**Indications**] Gastric pain, vomiting, poor appetite, abdominal distention, diarrhea.

[**Needling method**] Perpendicular insertion 0. 8 ~ 1. 2 *cun*.

3. 3. 8 Tianshu (ST 25 , front-*mu* acupoint)

[**Location**] This point is located on the center of the abdomen, and 2 *cun* lateral to anterior midline. (Fig. 2 – 4 – 22)

[**Indications**] (1) Abdominal distention, borborygmus, pain around the umbilicus, constipation, diarrhea, dysentery. (2) Irregular menstruation, mass and gathering in the abdomen, dysmenorrhea, amenorrhea.

[**Needling method**] Perpendicular insertion 1 ~ 1. 5 *cun*.

3. 3. 9 Shuidao(ST 28)

[**Location**] This point is located 3 *cun* below the umbilicus and 2 *cun* laterals to anterior midline. (Fig. 2 – 4 – 22)

[**Indications**](1) Edema, dysuria, lower abdominal distention, dysmenorrhea, hernia. (2) Constipation.

[**Needling method**] Perpendicular insertion 1 ~ 1. 5 *cun*.

3. 3. 10 Guilai(ST 29)

[**Location**] This point is located 4 *cun* below the umbilicus and 2 *cun* lateral to anterior midline. (Fig. 2 – 4 – 22)

[**Indications**] (1) Prolapse of uterus, irregular menstruation, amenorrhea, and leucorrhea, hernia, abdominal pain. (2) Constipation.

[**Needling method**] Perpendicular insertion 1 ~ 1. 5 *cun*.

3. 3. 11 Futu(ST 32)

[**Location**] This point is located in the front of the thigh, on the line connecting the anterior superior iliac spine and lateral border of the patella, 6 *cun* above the laterosuperior border of the patella. (Fig. 2 – 4 – 23)

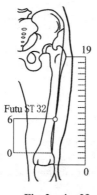 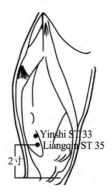

Fig. 2 – 4 – 23 Fig. 2 – 4 – 24

[**Indications**] Paralysis or weakness of the lower extremities, coldness and pain of the lower back and knee.

[**Needling method**] Perpendicular insertion 1 ~ 2 *cun*.

3. 3. 12 Liangqiu (ST 34 , *xi*-cleft acupoint)

[**Location**] When the knee is flexed, the acupoint is in the front of thing, on the line connecting the anterior superior iliac spine and lateral

border of the patella, 2 *cun* above the laterosuperior border of the patella.
(Fig. 2 – 4 – 24)

[**Indications**] (1) Acute stomach, vomiting, mastitis. (2) Pain in the knee joint and paralysis of the lower limbs.

[**Needling method**] Perpendicular insertion 0. 5 ~ 1 *cun*. Moxibustion is applicable.

3. 3. 13 Dubi(ST 35)

[**Location**] This acupoint is located in the depression lateral to the patellar ligament when the knee is flexed. (Fig. 2 – 4 – 25)

[**Indications**] Pain of the knee, paralysis of the lower limbs, inflexibility and beriberi.

[**Needling method**] Obliquely insertion toward the medial back 0. 5 ~ 1 *cun*.

3. 3. 14 Zusanli (ST 36 *he*-sea acupoint, lower *he*-sea acupoint, tonifaction acupoint)

[**Location**] This point is located on the lateral side of the shank, 3 *cun* below Dubi(ST35), one finger-breadth (midfinger) from the anterior crest of the tibia in m. tibialis anterior. (Fig. 2 – 4 – 25)

[**Indications**] (1) Stomachache, vomiting, dysphagia, abdominal pain, abdominal distention, borborygmus, diarrhea, dysentery, constipation, acute mastitis. (2) Dizziness, insomnia, manic depression. (3) Cough and asthma, palpitation, shortness of breath, emaciation due to general deficiency. (4) Pain in the knee joint, hemiplegia, beriberi, edema.

[**Needling method**] Perpendicular insertion 1 ~ 2 *cun*.

3. 3. 15 Shangjuxu (ST 37, lower-*he* sea point of large intestine meridian)

[**Location**] This point is located on the lateral side of the shank, 6 *cun* below Dubi (ST 35), one finger-breadth (midfinger) from the anterior crest of the tibia in m. tibialis anterior. (Fig. 2 – 4 – 25)

[**Indication**] (1) Abdominal pain, abdominal distention, borborygmus, diarrhea, dysentery, constipation. (2) Flaccidity and obstruction syndrome of lower limbs and beriberi.

[**Needling method**] Perpendicular insertion 1 ~ 1. 5 *cun*.

3. 3. 16 Tiaokou(ST 38)

[**Location**] This point is located on the lateral side of the shank, 8 *cun* below Dubi (ST 35), one finger-breadth (midfinger) from the anterior crest of the tibia in m. tibialis anterior. (Fig. 2 – 4 – 25)

[**Indications**] (1) Coldness, pain, and weakness of the shoulder. (2) Flaccidity and obstruction syndrome of lower limbs, swelling of foot.

[**Needling method**] Perpendicular insertion 1 ~ 1. 5 *cun*.

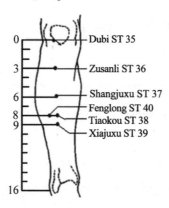

Fig. 2 – 4 – 25

3. 3. 17 Xiajuxu (ST 39)

[**Location**] This point is located on the lateral side of the shank, 9 *cun* below Dubi (ST 35), one finger-breadth (midfinger) from the anterior crest of the tibia in m. tibialis anterior. (Fig. 2 – 4 – 25)

[**Indications**] (1) Lower abdominal pain, pain in the lower back referring to pain in the testicles. (2) Diarrhea, dysentery. (3) Flaccidity and obstruction syndrome of lower limbs, swelling of the foot.

[**Needling method**] Perpendicular insertion 1 ~ 1. 5 *cun*.

3. 3. 18 Fenglong(ST 40)

[**Location**] This point is located on the lateral side of the shank, 8 *cun* above the tip of the external malleolus, lateral to the Tiaokou (ST 38) and two finger-breadth (midfinger) from the anterior crest of the tibia in m. tibialis anterior. (Fig. 2 – 4 – 25)

[**Indications**] (1) Cough, excessive phlegm, asthma. (2) Headache, dizziness, manic depression, epilepsy. (3) Flaccidity and obstruction syndrome of lower limbs.

[**Needling method**] Perpendicular insertion 1 ~ 1. 5 *cun*.

3. 3. 19 Jiexi (ST 44, *jing*-river acupoint)

[**Location**] This point is located in the depression at the midpoint of the transverse crease of the dorsum of foot and shank, between the tendons of m. extensor digitorum longus and hallucis longus. (Fig. 2 – 4 – 26)

[**Indications**] (1) Headache, dizziness, manic depression. (2) Abdominal distention, constipation. (3) Flaccidity and obstruction syndrome of lower limbs, pain of the ankle joint.

[**Needling method**] Perpendicular insertion 0. 5 ~ 1 *cun*.

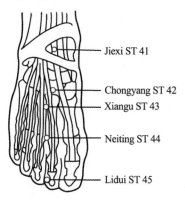

Jiexi ST 41

Chongyang ST 42
Xiangu ST 43

Neiting ST 44

Lidui ST 45

Fig. 2 – 4 – 26

3. 3. 20 Neiting (ST 44, *ying*-spring acupoint)

[**Location**] This point is located on the dorsum of foot, in the red and white part posterior to the birder of toe webs, proximal to the web margin between the second and the third toes. (Fig. 2 – 4 – 26)

[**Indications**] (1) Febrile disease, headache, toothache, sore throat, facial paralysis, epistaxis. (2) Abdominal distention, constipation, gastric pain. (3) Swelling and pain of the dorsum of the foot.

[**Needling method**] Perpendicular or oblique insertion 0. 5 ~ 0. 8 *cun*.

4. The Spleen Meridian of Foot-*taiyin*

4. 1 The course of the Spleen Meridian of Foot-*taiyin*

The spleen meridian foot-*taiyin* starts from the tip of the great toe, runs along the medial aspect of the foot at the junction of the red and white skin, ascends in front of the medial malleolus, up to the leg, follows the posterior aspect of the tibia, crosses and going in front of the liver meridian of foot-*juey-in*, passes through the anterior medial aspect of the knee and thigh, entering the abdomen, relates to the spleen, its pertaining organ, and connecting with the stomach, ascends and traversing the diaphragm, runs along the esophagus, reaches the root of the tongue and spreading over its lower surface, the branch from the stomach goes upward through the diaphragm, and flows into the heart to link with the heart meridian of hand-*shaoyin*. (Fig. 2 – 4 – 27)

[**Associated viscera**] Spleen, stomach and heart.

[**Associated organs**] Throat and tongue.

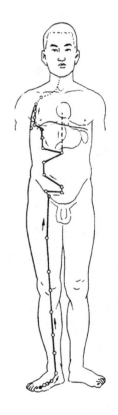

Fig. 2 – 4 – 27 The coures of the spleen meridian of foot-*taiyin*

4. 2 Indications

Disorders of the spleen and stomach, gynecological diseases, genital problems and diseases involving the areas through which the meridians flow.

4. 3 Commonly used acupoints of the Spleen Meridian of Foot-*taiyin*

This meridian starts at Yinbai(SP 1)and ends at Dabao(SP 2), bilaterally each consisting of 21 acupoints.

4. 3. 1 Yinbai (SP 1, *jing*-well acupoint)

[**Location**] The acupoint is located onThe medial side of the great toe, 0. 1 *cun* lateroposterior to the corner of the nail. (Fig. 2 −4 −28)

[**Indication**] (1) Manic depression, apoplexy, infantile convulsion, nightmares. (2)Metrorrhagia and metrostaxis, hematuria, hematochezia, epistaxis.

[**Needling method**] Subcutaneous insertion 0. 1 *cun* or prick to cause bleeding.

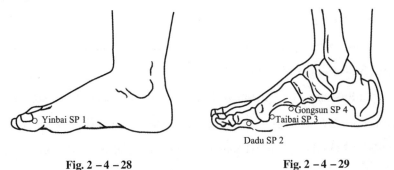

Fig. 2 −4 −28　　　　　　　Fig. 2 −4 −29

4. 3. 2 Taibai (SP 3, *shu-stream* and *yuan*-source acupoints of the spleen meridian of foot-*taiyin*)

[**Location**]The acupoint is located on the medial side the of great toe, in the depression proximal and inferior to the first metatarsodigital joint and the junction of the red and white skin. (Fig. 2 – 4 – 29)

[**Indications**] (1) Stomachache, abdominal distension, vomiting, diarrhea, constipation, edema. (2) Heaviness of the body, pain of joints and flaccidity syndrome.

[**Needling method**] Perpendicular insertion 0. 5 ~ 1 *cun*.

4. 3. 3 Gongsun(SP 4, *luo*-connecting acupoint and one of the eight convergent points associating with the throughfare vessel)

[**Location**] The acupoint is located on the medial border of the foot, in the depression distal and inferior to the base of the first metatarsal bone, at the junction of the red and white skin. (Fig. 2 – 4 – 29)

[**Indications**] (1) Acute and chronic stomachache, vomiting, abdominal distension diarrhea, dysentery. (2) Insomnia.

[**Needling method**] Perpendicular insertion 0. 5 ~ 1 *cun*.

4. 3. 4 Sanyinjiao (SP 6, crossing acupoint of the foot-*taiyin*, foot-*shaoyin* and foot-*jueyin*)

[**Location**] The point is located on the medial side of the shank, 3 *cun* directly above the tip of the medial malleolus, on the posterior border of the medial aspect of the tibia. (Fig. 2 – 4 – 30)

[**Indications**] (1) Irregular menstruation, dysmenorrhea, metrorrhagia and metrostaxis, leukorrhea, amenorrhea, dystocia, enuresis, anuria, edema, dysuria. (2) Borborygmus, abdominal distention, abdominal distension, diarrhea, constipation. insomnia, headache, dizziness, hypertention. (3) Eczema, urticaria. (4) Flaccidity and obstruction syndromes of lower limbs, beriberi.

[**Needling method**] Perpendicular insertion 1 ~ 1. 5 *cun*. This point is contraindicated to puncture in pregnancy.

4. 3. 5 Diji (SP 8, *xi*-cleft acupoint)

[**Location**] The point is located on the medial side of the shank, on the line joining the tip of the medial malleolus and yinlingquan (SP 9). (Fig. 2 – 4 – 30)

[**Indications**] (1) Abdominal pain, diarrhea. (2) Dysuria, edema, irregular menstruation, dysmenorrheal. (3) Flaccidity and obstruction syndromes of the lower limbs.

[**Needling method**] Perpendicular insertion 1 ~ 2 *cun*.

4. 3. 6 Yinlingquan(SP 9, *he*-sea acupoint)

[**Location**] The point is located on the medial side of the shank, on the lower border of the medial condyle of the tibia and in the depression on the medial border of the tibia. (Fig. 4 – 30)

[**Indications**] (1) Pain in the penis, dysmenorrhea, dysuria, enuresis, anuria, edema. (2) Abdominal distention, diarrhea, jaundice. (3) Pain in the medial aspect of the knee, flaccidity and obstruction syndromes of lower limbs.

[**Needling method**] Perpendicular insertion 1 ~ 2 *cun*.

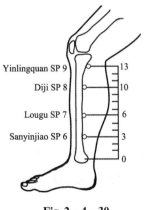

Fig. 2 – 4 – 30

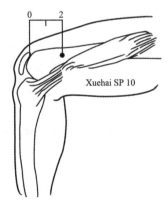

Fig. 2 – 4 – 31

4. 3. 7 Xuehai(SP 10)

[**Location**] When the knee is flexed, the point is located 2 *cun* above the mediosuperior border of the patella, on the bulge of the medial portion of m. quadriceps femoris. (Fig. 2 – 4 – 31)

[**Indications**] (1) Irregular menstruation, metrorrhagia and metrostaxis, amenorrhea. (2) Urticaria, eczema, erysipelas. (3) The tumescent pain of the knee joint.

[**Needling method**] Perpendicular insertion 1 ~ 1. 5 *cun*.

4. 3. 8 Dabao (SP 21, major *luo*-connecting acupoint)

[**Location**] The point is located on the lateral side of the chest, on the mid-axillary line and at the sixth costal interstice. (Fig. 2 – 4 – 32)

[**Indications**] (1) Chest and hypochondriac pain, cough, asthma. (2) General pain and flaccidity of the four limbs.

[**Needling method**] Oblique or subcutaneous insertion towards the posterior direction 0. 5 ~ 0. 8*cun*.

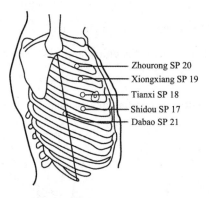

Zhourong SP 20
Xiongxiang SP 19
Tianxi SP 18
Shidou SP 17
Dabao SP 21

Fig. 2 – 4 – 32

5. The Heart Meridian of Hand-*shaoyin*

5. 1 The course of the Heart Meridian of Hand-*shaoyin*

The course of the heart meridian originates from the heart. It emerges and spreads over the heart system. It passes through the diaphragm to connect with the small intestine. The branch is from the heart system. Runs alongside the esophagus. Connects with the "eye system" (the tissues connecting the eyes with the brain). The straight portion of the meridian from the heart system goes upwards to the lung. Then it turns downward and emerges from the axilla. From there it goes along the posterior border of the medial aspect of the upper arm. Comes down to the cubital fossa. Then it descends along the posterior border of the medial aspect of the forearm. To the pisiform region proximal to the palm. Enters the palm. Then it follows the medial aspect of the little finger to its tip and links with the small intestine meridian. (Fig. 2 - 4 - 33)

[**Associated viscera**] Heart, small intestine and lung.

[**Associated organs**] Eye system, tongue, throat and larynx.

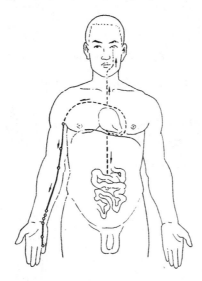

Fig. 2 - 4 - 33 The coures of the heart merdian of hand-*shaoyin*

5. 2 Indications

Diseases of the heart and chest, the mental diseases as well as diseases involving the regions the meridian running by.

5. 3 Commonly used acupoints of the Heart Meridian of Hand-*shaoyin*

The heart meridian starts at *Jiquan* (HT 1) and ends at *Shaochong* (HT 9), bilaterally each of consisting 9 acupoints.

5. 3. 1 Shaohai (HT 3, *he*-sea acupoint of the heart meridian of hand-*shaoyin*)

[**Location**] When the elbow is bent, the acupoint is in the depression between the medial end of the transverse and cubital crease and the medial epicondyle of humerus. (Fig. 2 - 4 - 34)

[**Indications**] (1) Angina pectoris, epilepsy. (2) Pain in the axilary and hypochondrium, spasmodic pain of the elbow and arm, tremor of hand.

[**Needling method**] Perpendicular insertion 0. 3 ~ 0. 5 *cun*.

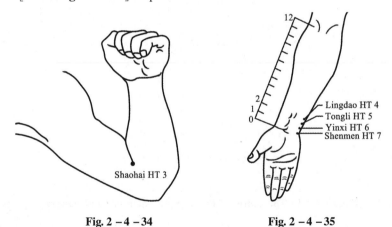

Fig. 2 - 4 - 34   Fig. 2 - 4 - 35

5. 3. 2 TongLi (HT 5, *luo*-connntcting acupoint)

[**Location**] When the palm is turned upward, the acupoint is on the radial side of the tendon of m. flexor carpi ulnaris, 1 *cun* above the transverse crease of the wrist. (Fig. 2 - 4 - 35)

[**Indications**] (1) Sudden loss of voice, stiffness of the tongue, aphasia due to stiff tongue. (2) Angina pectoris, palpitation and severe palpitation.

(3) Pain in the wrist and arm.

[**Needling method**] Perpendicular insertion 0. 3 ~ 0. 5 *cun*.

5. 3. 3 Yinxi (HT 6, *xi*-cleft acupoint)

[**Location**] When the palm is turned upward, the acupoint is on the radial side of the tendon of m. flexor carpi ulnaris, 0. 5 *cun* above the transverse crease of the wrist. (Fig. 2 – 4 – 35)

[**Indications**] (1) Angina pectoris, palpation due to fright. (2) Hematemesis, epistaxis. (3) Hectic fever and night sweating.

[**Needling method**] Perpendicular insertion 0. 3 ~ 0. 5 *cun*.

5. 3. 4 Shenmen (HT 7, *shu*-stream and *yuan*-source acup oint)

[**Location**] When the palm is turned upward, the point is at the ulnar end of the transverse crease of the wrist, in the depression on the radial side of the tendon of m. flexor carpi ulnaris. (Fig. 2 – 4 – 35)

[**Indications**] (1) Dysphoria, insomnia, amnesia, manic depression, epilepsy, stupor. (2) Angina pectoris, palpitation and severe palpitation. (3) Wrist pain and finger numbness.

[**Needling method**] Perpendicular insertion 0. 3 ~ 0. 5 *cun*.

5. 3. 5 Shaofu (HT 8, *ying*-spring acupoint)

[**Location**] When the palm is turned upward, the point is located between the fourth and fifth metacarpal bones. when the fist is formed, this point is where the tip of thelittle finger touches. (Fig. 2 – 4 – 36)

[**Indications**] (1) Pruritus and pain of the external genitalia, dysuria, and enuresis. (2) Cardic pain, palpation, chest

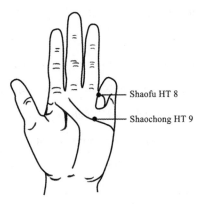

Shaofu HT 8

Shaochong HT 9

Fig. 2 – 4 – 36

pain. (3)Spasmodic pain of the little finger.

[**Needling method**]Perpendicular insertion 0. 3 ~ 0. 5 *cun*.

5. 3. 6 Shaochong (HT 9, *jing*-well acupoint)

[**Location**] The point is located on the radial side of the little finger, about 0. 1 *cun* latero-posterior to the corner of the nail. (Fig. 2 – 4 – 36)

[**Indications**] (1) Angina pectoris, palpitation. (2) Febrile disease. manic depression, epilepsy, coma.

[**Needling method**] Subcutaneous insertion 0. 1 *cun* or prick to cause bleeding.

6. The Meridian of the Small Intestine of Hand-*taiyang*

6. 1 The course of the Small Intestine of Hand-*taiyang* (Fig. 2 – 4 – 37)

The small intestine meridian starts from the ulnar side of the tip of the little finger. Following the ulnar side of the dorsum of the hand, it reaches the wrist where it emerges from the styloid process of the ulna. From there it ascends along the posterior aspect of the forearm, passes between the olecranon of the ulna and the medial epicondyle of the humerus, and runs along the posterior border of the lateral aspect of the upper arm to the shoulder joint. Circling around the scapular region, it converges over the shoulder, turns downward to the supraclavicular fossa to connect with the heart. From there it descends along the esophagus, passes through the diaphragm, reaches the stomach, and finally enters the small intestine. The branch from the supraclavicular fossa ascends to the neck, and further to the cheek. Then it reaches the outer canthus and enters the ear. The other branch from the cheeks runs upward to the infraorbital region and further to the lateral side of the nose and inner canthus to connect with the Urinary Bladder Meridian.

[**Associated viscera**]Small intestine and stomach.

[**Associated organs**]Throat, ears, nose and eyes.

6. 2 Indications

Disorders of the organs on the face and throat, febrile diseases and pathological changes of the lateral side of the upper limbs, scapula and neck.

6. 3 Commonly used acupoints of the Small Intestine of Hand-*taiyang*

The small Intestine meridian starts at Shaoze (SI 1)and ends at Tinggong (SI 19)bilaterally each of consisting 19 acupoints.

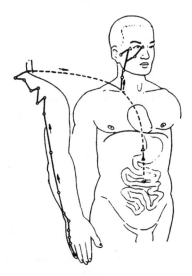

Fig. 2 – 4 – 37 The coures of the samall intestine meridian of hand-*taiyang*

6. 3. 1 Shaoze(SI 1,*jing*-well acupoint)

[**Location**]The point is located on the ulnar side of the little finger, about 0. 1 *cun* lateroposterior to the corner of the nail. (Fig. 2 – 4 – 38)

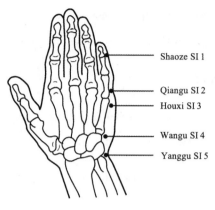

Shaoze SI 1

Qiangu SI 2
Houxi SI 3

Wangu SI 4

Yanggu SI 5

Fig. 2 - 4 - 38

[**Indication**] (1) Insufficient lactation, acute mastitis. (2) Febrile diseases, apoplexy, loss of consciousness.

[**Needling method**] Subcutaneous insertion 0. 1 *cun* or prick to cause bleeding.

6. 3. 2 Houxi(SI 3, *shu*-stream acupoint and one of the eight convergent points associating with governor vessel)

[**Location**] When the hand is slightly clenched, the point is located on the ulnar side, proximal to the fifth metacarpophalangeal joint, at the end of the transverse crease and the junction of the red and white skin. (Fig. 2 - 4 - 38)

[**Indications**] (1) Febrile diseases. Malaria, manic depression, epilepsy. (2) Pain and swelling of eye, deafness, sore throat. (3) Pain and rigidity of the head and neck, pain in the lumbar and sacrum, spasmodic pain in the elbow and arm, numbness of fingers.

[**Needling method**] Perpendicular insertion 0. 5 ~ 1 *cun.*

6. 3. 3 Yanglao(SI 6)

[**Location**] The acupoint is located at the dorsal and ulnar side of the arm and in the depression at the radial side proximal to ulnar head. (Fig. 2 - 4 - 39)

[**Indications**] (1) Blurred vision, headache. (2) Pain in the shoulder, back, elbow and arm.

[**Needling method**] Oblique insertion towards the elbow 0. 5 ~ 0. 8 *cun*.

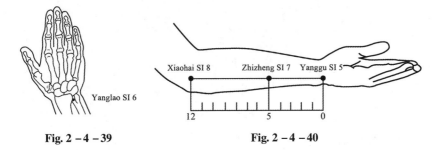

Fig. 2 – 4 – 39　　　　　　　　　　Fig. 2 – 4 – 40

6. 3. 4 Xiaohai (SI 8, *he*-sea point of the small intestine of hand-*taiyang*)

[**Location**] The acupoint is located in the depression between the olecranon of the ulna and the medial epicondyle of the humerus when the elbow is flexed. (Fig. 2 – 4 – 40)

[**Indications**] (1) Headache, dizziness, tinnitus, deafness, epilepsy. (2) Spasmodic pain in the elbow and arm.

[**Needling method**] Perpendicular insertion 0. 3 ~ 0. 5 *cun*.

6. 3. 5 Tianzong(SI 11)

[**Location**] The acupoint is in the infrascapular fossa, at the junction of the upper 1/3 and middle 1/3 of the distance between the lower border of the scapular spine and the inferior angle of the scapula. (Fig. 2 – 4 –41)

[**Indications**] (1) Cough, asthma, acute mastitis. (2) Pain in the scapula and back.

[**Needling method**] Perpendicular or oblique insertion 0. 5 ~ 1 *cun*.

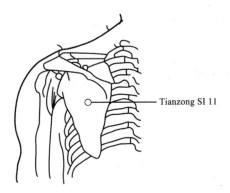

Tianzong SI 11

Fig. 2 – 4 – 41

6. 3. 6 Quanliao(SI 18)

[**Location**]The point is located directly below the outer canthus, in the depression on the lower border of zygoma. (Fig. 2 – 4 – 42)

[**Indications**]Facial paralysis, twitching of eyelids, toothache and swelling of cheeks.

[**Needling method**] Perpendicular insertion 0. 3 ~ 0. 5 *cun*, oblique or subcutaneous insertion 0. 5 ~ 0. 8 *cun*.

6. 3. 7 Tinggong(SI 19)

[**Location**]The point is located anterior to the tragus and posterior to the condyloid process of the mandible and in the depression formed when the mouth is open. (Fig. 2 – 4 – 43)

[**Indications**]Tinnitus, deafness, otorrhea, toothache.

[**Needling method**] Perpendicular insertion 1 ~ 1. 5 *cun* with mouth open.

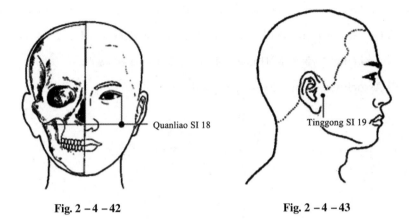

Fig. 2 - 4 - 42　　　　　　　Fig. 2 - 4 - 43

7. The Urinary Bladder Meridian of Foot-*taiyang*

7. 1 The course of the Urinary Bladder Meridian of Foot-*taiyang*

The urinary bladder meridian of foot-*taiyang* starts from the inner canthus. Ascend to the forehead. It joins the governor vessel at the vertex. From
the vertex, a branch arises, running to the temple.

The straight portion of the Meridian enters and communicates with the
brain from the vertex. It then emerges and bifurcates to descend along the posterior aspect of the neck. Running downward along the medial aspect of the
scapular region and parallel to the vertebral column, it reaches the lumbar region, where it enters the body cavity via the paravertebral muscle to connect
with the kidney and joins its pertaining organ, the urinary bladder. The branch
of the lumbar region descends through the gluteal region and ends in the popliteal fossa. The branch from the posterior aspect of the neck runs straight
downward along the medial border of the scapula, passing through the gluteal
region and going downward along the lateral aspect of the thigh, it meets the
preceding branch descending from the lumbar region in the popliteal fossa. From there, it descends through the gastrocnemius muscle to the posterior

aspect of the external malleolus. It reaches the lateral side of the tip of the little toe, where it links with the kidney meridian of foot-*shaoyin*. (Fig. 2 – 4 – 44)

[**Associated viscera**] Urinary bladder, kidney and brain.

[**Associated organ**] Eyes, nose and ears.

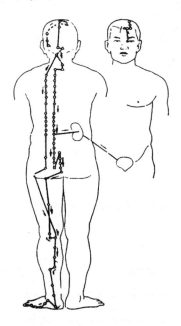

Fig. 2 – 4 – 44 The coures of the bladder meridian of foot-*taiyang*

7. 2 Indications

Diseases of the five sensory organs, problems of neck, back, waist and lower limbs as well as mental problems. The indication of the Back-*Shu* acupoints on the first lateral line of the back and the acupoints on the second line parallel to the first lateral line include the disorders of the related viscera, tissues and organs.

7. 3 Commonly used acupoints of the Urinary Bladder of the Foot-*taiyang*

The urinary bladder meridian starts at Jingming(BL 1) and ends at Zhiyin(BL 67), bilaterally each of consisting 67 acupoints.

7. 3. 1 Jingming(BL 1)

[**Location**] The point is located in the depression slightly superior to the inner canthus. (Fig. 2 – 4 – 45)

[**Indications**] Redness, swelling and pain of eyes, epiphora, blurred vision, dizziness, near sightedness (myopia).

[**Needling method**] Ask the patient to close eyes. with the left hand gently push the eyeball toward the lateral side with the right hand slowly insert the needle perpendicularly 0. 5 ~ 1 *cun* along the orbital wall. It is not advisable to rotate or lift and thrust the needle (or only rotate or lift and thrust slightly). to avoid bleeding, press the punctured site momentarily after withdrawing the needle.

7. 3. 2 Cuanzhu(BL 2)

[**Location**] The point is located in the depression of the eyebrow or on the superaorbital notch. (Fig. 2 – 4 – 45)

[**Indications**] Facial paralysis, blurred vision, epiphora, redness, swelling and pain of the eyes, twitching of the eyelids. pain in the supraorbital region and headache.

[**Needling method**] Subcutaneous insertion 0. 5 ~ 0. 8 *cun* or prick to cause bleeding.

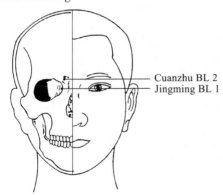

Cuanzhu BL 2
Jingming BL 1

Fig. 2 – 4 – 45

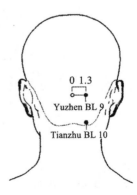

0 1.3

Yuzhen BL 9

Tianzhu BL 10

Fig. 2 – 4 – 46

7. 3. 3 Tianzhu(BL 10)

[**Location**]The point is located in the depression on the lateral aspect of m. trapezious and 1. 3 *cun* laterals to the midline of the posterior hairline. (Fig. 2 −4 −46)

[**Indications**](1)Febrile diseases, headache, dizziness, nasal bstruction. (2)Stiff neck, pain in the shoulder and back. (3)Manic depression, epilepsy.

[**Needling method**] Perpendicular or oblique insertion 0. 5 ~ 0. 8 *cun*. Do not insert the needle medial deeply upwards to avoid injuring medulla oblongata.

7. 3. 4 Dazhu(BL 11, one of the eight confluent acupoint associating with bones)

[**Location**]This point is located below and 1. 5 *cun* lateral to the spinous process of the first thoracic vertebral. (Fig. 2 −4 −47)

[**Indications**](1)All kinds of bone diseases such as pain in the shoulder, lumbar, sacrum and knees. (2)Headache, stiffness, nasal obstruction, sore throat, cough and fever.

[**Needling method**]Oblique insertion 0. 5 ~0. 8 *cun*.

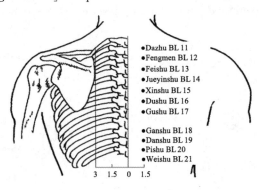

●Dazhu BL 11
●Fengmen BL 12
●Feishu BL 13
●Jueyinshu BL 14
●Xinshu BL 15
●Dushu BL 16
●Gushu BL 17

●Ganshu BL 18
●Danshu BL 19
●Pishu BL 20
●Weishu BL 21

3　1.5　0　1.5

Fig. 2 −4 −47

7. 3. 5 Fengmen(BL 12)

[**Location**]This point is located below and 1. 5 *cun* lateral to the spinous process of the second thoracic vertebral. (Fig. 2 – 4 – 47)

[**Indications**] (1) Common cold, cough, nasal obstruction, sore throat, fever, headache. (2) Stiff neck, pain in the shoulder and back.

[**Needling method**] Oblique insertion 0. 5 ~0. 8 *cun*.

7. 3. 6 Feishu (BL13, back-*shu* acupoint)

[**Location**] This point is located below and 1. 5 *cun* lateral to the spinous process of the third thoracic vertebral. (Fig. 2 – 4 – 47)

[**Indications**] (1) Fever, nasal obstruction, cough, hemoptysis, night sweating. (2) Skin diseases such as urticaria, acne.

[**Needling method**] Oblique insertion 0. 5 ~0. 8 *cun*.

7. 3. 7 Jueyinshu(BL 14, back-*shu* acupoint)

[**Location**] This point is located below and 1. 5 *cun* lateral to the spinous process of the fourth thoracic vertebral. (Fig. 2 – 4 – 47)

[**Indications**] (1) Cardiac pain, palpitation. (2) Cough, chest oppression.

[**Needling method**] Oblique insertion 0. 5 ~0. 8 *cun*.

7. 3. 8 Xinshu(BL 15, back-*shu* acupoint)

[**Location**] This point is located below and 1. 5 *cun* lateral to the spinous process of the fifth thoracic vertebral. (Fig. 2 – 4 – 47)

[**Indications**] (1) Cardiac pain, palpitation. (2) Cough, asthma, night sweeting. (3) Insomnia, bad memory, dreaminess, epilepsy.

[**Needling method**] Oblique insertion 0. 5 ~0. 8 *cun*.

7. 3. 9 Geshu (BL 17, one of the eight confluent acupoints associating with blood)

[**Location**] This point is located below and 1. 5 *cun* lateral to the spinous process of the seventh thoracic vertebral. (Fig. 2 – 4 – 47)

[**Indications**] (1) Stomachache, hiccup, vomiting, dysphagia. (2) Cough, asthma, hematemesis, hectic fever and night sweating. (3) Skin diseases such as urticaria, acne.

[**Needling method**] Oblique insertion 0. 5 ~ 0. 8 *cun.*

7. 3. 10 Ganshu(BL 18, back-*shu* acupoint)

[**Location**] This point is located below and 1. 5 *cun* lateral to the spinous process of the ninth thoracic vertebral. (Fig. 2 – 4 – 47)

[**Indications**] (1) Pain in the hypochondrium, jaundice, vomiting. (2) Red and pain of eye, blurred eye. (3) Manic depression epilepsy.

[**Needling method**] Oblique insertion 0. 5 ~ 0. 8 *cun.*

7. 3. 11 Danshu(BL 19, back-*shu* acupoint)

[**Location**] This point is located below and 1. 5 *cun* lateral to the spinous process of the tenth thoracic vertebral. (Fig. 2 – 4 – 47)

[**Indications**] (1) Jaundice, bitter taste in the mouth, pain in the hypochondrium. (2) Pulmonary tuberculosis, hectic fever.

[**Needling method**] Oblique insertion 0. 5 ~ 0. 8 *cun.*

7. 3. 12 Pishu(BL 20, back-*shu* acupoint)

[**Location**] This point is located below and 1. 5 *cun* lateral to the spinous process of the eleventh thoracic vertebral. (Fig. 2 – 4 – 47)

[**Indications**] Abdominal distention, jaundice, vomiting, diarrhea, dysentery.

[**Needling method**] Oblique insertion 0. 5 ~ 0. 8 *cun.*

7. 3. 13 Weishu(BL 21, back-*shu* acupoint)

[**Location**] This point is located below and 1. 5 *cun* lateral to the spinous process of the twelfth thoracic vertebral. (Fig. 2 – 4 – 47)

[**Indications**] Stomachache, vomiting, abdominal distention, borborygmus.

[**Needling method**] Oblique insertion 0. 5 ~ 0. 8 *cun.*

7. 3. 14 Shenshu(BL 23, back-*shu* acupoint)

[**Location**] This point is located below and 1. 5 *cun* lateral to the spinous process of the second lumbar vertebral. (Fig. 2 –4 –48)

[**Indications**] (1) Enuresis, dysuria, edema, spermatorrhea, impotence, irregular menstruation, leucorrhea. (2) Dizziness, blurred eye deafness, tinnitus, deafness. (3) Cough, asthma. (4) Lumbar pain.

[**Needling method**] Perpendicular insertion 0. 5 ~ 1 *cun*.

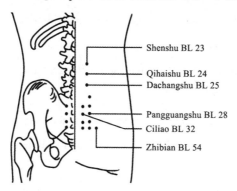

Shenshu BL 23

Qihaishu BL 24
Dachangshu BL 25

Pangguangshu BL 28
Ciliao BL 32

Zhibian BL 54

Fig. 2 –4 –48

7. 3. 15 Qihaishu(BL 24)

[**Location**] This point is located below and 1. 5 *cun* lateral to the spinous process of the third lumbar vertebral. (Fig. 2 –4 –48)

[**Indications**] (1) Abdominal distention, borborygmus. (2) Enuresis, dysuria, edema. (3) Lumbar pain.

[**Needling method**] Perpendicular insertion 0. 5 ~ 1 *cun*.

7. 3. 16 Dachangshu (BL 25, back-*shu* acupoint)

[**Location**] This point is located below and 1. 5 *cun* lateral to the spinous process of the fouth lumbar vertebral. (Fig. 2 –4 –48)

[**Indications**] (1) Abdominal distention, diarrhea, constipation, hemorrhoids. (2) Lumbar pain.

[**Needling method**] Perpendicular insertion 0. 8 ~ 1. 2 *cun*.

7. 3. 17 Pangguangshu(BL 28 , back-*shu* acupoint)

[**Location**] This point is located 1. 5 *cun* lateral to bedial sacral crest and on the level with the second posterior sacral foramen. (Fig. 2 – 4 – 48)

[**Indications**] (1) Enuresis, dysuria, edema. (2) Lumbosacral pain, weakness, and numbness of the lower extremities.

[**Needling method**] Perpendicular insertion 0. 8 ~ 1. 2 *cun*.

7. 3. 18 Ciliao(BL 32)

[**Location**] This point is located medial and inferior to the posterior superior iliac and the posterior midline, in the second sacral foramen and approximately the midpoint of Pangguangshu (BL 28) and the midline on the back. (Fig. 2 – 4 – 48)

[**Indications**] (1) Spermatorrhea, impotence, irregular menstruation, dysmenorrhea, leucorrhea. (2) Lumbosacral pain, weakness, and numbness of the lower extremities.

[**Needling method**] Perpendicular insertion 1 ~ 1. 5 *cun*.

7. 3. 19 Weizhong (BL 40 , lower-*he*-sea acupoint)

[**Location**] This point is located on the midpoint of the popliteal transverse crease and between the tendons of the m. biceps femoris and m. semitendinosus. (Fig. 2 – 4 – 49)

[**Indications**] (1) Lumbar pain, spasm of the popliteal tendons, hemiplegia, pain, numbness and weakness of the lower extremities. (2) Erysipelas, rash, general pruritus, furuncle, carbuncle on the back. (3) Abdominal pain, vomiting, diarrhea. (4) Enuresis, dysuria.

[**Needling method**] Perpendicular insertion 1 ~ 1. 5 *cun*, or prick the popliteal vein with the three-edged needle to cause bleeding.

7. 3. 20 Gaohuang(BL 43)

[**Location**] This point is located below and 3 *cun* lateral to the spinous process of the fouth thoracic vertebral. (Fig. 2 – 4 – 50)

[**Indications**] (1) Pulmonary tuberculosis, cough, asthma, poor appetite, emaciation and weakness. (2) Pain in the shoulder and back.

[**Needling method**] Oblique insertion 0. 5 ~0. 8 *cun*.

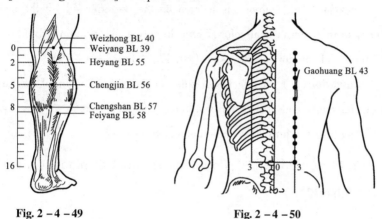

Fig. 2 −4 −49	**Fig. 2 −4 −50**

7. 3. 21 Zhibian(BL 54)

[**Location**] The acupoint is located at the level of the fouth posterior sacral foramen and 3 *cun* lateral to the median sacral crest. (Fig. 2 − 4 − 48)

[**Indications**] (1) Lumbosacral pain, weakness, and numbness of the lower extremities. (2) Dysuria, constipation, hemorrhoids.

[**Needling method**] Perpendicular insertion 1 ~2 *cun*.

7. 3. 22 Chengshan(BL 57)

[**Location**] This point is located directly below the belly of m. gastrocnemius, between Weizhong (BL 40) and Kunlun (BL 60) and in the depression below the belly of the m. gastrocnemius when the shank stretches out or when the heel lifts up, approximately at the midpoint between Weizhong (BL 40) and tendo calcaneus. (Fig. 2 −4 −49)

[**Indications**] (1) Hemorrhoids, constipation. (2) Spasm and pain of the lumbar and leg. (3) Beriberi.

[**Needling method**] Perpendicular insertion 1 ~2 *cun*.

7. 3. 23 Feiyanng (BL 58, *luo*-connecting acupoint of bladder meridian of foot-*taiyang*)

[**Location**] This acupoint is located on the posterior side of the shank, posterior to the external malleolus, 7 *cun* directly above Kunlun(BL 60) and 1 *cun* lateral and inferior to Chengshan(BL 57). (Fig. 2 – 4 – 49)

[**Indications**] (1) Headache, dizziness, epistaxis. (2) Pain of the lumbar and leg, flaccidity and obstruction syndromes of lower limbs.

[**Needling method**] Perpendicular insertion 1 ~ 2 *cun*.

7. 3. 24 Kunlun(BL 60, *jing*-river acupoint of bladder meridian of foot-*taiyang*)

[**Location**] This point is located posterior to the external malleolus and in the depression between the external malleolus and tendo calcaneus. (Fig. 2 – 4 – 51)

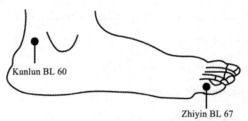

Kunlun BL 60

Zhiyin BL 67

Fig. 2 – 4 – 51

[**Indications**] (1) Headache, neck stiffness, dizziness, epistaxis. (2) Acute lumbar pain, swelling and pain of the heel. (3) Dystocia.

[Needling method] Perpendicular insertion 0. 5 ~ 1 *cun*.

7. 3. 25 Zhiyin(BL 67, *jing*-well acupoint)

[**Location**] The point is located on the lateral side of the small toe, about 0. 1 *cun* posterior to the corner of the nail. (Fig. 2 – 4 – 51)

[**Indications**] (1) Headache, pain of eyes, nasal obstruction, epistaxis. (2) Malposition of the fetus and dystocia.

[**Needling method**] Superficial insertion 0. 1 *cun* or prick to cause bleeding. Use moxibustion for malposition of fetus.

8. The Kidney Meridian of Foot-*shaoyin*

8. 1 The course of the Kidney Meridian of Foot-*shaoyin* (Fig. 2 −4 −52)

The kidney meridian of foot-*shaoyin* starts from the inferior aspect of the small toe and runs oblique lee towards the sole Yongquan (KI 1). Emerging from the lower aspect of the tuberosity of the navicular bone and running behind the medial malleolus, it enters the heel. Then it ascends along the medial side of the leg to the medial side of the popliteal fossa and goes further upward along the posteromedial aspect of the thigh towards the vertebral column (Changqiang, GV 1) , where it enters the kidney, its pertaining organ, and connects with the urinary bladder. The straight portion of the meridian reemerges from the kidney. Ascending and passing through the liver and diaphragm, it enters the lung, runs along the throat, and terminates at the root of the tongue. A branch stems from the lung, joins the heart and runs into the chest to link with the pericardium meridian of hand-*jueyin*.

[**Associated viscera**] Kidney, urinary bladder, heart, lung, liver and marrow

[**Associated organs**] Throat and tongue root.

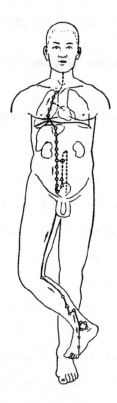

Fig. 2 – 4 – 52 The course of the kidney meridian of foot-*shaoyin*

8. 2 Indications

Gynecological diseases, external genitalia diseases, disorders of kidney, lung and throat as well as diseases involving the regions through which the meridian passes.

8. 3 Commonly used acupoints of the Kidney of Foot-*shaoyin*

The kidney meridian starts at Yongquan (KI 1) and ends at Shufu (KI 27) , bilaterally each of consisting 27 acupoints.

8. 3. 1 Yongquan(KI 1, *jing*-well acupoint)

[**Location**] This point is located on the sole and in the depression when the foot is in plantar flexion, in the anterior depression when the foot flexed, approximately at the junction of the anterior one third and posterior two thirds of the sole. (Fig. 2 – 4 – 53)

[**Indications**] (1) Parietal headache, vertigo, syncope, infantile convulsion, manic and depressive psychosis, insomnia. (2) Dysuria, and constipation. (3) Sore throat, dryness of the tongue, aphonia. (4) Hot sensation in the sole.

[**Needling method**] Perpendicular insertion 0. 5 ~ 1 *cun*.

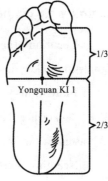

Fig. 2 – 4 – 53

8. 3. 2　Taixi (KI 3, *shu-stream* and *yuan-source* acupoint)

[**Location**] This point is located on the medial side of the foot, posterior to the medial malleolus and in the depression between the medial malleolus and tendo calcaneus. (Fig. 2 – 4 – 54)

[**Indications**] (1) Irregular menstruation, impotence, spermatorrhea, frequent urination. (2) Headache, dizziness. (3) Blurred vision, deafness, tinnitus, toothache, soreness and dryness throat. (4) Cough, asthma. (5) Insomnia, amnesia. (6) Diabetes, diarrhea.

[**Needling method**] Perpendicular insertion 0. 5 ~ 1 *cun*.

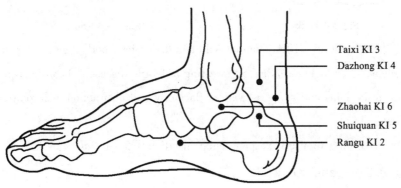

Fig. 2 – 4 – 54

8. 3. 3 Zhaohai(KI 6 , one of the eight convergent points asso-
ciating with *yin*-heel vessel)

[**Location**] The point is located on the medial side of the side and in the depression below the tip of the medial malleolus. (Fig. 2 – 4 – 54)

[**Indications**] (1) Dryness and soreness of throat. (2) Irregular menstruation, leukorrhea, prolapse of uterus, frequent urination, difficult urination. (3) Insomnia, epilepsy.

[**Needling method**] Perpendicular insertion 0. 3 ~ 0. 5 *cun*.

8. 3. 4 Fuliu(KI 7 , *jing*-river acupoint)

[**Location**] This acupoint is located on the medial side of the shank , 2 *cun* directly above Taixi(KI 3) and on the anterior border of tendo calcaneus. (Fig. 2 – 4 – 55)

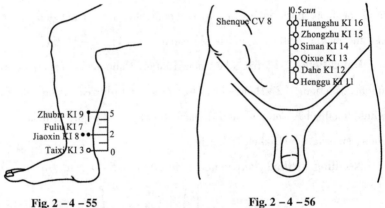

Fig. 2 – 4 – 55   Fig. 2 – 4 – 56

[**Indications**] (1) Abdominal pain and distension , borborygmus , diarrhea , edema. (2) Night sweating , no sweating in febrile disease. (3) Stiffness and pain in the loins and spine as well as flaccidity and obstruction syndromes of lower limbs.

[**Needling method**] Perpendicular insertion 0. 5 ~ 1 *cun*.

8. 3. 5 Dahe(KI 12)

[**Location**] This acupoint is located on the abdomen , 4 *cun* below umbilicus and 0. 5 *cun* lateral to the anterior midline. (Fig. 2 – 4 – 56)

[**Indications**] (1) Lower abdominal pain. (2) Irregular menstruation, leukorrhea, prolapse of uterus. (3) Impotence, spermatorrhea, hernia.

[**Needling method**] Perpendicular insertion 1 ~ 1. 5 *cun*.

8. 3. 6 Huangshu(KI 16)

[**Location**] This acupoint is located on the center of the abdomen, 0. 5 *cun* lateral to the anterior midline. (Fig. 2 – 4 – 56)

[**Indications**] (1) Abdominal pain around the umbilicus, abdominal distension, diarrhea, dysentery, constipation. (2) Irregular menstruation. (3) Hernia.

[**Needling method**] Perpendicular insertion 1 ~ 1. 5 *cun*.

8. 3. 7 Shufu(KI 27)

[**Location**] This acupoint is located on the chest, at the lower border of the clavicle and 2 *cun* lateral to the anterior midline. (Fig. 2 – 4 – 57)

[**Indications**] (1) Cough, asthma, chest pain. (2) Vomiting and anorexia.

[**Needling method**] Oblique or subcutaneous insertion 0. 5 ~ 0. 8 *cun*.

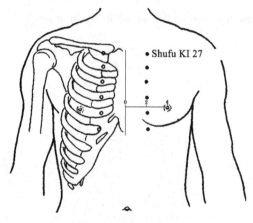

Fig. 2 – 4 – 57

9. The Pericardium Meridian of Hand-*jueyin*

9. 1 The course of the Pericardium Meridian of Hand-*jueyin* (Fig. 2 – 4 – 58)

The pericardium meridian originates from the chest. On emerging it enters its pertaining organ the pericardium. Then it descends through the diaphragm to the abdomen, connecting successively with the upper, middle and lower energizers. A branch arising from the chest runs inside the chest, emerges from the costal region at a point 3 *cun* below the anterior axillary fold and ascends to the axilla. Following the medial aspect of the upper arm, it runs between the lung meridian of hand-*taiyin* and the heart meridian of hand-*shaoyin* to the cubital fossa, further downwards to the forearm between the tendons of m. palmaris longus and m. flexor carpi radialis, entering the palm. From there it passes along the middle finger right down to its tip. Another branch stems from the palm and runs along the ring finger to its tip and links with the triple energizer meridian.

[**Associated viscera**] Pericardium and triple energizer.

9. 2 Indications

Diseases of the heart, chest and the stomach, mental diseases as well as diseases involving the regions the meridian running by.

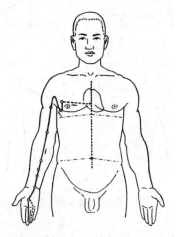

Fig. 2 −4 −58 The course of the pericardium meridian of hand-*jueyin*

9. 3 Commonly used acupoints of the Pericardium Meridian of the Hand-*jueyin*

The pericardium meridian starts at Tianchi (PC 1) and ends at Zhongchong(PC 9) , bilaterally each of consisting 9 acupoints.

9. 3. 1 Quze(PC 3, *he*-sea acupoint)

[**Location**] This acupoint is located on the medial side of the forearm, on the transverse cubital crease and at the ulnar side of the tendon of m. biceps brachii. (Fig. 2 – 4 – 59)

[**Indications**] (1) Cardiac pain, palpitation, manic and depressive psychosis, epilepsy. (2) Stomachache, vomiting, diarrhea. (3) Febrile disease, sunstroke. (4) Spasmodic pain of elbow and arm.

[**Needling method**] Perpendicular insertion 1 ~ 1. 5 *cun*, or prick to cause bleeding.

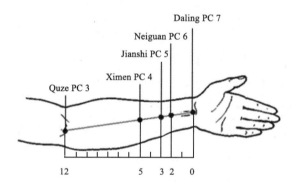

Fig. 2 – 4 – 59 The points of the pericardium meridian of hand-*jueyin*

9. 3. 2 Ximen(PC 4, *xi*-cleft acupoint)

[**Location**] The palm is turned up. The point is 5 *cun* above the transverse crease of the wrist, between the two tendons of the m. palmaris longus and m. flexor carpi radialis. (Fig. 2 – 4 – 59)

[**Indications**] (1) Cardiac pain, palpitation, manic and depressive psychosis, epilepsy. (2) Hemoptysis, hematemesis, epistaxis. (3) Furuncle.

[**Needling method**] Perpendicular insertion 0. 5 ~ 1 *cun*.

9. 3. 3 Jianshi(PC 5, *jing*-river acupoint)

[**Location**] The palm is turned up. The point is 3 *cun* above the transverse crease of the wrist, between the two tendons of the m. palmaris longus and m. flexor carpi radialis. (Fig. 2 – 4 – 59)

[**Indications**] (1) Cardiac pain, palpitation, manic and depressive psychosis, epilepsy. (2) Stomachache, vomiting, hiccup. (3) Febrile disease, malaria.

[**Needling method**] Perpendicular insertion 0. 5 ~ 1 *cun*.

9. 3. 4 Neiguan (PC 6, *luo*-connecting and one of the eight convergent acupionts associating with *yinwei* meridian)

[**Location**] The palm is turned up. The point is 2 *cun* above the transverse crease of the wrist between the two tendons of the m. palmaris longus and m. flexor carpi radialis. (Fig. 2 – 4 – 59)

[**Indications**] (1) Angina pectoris, palpitation, arrhythmia. (2) Manic and depressive psychosis, epilepsy, postpartum bleeding and dizziness. (3) Stomachache, vomiting, hiccup. (4) Melancholia, insomnia, migraine, vertigo. (5) Apoplexy, hemiplegia, spasm and pain of the upper extremities.

[**Needling method**] Perpendicular insertion 0. 5 ~ 1 *cun*.

9. 3. 5 Laogong (PC 8, *ying*-spring acupoint)

[**Location**] The palm is turned up. The acupoint is located on the transverse crease of the palm, between the second and third metacarpal bones. When the fist is clenched, the point is just below the tip of the middle finger. (Fig. 2 – 4 – 60)

[**Indications**] (1) Angina pectoris, palpitation, apoplectic coma, manic and depressive psychosis, epilepsy, sunstroke. (2) Vomiting, bad breath, aphtha. (3) Tinea manuum.

[**Needling method**] Perpendicular insertion 0. 3 ~ 0. 5 *cun*.

9. 3. 6 Zhongchong (PC 9, *jing*-well acupoint)

[**Location**] The point is located in the center of the tip of the middle finger. (Fig. 2 – 4 – 60)

[**Indications**] (1) Angina pectoris, coma, sunstroke, syncope. (2) Infantile convulsion. (3) Stiffness and swelling of the tongue and febrile diseases.

[**Needling method**] Superficial insertion 0. 1 *cun*, or prick to cause bleeding.

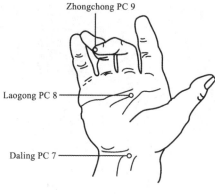

Fig. 2 –4 –60

10. The Triple Energizer Meridian of Hand-*shaoyang*

10. 1 The course of the Triple Energizer Meridian of Hand-*shaoyang* (Fig. 2 –4 –61)

The triple energizer meridian originates from the tip of the ring finger and runs upward between the fourth and fifth metacarpal bones along the dorsal aspect of the wrist to the lateral aspect of the forearm between the radius and ulna. Then it passes through the olecranon along the lateral aspect of the upper arm. It reaches the shoulder region. It moves forward into the supraclavicular fossa and spreads in the chest to connect with the pericardium. Then it descends through the diaphragm down to the abdomen to join the upper, middle and lower energizers. A branch originates from the chest nd emerges from the supraclavicular fossa. From there it ascends to the neck and runs along the posterior border of the ear and to the corner of the anterior hairline. Then it turns downward to join the other branch at the cheek and terminates in the infraorbital region. The other branch arises from the retroauricular region and enters the ear. Then it emerges in front of the ear, crosses the previous branch at the cheek and reaches the outer canthus to link with the gall bladder meridian.

[**Associated viscera**] Triple energizer and pericardium.

[**Associated organs**] Eyes and ears.

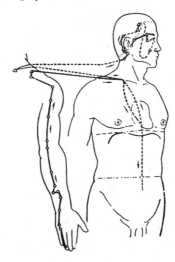

Fig. 2 –4 –61 The course of the triple triple energizer meridian of hand-*shaoyang*

10. 2 Indications

Disorders of the side of the head, ears, eyes and throat, as well as diseases involving the regions through which the meridian runs.

10. 3 Commonly used acupoints of the Triple Energizer Meridian of Hand-*shaoyang*

The triple energizer meridian starts at Guanchong (TE 1) and ends at Sizhukong(TE 23) , bilaterally each of consisting 23 acupoints.

10. 3. 1 Guanchong(TE 1 , jing-well acupoint)

[**Location**] The acupoint is located on the lateral side of the ring finger, 0. 1 *cun* latero-posterior to the corner of the nail. (Fig. 2 –4 –62)

[**Indications**] (1) Febrile disease, apoplexy, coma. (2) Sore throat, redness, swelling and pain of eyes, tinnitus and deafness.

[**Needling method**] Superficial insertion 0. 1 *cun*, or prick to cause Bleeding.

10. 3. 2 Zhongzhu(TE 3, *shu*-stream acupoint)

[**Location**] When the fist is clenched, the point is in the depression between the posterior borders of the small ends of the 4th and 5th metacarpal bones, 1 *cun* posterior to Yemen (TE 2). (Fig. 2 – 4 – 62)

[**Indications**] (1) Tinnitus, deafness, headache, redness, swelling and pain of the eye, sore throat. (2) Pain in the scapula, back, elbow and armas well as spasmodic pain of fingers.

[**Needling method**] Perpendicular insertion 0. 3 ~ 0. 5 *cun*.

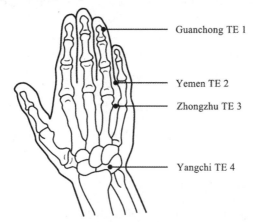

Guanchong TE 1

Yemen TE 2

Zhongzhu TE 3

Yangchi TE 4

Fig. 2 – 4 – 62

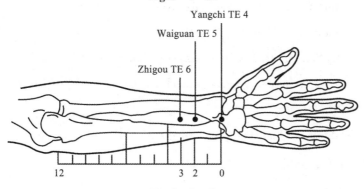

Yangchi TE 4

Waiguan TE 5

Zhigou TE 6

12　　　　　3 2　0

Fig. 2 – 4 – 63

10. 3. 3 Yangchi(TE 4, *yuan*-source acupoint of the triple energizer meridian of hand-*shaoyang*)

[**Location**]The acupoint is located on the transverse crease of the dorsum of wrist and in the depression lateral to the tendon of m. extensor digitorum communis. (Fig. 2 – 4 – 63)

[**Indications**] (1) Tinnitus, deafness and sore throat. (2) Diabetes and malaria. (3) Pain of the wrist joint, flaccidity and obstruction syndromes of upper limbs.

[**Needling method**] Perpendicular insertion 0. 3 ~ 0. 5 *cun*.

10. 3. 4 Waiguan (TE 5, *luo*-connecting acupoint and one of the eight convergent acupoints associating with *yang* heel link vessel)

[**Location**]2 *cun* above the transverse crease of the dorsum of wrist, between the radius and ulna. (Fig. 2 – 4 – 63)

[**Indications**] (1) Febrile disease, headache, redness, swelling and pain of the eye, tinnitus, deafness. (2) Pain in the hypochondrium. (3) Spasmodic pain of the upper extremities.

[**Needling method**] Perpendicular insertion 0. 5 ~ 1 *cun*.

10. 3. 5 Zhigou(TE 6, *jing*-river acupoint)

[**Location**]3 *cun* above the transverse crease of the dorsum of wrist, between the radius and ulna. (Fig. 2 – 4 – 63)

[**Indications**] (1) Febrile disease, constipation. (2) Sudden loss of voice, deafness, tinnitus. (3) Hypochondriac pain, pain in the shoulder and back.

[**Needling method**] Perpendicular insertion 0. 8 ~ 1. 2 *cun*.

10. 3. 6 Jianliao(TE 14)

[**Location**]Posterior and inferior to the acromion, in the depression a-

bout 1 *cun* posterior to Jianyu (LI 15) when the arm is abducted. (Fig. 2 –
4 – 64)

[**Indicatios**] Pain and limitation of the shoulder and arm.

[**Needling method**] Perpendicular insertion toward the shoulder joint
1 ~ 1. 5 *cun*.

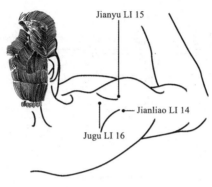

Fig. 2 – 4 – 64

10. 3. 7 Yifeng(TE 17)

[**Location**] Antero-inferior to the mastoid process, in the depression posterior to the inferior border of the lobule of the ear. (Fig. 2 – 4 – 65)

[**Indications**] (1) Tinnitus, deafness, facial paralysis. (2) Swelling of
the cheek (mumps), toothache, scrofula.

[**Needling method**] Perpendicular insertion 0. 8 ~ 1. 2 *cun*.

10. 3. 8 Jiaosun(TE 20)

[**Location**] The acupoint is located directly above the ear apex, within
the hair line. (Fig. 2 – 4 – 65)

[**Indications**] (1) Migraine, swelling of cheek (mumps). (2) Tinnitus,
deafness.

[**Needling method**] Subcutaneous insertion 0. 3 ~ 0. 5 *cun*.

10. 3. 9 Ermen(TE 21)

[**Location**] In front of the superior notch of the auricula, in the depression on the posterior border of the mandibular condyloid process. (Fig. 2 – 4 –

65)

[**Indications**]Tinnitus, deafness, facial paralysis, toothache.

[**Needling method**]Perpendicular insertion 0. 5 ~ 1 *cun* with the mouth open.

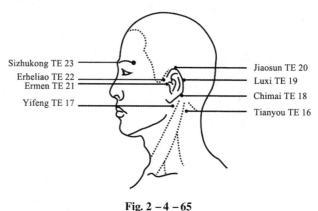

Sizhukong TE 23
Erheliao TE 22
Ermen TE 21
Yifeng TE 17

Jiaosun TE 20
Luxi TE 19
Chimai TE 18
Tianyou TE 16

Fig. 2 – 4 – 65

10. 3. 10 Sizhukong(TE 23)

[**Location**]In the depression at the lateral end of the eyebrow. (Fig. 2 – 4 – 65)

[**Indications**]Redness, swelling and pain of the eye, twitching of the eyelids.

[**Needling method**]Avoiding the artery, oblique or subcutaneous insertion 0. 3 ~ 0. 5 *cun*.

11. The Gallbladder Meridian of Foot-*shaoyang*

11. 1 The course of the Gallbladder Meridian of Foot-*shao yang* (Fig. 2 – 4 – 66)

The gallbladder meridian of foot-*shaoyang* originates from the outer canthus (Tongziliao, GB 1), ascends to the corner of the forehead (Hanyan, GB 4), then curves downwards to the retroauricular region (Fengchi, GB 20) and runs along the side of the neck in front of the san jiao meridian of *hand-shaoyang* to the shoulder. Turning back, it traverses and passes behind the triple energizer meridian of hand-*shaoyang* down to the supraclavicular fossa.

The retroauricular branch stemsn from the retroauricular region and enters into the ear. Emerging before the ear, it runs to the posterior aspect of the outer canthus.

The second branch stems from the outer canthus and runs downwards to Daying (ST 5) and meets the triple energizer meridian of hand-*shaoyang* in the infraorbital region. Then, passing through Jiache (ST 6), it descends to the neck and enters the supraclavicular fossa where it meets. The branch which has already reached the place previously. From there, it further descends into the chest, passes through the diaphragm to connect with the liver and enters its pertaining organ, the gallbladder. Then it runs inside the hypochondriac region, comes out from the lateral side of the lower abdomen near the femoral artery at the inguinal region. From there it

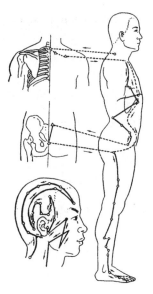

Fig. 2 – 4 – 66 The

course the gallbladder

meridian of foot-*shaoyang*

runs superficially along the margin of the pubic hair and goes transversely into the hip region (Huantiao, GB 30).

The straight portion of the meridian runs downward from the supraclavicular fossa, passes in front of the axlla along the lateral aspect of the chest and through the floating ribs to the hip region where it meets the previous meridian. Then it descends along the lateral aspect of the thigh to the lateral side of the knee. Going further downward along the anterior aspect of the fibula all the way to its lower end, it reaches the anterior aspect of the external malleolus. It then follows the dorsum of the foot to the lateral side of the 4th toe.

The branch of the dorsum of the foot stems from Zulinqi (GB 41), runs between the first and second metatarsal bones to the distal portion of the great toe and passes through the nail, and terminates at its hairy region, where it links with the liver meridian of foot-*jueyin*.

[**Associated viscera**] Gallbladder and liver.

[**Associated organs**] Eyes and ears.

11. 2 Indications

Disorders of the lateral side of the head, eyes, ears and throat as well as mental problems, febrile diseases and other diseases involving the areas through which the meridian passes.

11. 3 Commonly used acupoints of the Gallbladder Meridian of Foot-*shaoyang*

This meridian starts at Tongziliao (GB 1) and ends at Zuqiaoyin (GB 44), bilaterally each of consisting of 44 acupoints.

11. 3. 1 Tongziliao(GB 1)

[**Location**] 0. 5 *cun* lateral to the outer canthus, in the depression on the lateral side of the orbit. (Fig. 2 – 4 – 67)

[**Indications**] (1) Redness, swelling and pain of eyes, cataract. (2) Glaucoma and headache.

[**Needling method**] Subcutaneous insertion 0. 3 ~ 0. 5 *cun*.

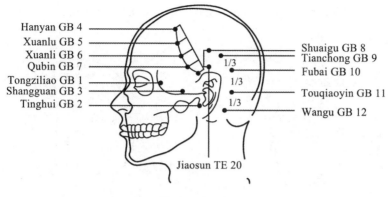

Hanyan GB 4
Xuanlu GB 5
Xuanli GB 6
Qubin GB 7
Tongziliao GB 1
Shangguan GB 3
Tinghui GB 2

Shuaigu GB 8
Tianchong GB 9
Fubai GB 10
Touqiaoyin GB 11
Wangu GB 12

1/3
1/3
1/3

Jiaosun TE 20

Fig. 2 – 4 – 67

11. 3. 2 Tinghui(GB 2)

[**Location**] Anterior to the intertragic notch, at the posterior border of the condyloid process of the mandible. The point is located when the mouth is open. (Fig. 2 – 4 – 67)

[**Indications**] (1) Tinnitus, deafness. (2) Facial paralysis.

[**Needling method**] Perpendicular insertion 0. 5 ~ 1 *cun* with mouth open.

11. 3. 3 Shuaigu(GB 8)

[**Location**] This acupoint is located 1. 5 *cun* from the tip of ear straightly into the hair line. (Fig. 2 – 4 – 67)

[**Indications**] (1) Migraine, vertigo. (2) Acute and chronic infantile convulsion.

[**Needling method**] Subcutaneous insertion 0. 5 ~ 0. 8 *cun*.

11. 3. 4 Yangbai(GB 14)

[**Location**] When the patient looks straight forward, the point is directly above the pupil, 1 *cun* superior to the eyebrow. (Fig. 2 – 4 – 68)

[**Indications**] (1) Redness, swelling and pain of eyes, ptosis of the lower eyelid, twitching of eyelids, blurred vision. (2) Facial paralysis forehead pain, vertigo.

[**Needling method**] Subcutaneous insertion 0. 3 ~ 0. 5 *cun*.

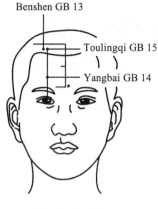

Benshen GB 13
Toulingqi GB 15
Yangbai GB 14

Fig. 2 – 4 – 68

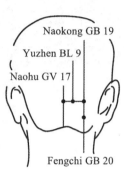

Naokong GB 19
Yuzhen BL 9
Naohu GV 17
Fengchi GB 20

Fig. 2 – 4 – 69

11. 3. 5 Fengchi(GB 20)

[**Location**] This acupoint is located below the occipital bone, parallel to Fengfu(GV 16) an din the depression between the upper portion of m. sterno-cleidomastoideus and m. trapezius. (Fig. 2 – 4 – 69)

[**Indications**] (1) Headache, redness, swelling and pain of the eye, nasal obstruction, epistaxis, tinnitus, deafness, vertigo, apoplexy and epilepsy. (2) Febrile disease, common cold, malaria. (3) Rigidity and pain of the neck, pain and limitation of the shoulder.

[**Needling method**] Oblique insertion 0. 8 ~ 1. 2 *cun* towards the tip of the nose with the tip of the needle slightly downwards, or subcutaneous insertion through Fengfu(GV 16). Towards the middle in the deeper layer, is the medulla oblongata. The angle and depth of the needle must be strictly controlled.

11. 3. 6 Jianjing(GB 21)

[**Location**] This point is located on the shoulder and at the midpoint between Dazhui (GV 14) and the acromion. (Fig. 2 – 4 – 70)

[**Indications**] (1) Stiffness and pain of neck, shoulder and back. (2) Paralysis of upper limbs. (3) Mastitis insufficiency of lactation.

[**Needling method**] Perpendicular insertion 0. 5 ~ 0. 8 *cun* below this point is apex of the lung, do not puncture deeply. Needling this point is contraindicated in pregnancy.

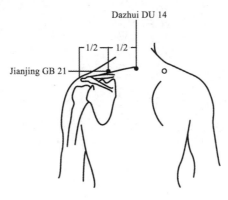

Fig. 2 – 4 – 70

11. 3. 7 Riyue(GB 24)

[**Location**] Below the nipple, in the 7th intercostal space. (Fig. 2 – 4 – 71)

[**Indications**] (1)Jaundice, hypochondriac pain. (2)Vomiting and acid regurgitation.

[**Needling method**] Oblique or subcutaneous insertion 0. 5 ~ 0. 8 *cun*.

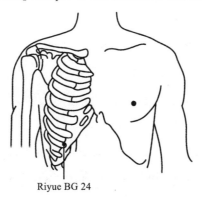

Riyue BG 24

Fig. 2 – 4 – 71

11. 3. 8 Daimai(GB 26)

[**Location**] Directly below the free end of the 11th rib, and level with the umbilicus. (Fig. 2 – 4 – 72)

[**Indications**] (1) Irregular menstruation, amenorrhea, leukorrhea, hernia. (2) Pain in the loins. (3) Hypochondria.

[**Needling method**] Perpendicular insertion 0.5 ~ 1 *cun*.

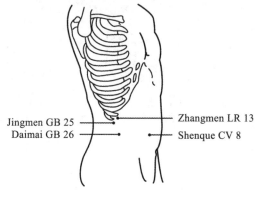

Jingmen GB 25 ——— Zhangmen LR 13
Daimai GB 26 ——— Shenque CV 8

Fig. 2 – 4 – 72

11. 3. 9 Huantiao(GB 30)

[**Location**] At the junction of the lateral 1/3 and medial 2/3 of the distance between the great trochanter of the femur and the hiatus of the sacrum. (Fig. 2 – 4 – 73)

[**Indications**] Flaccidity and obstruction syndromes of lower limbs, pain of the lumbar and leg, hemiplegia.

[**Needling method**] Perpendicular insertion 2 ~ 3 *cun*.

11. 3. 10 Fengchi(GB 31)

[**Location**] On the midline of the lateral aspect of the thigh, 7 *cun* above the transverse popliteal crease. (Fig. 2 – 4 – 74)

[**Indications**] (1) Flaccidity and obstruction of lower extremities, beriberi. (2) Hemiplegia, general pruritus. (3) Sudden deafness.

[**Needling method**] Perpendicular insertion 1 ~ 2 *cun*.

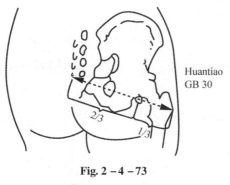

Huantiao
GB 30

Fig. 2 – 4 – 73

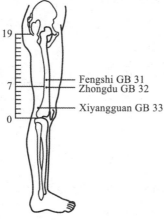

Fengshi GB 31
Zhongdu GB 32

Xiyangguan GB 33

Fig. 2 – 4 – 74

11. 3. 11 Yanglingquan(GB 34, *he*-sea acupoint and lower-He-sea acupoint as well as one of the eight convergent acupoints associating with tendons)

[**Location**] In the depression anterior and inferior to the small head of the fibula. (Fig. 2 – 4 – 75)

[**Indications**] (1) Pain in the hypochondrium, bitter taste in the mouth, vomiting, jaundice. (2) Hemiplegia, pain of the shoulder, weakness, numbness and pain of lower extremities, swelling and pain of the knee, beriberi. (3) Infantile convulsion.

[**Needling method**] Perpendicular insertion 1 ~ 1. 5 *cun*.

11. 3. 12 Guangming(GB 37, *luo*-connecting acupoint)

[**Location**] 5 *cun* above the tip of the external malleolus, on the anterior border of the fibula. (Fig. 2 – 4 – 75)

[**Indications**] (1) Pain of the eyes, night blindness, nearsightedness, epiphora. (2) Distending pain in the breast. (3) Flaccidity and obstruction syndromes of the lower limbs.

[**Needling method**] Perpendicular insertion 1 ~ 1. 5 *cun*.

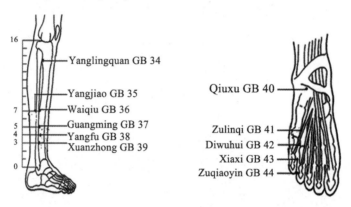

Fig. 2 – 4 – 75   Fig. 2 – 4 – 76

11. 3. 13 Xuanzhong (GB 39, one of the eight confluent acupoints associating with marrow)

[**Location**] 3 *cun* above the tip of the external malleolus, on the anterior border of the fibula. (Fig. 2 – 4 – 75)

[**Indications**] (1) Headache, dizziness, tinnitus and deafness. (2) Hemiplegia, rigidity and pain of the neck, pain in the hypochondrium, flaccidity and obstruction syndromes of lower limbs, beriberi.

[**Needling method**] Perpendicular insertion 1 ~ 1. 5 *cun*.

11. 3. 14 Qiuxu (GB 40, *yuan*-source acupoint)

[**Location**] Anterior and inferior to the external malleolus, in the depression on the lateral side of the tendon of m. extensor digitorum longus. (Fig. 2 – 4 – 76)

[**Indications**] (1) Redness, swelling and pain of eyes, cataract. (2) Malaria. (3) Distending pain in the chest and hypochondria, swelling in the axillary region, flaccidity and obstruction syndromes of the lower limbs, swelling and pain of the external malleolus.

[**Needling method**] Perpendicular insertion 0. 3 ~ 0. 5 *cun*.

11. 3. 15 Zulingqi(GB 41, *shu*-stream acupoint and one of the eight convergent acupoints associating with Belt Vessel)

[**Location**] Anterior to the junction of the 4th and 5th metatarsal bones, in the depression on the lateral side of the tendon of m. extensor digiti minimi of the foot. (Fig. 2 - 4 - 76)

[**Indications**] (1) Migraine and redness, swelling and pain of eyes. (2) Hypochondriac pain, pain of foot dorsum, numbness of toes. (3) Irregular menstruation, distension in the breast.

[**Needling method**] Perpendicular insertion 0. 3 ~ 0. 5 *cun*.

12. The Liver Meridian of Foot-*jueyin*

12. 1 The course of the Liver Meridian of Foot-*jueyin* (Fig. 2 - 4 - 77)

The liver meridian of foot-*jueyin* starts from the dorsal hair of the great toe, running upward along the dorsum of the foot, passing through a point, 1 *cun* in front of the medial malleolus, it ascends to an area 8 *cun* above the medial malleolus, where it runs across and behind the spleen meridian of foot-*taiyin*. Then it runs further upward to the medial side of the knee and along the medial side of the thigh to the pubic hair region, where it curves around the external genitalia and goes up to the lower abdomen. It then runs upward and curves around the stomach to enter the liver, its pertaining organ, and connects with the gallbladder. From there it continues to ascend, passing through the diaphragm, and branching out in the costal and hypochondriac region. Then it ascends along the posterior aspect of the throat to the nasopharynx and connects with the "eye system" (the area where the eyeball links with the brain). Running further upward, it emerges from the forehead and meets the governor vessel at the vertex.

The branch which arises from the "eye system" runs downward into the cheek and curves around the inner surface of the lips.

The branch arising from the liver passes through the diaphragm, runs upward into the lung and links with the lung meridian of hand-*taiyin*.

[Associated viscera] Liver, gallbladder, lung and stomach.

[Associated organs] Genitalia, throat, pharynx, eyes and mouth.

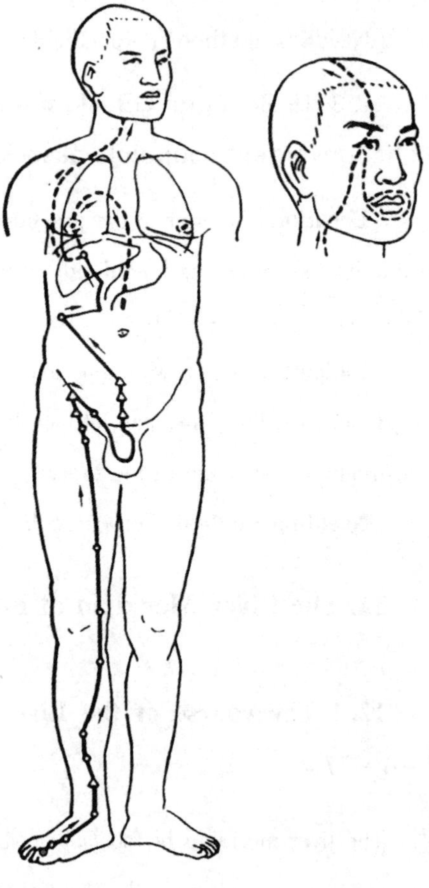

Fig. 2 −4 −77 The coures of the liver
meridian of foot-*jueyin*

12. 2 Indications

Liver disease, gynecological disease, genitalia disorder and other diseases involving the areas through which the meridian flows.

12. 3　Commonly used acupoints of the Liver Meridian of Foot-*jueyin*

This meridian starts at Dadun(LR 1) and ends at Qimen(LR 14) , bilaterally each of consisting of 14 acupoints.

12. 3. 1　Dadun(LR 1 , *jing*-well acupoint)

[**Location**] This acupoint is located on the lateral side of the dorsum of the great toe , about 0. 1 *cun* lateral to the corner of the nail. (Fig. 2 – 4 – 78)

[**Indications**] (1) Apoplexy , coma , epilepsy. (2) Hernia , enuresis , difficulty in urination irregular menstruation , metrorrhagia and metrostaxis.

[**Needling method**] Oblique insertion 0. 1 ~ 0. 2 *cun* , or prick to the cause of bleeding.

12. 3. 2　Xingjian(LR 2 , *ying*-spring acupoint)

[**Location**] This acupoint is located on the dorsum of the foot between the first and second toes , proximal to the margin of the web. (Fig. 2 – 4 – 78).

[**Indications**] (1) Headache , vertigo , redness , swelling and pain of the eyes , glaucoma , pacial paralysis. (2) Hypochondriac pain , bitter taste in the mouth , jaundice. (3) Insomnia , epilepsy. (4) Hernia , dysuria , irregular menstruation , dysmenorrhea , metrorrhagia and menostaxis.

[**Needling method**] Oblique insertion 0. 5 ~ 0. 8 *cun*.

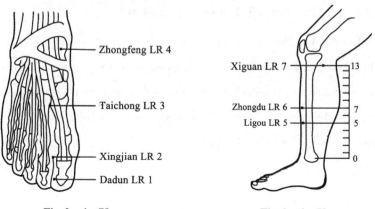

Zhongfeng LR 4

Taichong LR 3

Xingjian LR 2

Dadun LR 1

Xiguan LR 7　13

Zhongdu LR 6　7

Ligou LR 5　5

0

Fig. 2 – 4 – 78　　　　　　　　Fig. 2 – 4 – 79

12. 3. 3 Taichong (LR 3, *shu-stream* and *yuan*-source acupoint)

[**Location**]This acupoint is located on the dorsum of the foot, in the depression anterior to the junction of the first and second metatarsal bones. (Fig. 2 − 4 − 78)

[**Indications**] (1) Headache, vertigo, redness, swelling and pain of the eye, facial paralysis. (2) Depression, pain in the hypochondrium, abdominal distention, stomachache, vomiting, hiccup. (3) Hernia, enuresis, irregular menstruation, metrorrhagia and metrostaxis. (4) Apoplexy, manic depression psychosis, epilepsy, infantile convulsion. (5) Flaccidity and obstruction of the lower limbs, difficulty in walking.

[**Needling method**]Perpendicular intertion 0. 5 ~ 0. 8 *cun*.

12. 3. 4 Ligou(LR 5, *luo*-connecting acupoint)

[**Location**]This acupoint is located on the medial side of the shank, 5 *cun* above the tip of the medial malleolus and on the middle of the medial aspect of the tibia. (Fig. 2 − 4 − 79)

[**Indications**] (1) Pruritus vulva, hernia, irregular menstruation, leucorrhea, dysuria. (2) Severe lumbago and lower abdominal pain.

[**Needling method**]Subcutaneous insertion 0. 5 ~ 0. 8 *cun*.

12. 3. 5 Ququan(LR 8, *he*-sea acupoint)

[**Location**] This acupoint is located on the medial side of the shank. When the knee is flexed, the acupoint is in the depression above the end of the transverse popliteal crease, posterior to the medial epicondyle of the femur, on the anterior part of insertion of m. semimembranousus and m. semitendinosus. (Fig. 2 − 4 − 80)

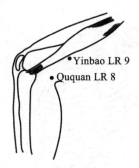

Fig. 2 – 4 – 80

[**Indications**] (1) Irregular menstruation, dysmenorrheal, leucorrhea, seminal emission, dysuria. (2) Swelling and pain of knee.

[**Needling method**] Perpendicular insertion 1 ~ 1. 5 *cun*.

12. 3. 6 Zhangmen(LR 13, front-*mu* acupoint of spleen. one of the eight convergent acupoints associating with *zang* organ)

[**Location**] This acupoint is located on the lateral side of the abdomen, below the free end of the eleventh floating rib. (Fig. 2 – 4 – 81)

[**Indications**] (1) Abdominal distention, abdominal mass, borborygmus, diarrhea, vomiting. (2) Pain in the hypochondrium and loins.

[**Needling method**] Oblique insertion 0. 5 ~ 0. 8 *cun*.

12. 3. 7 Qimen(LR 14, front-*mu* acupoint of the liver)

[**Location**] This acupoint is located on the chest, directly below the nipple, in the sixth intercostal space. (Fig. 2 – 4 – 82)

[**Indications**] Hypochondriac pain, bitter taste in the mouth, vomiting, hiccup and mastitis.

[**Needling method**] Oblique insertion 0. 5 ~ 0. 8 *cun*.

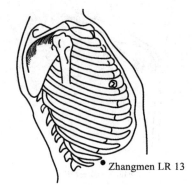

Zhangmen LR 13

Fig. 2 – 4 – 81

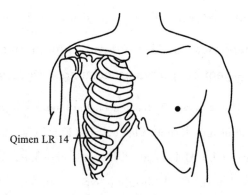

Qimen LR 14

Fig. 2 – 4 – 82

13. The Governor Vessel

13. 1 The course of the Governor Vessel (Fig. 2 – 4 – 83)

The governor vessel starts from the uterus, runs downward to the central region of the pelvis around the genitals and into the external orifice of the urethra in women and around penis in men, it joins the conception and thoroughfare vessels over perineum, passes by the anus, moves upward from inside the coccyx and sacrum and enters the brain from Fengfu (GV 16). The external portion runs to the end of the nose bridge from the vertex through the forehead and ends at the gum.

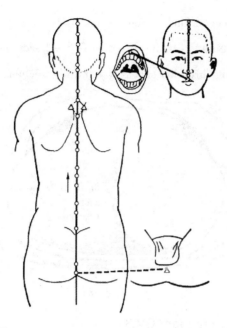

Fig. 2 −4 −83 The coures of the governor vessel

13. 2 Indications

Mental problems, febrile diseases, disorders of the lumbosacral region, back and head as well as diseases of the related viscera.

13. 3 Commonly used acupoints of the Governor Vessel

This vessel starts at Changqiang(GV 1) and ends at *Yinjiao* (GV 28), consisting of 28 acupoints.

13. 3. 1 Changqiang(GV 1, *luo*-connecting acupoint of gover-nor vessel)

[**Location**] This acupont is at the midpoint between the tip of the coccyx and the anus in prone position when patient touches the knees with the chest. (Fig. 2 −4 −84)

[**Indications**] (1) Diarrhea, constipation, hemorrhoids, prolapses of the rectum. (2) Manic-depressive psychosis, epilepsy. (3) Rigid and arched back, pain in the coccyx and sacrum region.

[**Needling method**] Oblique insertion 0. 8 ~ 1 *cun* right in front of the coccyx. Perpendicular insertion caneasily injure the rectum.

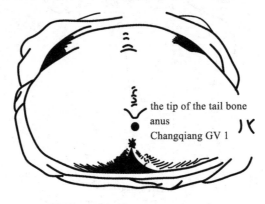

the tip of the tail bone
anus
Changqiang GV 1

Fig. 2 − 4 − 84

13. 3. 2 Yaoyangguan(GV 3)

[**Location**] This acupont is located on the posterior midline and in the depression below the spinous process of the fourth lumbar vertebra in prone position, at the level with the iliac crest. (Fig. 2 − 4 − 85)

[**Indications**] (1) Irregular menstruataion, spermatorrhea, impotence. (2) Lumbosacral pain, pain, flaccidity and obstruction syndromes of lower limbs.

[**Needling method**] Oblique insertion upward 0. 5 ~ 1 *cun*.

13. 3. 3 Mingmen(GV 4)

[**Location**] This acupont is located on the posterior midline and in the depression below the spinous process of the second lumbar vertebrain pronr position. (Fig. 2 − 4 − 85)

[**Indications**] (1) Irregular menstruation, leukorrhea, sterility, spermatorrhea, impotence. (2) Morning diarrhea. (3) Stiffness and pain in the loins and spine, flaccidity and obstruction syndromes of lower limbs.

[**Needling method**] Oblique insertion upward 0. 5 ~ 1 *cun*.

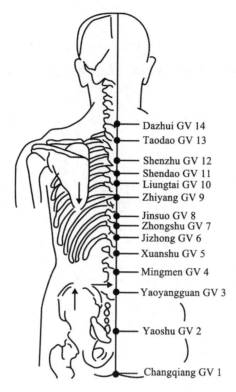

Dazhui GV 14
Taodao GV 13
Shenzhu GV 12
Shendao GV 11
Liungtai GV 10
Zhiyang GV 9
Jinsuo GV 8
Zhongshu GV 7
Jizhong GV 6
Xuanshu GV 5
Mingmen GV 4
Yaoyangguan GV 3
Yaoshu GV 2
Changqiang GV 1

Fig. 2 - 4 - 85

13. 3. 4 Shenzhu(GV 12)

[**Location**]This acupont is located on the posterior midline and in the depression below the spinous process of the seventh thoracic vertebra in prone position. (Fig. 2 - 4 - 85)

[**Indications**](1) Distending pain in the chest and hypochondria, jaundice, stomachache. (2) Cough, asthma. (3) Stiffness of spine and pain in the back.

[**Needling method**] Oblique insertion upward 0. 5 ~ 1 *cun*. Moxibustion is applicable.

13. 3. 5 Shenzhu(GV 12)

[**Location**]This acupont is located on the posterior midline and in the depression below the spinous process of the third thoracic vertebra. (Fig. 2 -

4 – 85)

[**Indications**] (1) Cough, asthma, dysponia. (2) Manic-depressive psychosis, epilepsy, infantile convulsion. (3) Stiffness and pain in the spine and back.

[**Needling method**] Oblique insertion upward 0. 5 ~ 1 *cun*. Moxibustion is applicable.

13. 3. 6 Dazhui(GV 14)

[**Location**] This acupont is located on the posterior midline and in the depression below the spinous process of the seventh cervical vertebra. (Fig. 2 – 4 – 85)

[**Indications**] (1) Febrile diseases, malaria, common cold, hectic fever and night sweat, cough, asthma. (2) Manic-depressive psychosis, epilepsy. (3) Neck rigidity and pain, pain in the shoulder and back.

[**Needling method**] Oblique insertion upward 0. 5 ~ 1 *cun*.

13. 3. 7 Yamen(GV 15)

[**Location**] This acupoint is located 0. 5 *cun* directly above the midpoint of the posterior hairline and below the first cervical vertebra when the patient sits upright. (Fig. 2 – 4 – 86)

[**Indications**] (1) Sudden loss of voice, stiff tongue due to apoplexy. (2) Headache, stiff neck. (3) Manic-depressive psychosis, epilepsy.

[**Needling method**] Perpendicular or oblique insertion downward to mandible 0. 5 ~ 1 *cun*, do not puncture obliquely upward or deep. Deeper is the medulla oblongata. Strict attention must be paid to the needle angle and depth.

13. 3. 8 Fengfu(GV 16)

[**Location**] This acupoint is located 1 *cun* directly above the midpoint of the posterior hairline and directly below the external occipital protuberance, in the depression between m. trapezius of both sides when the patient sits upright. (Fig. 2 – 4 – 86)

[**Indications**] (1) Manic-depressive psychosis, epilepsy, inability to speak after apoplexy. (2) Headache, stiff neck, dizziness.

[**Needling method**] Perpendicular or oblique insertion downward to mandible 0. 5 ~ 1 *cun*, do not puncture obliquely upward or deep. Deeper is the medulla oblongata. attention should be given to needling method.

13. 3. 9 Baihui(GV 20)

[**Location**] This point is located 7 *cun* directly above the posterior hairline when the patient sits upright. (Fig. 2 − 4 − 86)

[**Indications**] (1) Headache, dizziness, nasosinusitis. (2) Insomnia, amnesia, manic-depressive psychosis, epilepsy, coma, apoplexy, hemiplegia, aphasia. (3) Prolapse of rectum, prolapse of uterus.

[**Needling method**] Subcutaneous insertion 0. 5 ~ 0. 8 *cun*.

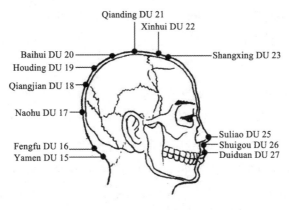

Qianding DU 21
Xinhui DU 22

Baihui DU 20
Houding DU 19
Qiangjian DU 18

Naohu DU 17

Fengfu DU 16
Yamen DU 15

Shangxing DU 23

Suliao DU 25
Shuigou DU 26
Duiduan DU 27

Fig. 2 − 4 − 86

13. 3. 10 Shangxing(GV 23)

[**Location**] This acupoint is located 1 *cun* directly above the anterior hairline when the patient sits with the back leaning against the chair. (Fig. 2 − 4 − 86)

[**Indications**] (1) Headache, vertigo, nasal obstruction, nasosinusitis, epistaxis, pain of eye, epiphora. (2) Febrile diseases, malaria. (3) Manic-depressive psychosis, epilepsy.

[**Needling method**] Subcutaneous insertion 0. 5 ~ 1 *cun*. Moxibustion is applicable.

13. 3. 11 Shenting(GV 24)

[**Location**] This acupoint is located 0. 5 *cun* directly above the anterior hairline when the patient sits with the back leaning against the chair. (Fig. 2 – 4 – 86)

[**Indications**] (1) Headache, vertigo, nasal obstruction, nasosinusitis, epistaxis, pain of eye, epiphora. (2) Insomnia, manic-depressive psychosis, epilepsy.

[**Needling method**] Subcutaneous insertion 0. 5 ~ 1 *cun*. Moxibustion is applicable.

13. 3. 12 Shuigou(GV 26)

[**Location**] This acupoint is located at the junction of the superior 1/3 and middle 1/3 of the philtrum when the patient sits with the back leaning a-gainst the chair. (Fig. 2 – 4 – 86)

[**Indications**] (1) Apoplexy, coma, trismus, manic-depressive psycho-sis, epilepsy, infantile convulsion. (2) Swelling of the face, deviation of the mouth and eye. (3) Pain and stiffness of the lower back.

[**Needling method**] Oblique insertion upward 0. 3 ~ 0. 5 *cun*.

14. The Conception Vessel

14. 1 The course of the Conception Vessel (Fig. 2 – 4 – 87)

The conception vessel starts from the uterus and emerges from the perine-um. It goes anteriorly to the pubic region and ascends along the interior of the abdomen, passing through Guanyuan (CV 4) and the other points along the front midline to the throat, ascending further, it curves around the lips, pas-ses through the cheek and enters the infraorbital region.

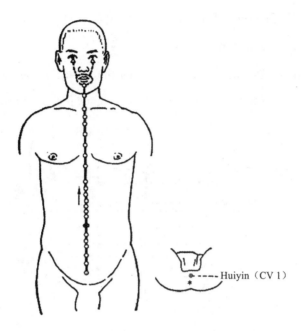

Huiyin（CV 1）

Fig. 2 - 4 - 87 The coures of the conception vessel

14. 2 Indications

Local disorders of the abdomen, chest, neck and head as well as diseases of related viscera. A few of the acupoints on the conception vessel are effective in strengthening the body.

14. 3 Commonly used acupoints of the Conception Vessel

This vessel starts at Huiyin(CV 1) and ends at Chengjiang(CV 24), consisting of 24 acupoints.

14. 3. 1 Zhongji(CV 3,front-*mu* acupoint of the bladder)

[**Location**]This acupoint is located on the lower abdomen,anterior midline and 4 *cun* directly below the umbilicus in supine position. (Fig. 2 -4 -88)

[**Indications**] (1) Enuresis, dysuria, hernia. (2) Irregular menstruation, metrorrhagia, leukorrhea, prolapse of uterus, sterility,spermatorrhea, impotence.

[**Needling method**] Perpendicular insertion 1 ~ 1. 5 *cun.*

14. 3. 2 Guanguan(CV 4)

[**Location**] This acupoint is located on the lower abdomen, anterior midline and 3 *cun* directly below the umbilicus in supine position. (Fig. 2 – 4 – 88)

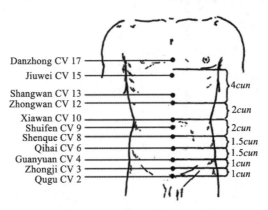

Danzhong CV 17
Jiuwei CV 15
4cun
Shangwan CV 13
Zhongwan CV 12
2cun
Xiawan CV 10
Shuifen CV 9
2cun
Shenque CV 8
1.5cun
Qihai CV 6
1.5cun
Guanyuan CV 4
1cun
Zhongji CV 3
1cun
Qugu CV 2

Fig. 2 – 4 – 88

[**Indications**] (1) Irregular menstruation, metrorrhagia, metrostaxis, leukorrhea, dysmenorrhea, prolapse of uterus, sterility, postpartum hemorrhage, impotence, spermatorrhea, enuresis, retention of urine. (2) Flaccidity of apoplexy, emaciation due to consumptive disease. (3) Diarrhea, prolapse of rectum. (4) This point has the function to tonify, as well as maintain health.

[**Needling method**] Perpendicular insertion 1 ~ 2 *cun.*

14. 3. 3 Qihai(CV 6)

[**Location**] This acupoint is located on the lower abdomen, anterior midline and 1. 5 *cun* below the umbilicus. (Fig. 2 – 4 – 88)

[**Indications**] (1) Abdominal pain, diarrhea, constipation. (2) Irregular menstruation, amenorrhea, enuresis, hernia, spermatorrhea, impotence. (3) Flaccidity of apoplexy, emaciation due to consumptive disease. (4) This point has the function to tonify, as well as maintain health.

[**Needling method**] Perpendicular insertion 1 ~ 2 *cun.*

14. 3. 4 Shenque(CV 8)

[**Location**] This acupoint is located on the center of the abdomen and the umbilicus. in supine position. (Fig. 2 – 4 – 88)

[**Indications**] (1) Abdominal pain, diarrhea, constipation, dysentery, prolapse of rectum. (2) Flaccidity of apoplexy, coldness of the four extremities, collapse. (3) Edema, difficult urination.

[**Needling method**] Indirect moxibustion with moxa stick, or moxibustion on some type of material (salt, ginger, etc.).

14. 3. 5 Shuifen(CV 9)

[**Location**] This acupoint is located on the upper abdomen and anterior midline and 1 *cun* above the umbilicus. (Fig. 2 – 4 – 88)

[**Indications**] (1) Abdominal pain, borborygmus, edema, retention of urine. (2) Stomachache, regurgitation, diarrhea.

[Needling method] perpendicular insertion 1 ~ 2 *cun*. moxibustion is applicable.

14. 3. 6 Zhongwan(CV 12, front-*mu* acupoint of the stomach and one of the eight convergent acupoints associating with *fu* organs)

[**Location**] This acupoint is located on the upper abdomen and anterior midline, 4 *cun* above the umbilicus. (Fig. 2 – 4 – 88)

[**Indications**] (1) Epigastric pain, vomiting, hiccup, acid regurgitation, adominal distention, diarrhea, dyspepsia. (2) Cough with phlegm. (3) Jaundice. (4) Insomnia, manic-depressive psychosis, epilepsy.

[**Needling method**] Perpendicular insertion 1 ~ 1. 5 *cun*.

14. 3. 7 Danzhong(CV 17, front-*mu* acupoint of pericardium and one of the eight convergent acupoints associating with *qi*)

[**Location**] This acupoint is located on the anterior midline, at the level with the fourth intercostals space. (Fig. 2 – 4 – 88)

[**Indications**] (1) Cough, asthma, pain and oppression of the chest.

(2) Angina pectoris, palpitation and dysphoria. (3) Insufficient lactation, mastitis. (4) Vomiting, hiccup, dysphagia.

[**Needling method**] Subcutaneous insertion 0. 3 ~ 0. 5 *cun*.

14. 3. 8 Tiantu(CV 22)

[**Location**] This acupoint is located on the anterior midline and in the center of the suprasternal fossa. (Fig. 2 – 4 – 89)

[**Indications**] (1) Cough, asthma, sore throat, sudden loss of voice, hoarseness of the voice. (2) Scrofula, goiter. (3) Plum pit sensation in the throat, dysphasia.

[**Needling method**] First, puncture perpendicularly 0. 2 *cun*, then insert the needle tip downward along the posterior aspect of the sternum 1 ~ 1. 5 *cun*. Strict attention must be paid to the needle angle and depth. The lung can easily be injured.

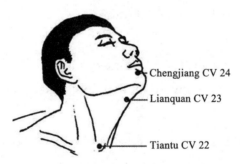

Chengjiang CV 24

Lianquan CV 23

Tiantu CV 22

Fig. 2 – 4 – 89

14. 3. 9 Lianquan(CV 23)

[**Location**] This acupoint is located on the anterior midline, above the Adam's apple and in the depression of the upper border of the hyoid bone. (Fig. 2 – 4 – 89)

[**Indications**] Subglossal swelling and pain, stiffness of tongue due to apoplexy, aphasia, sudden loss of voice, difficulty in swallowing.

[**Needling method**] Oblique insertion 0. 5 ~ 1 *cun* toward the tongue root. Moxibustion is applicable.

14. 3. 10 Chengjiang(CV 24)

[**Location**] This acupoint is located in the center of the mentolabial groove. (Fig. 2 – 4 – 89)

[**Indications**] (1) Deviation of the mouth, swelling of the face, swelling of the gums, salivation, sudden loss of voice. (2) Manic-depressive psychosis, epilepsy.

[**Needling method**] Subcutaneous insertion 0. 3 ~ 0. 5 *cun*. Moxibustion is applicable.

15. Extraordinary acupoints

15. 1 Acupoints on the head and neck

15. 1. 1 Sishencong(EX-HN 1)

[**Location**] A group of four acupoints, at the vertex, 1 *cun* respectively posterior, anterior, and lateral to Baihui(GV 20). (Fig. 2 – 4 – 90)

[**Indications**] Headache, vertigo, insomnia, amnesia and epilepsy.

[**Needling method**] Subcutaneous insertion 0. 5 ~ 0. 8 *cun*.

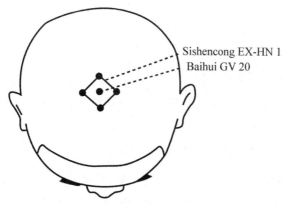

Sishencong EX-HN 1
Baihui GV 20

Fig. 2 – 4 – 90

15. 1. 2 Yintang(EX-HN 3)

[**Locatioin**] This acupoint is located midway between the medial ends of the two eyebrows. (Fig. 2 – 4 – 91)

[**Indications**] (1) Headache, vertigo, epistaxis, nasosinusitis. (2) Infantile convulsion, insomnia and sunstroke.

[**Needling method**] Lifting and pinching the local skin and subcutaneous insertion 0. 3 ~ 0. 5 *cun*.

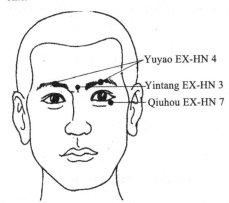

Fig. 2 – 4 – 91

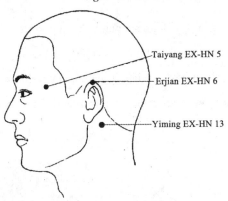

Fig. 2 – 4 – 92

15. 1. 3 *Taiyang* (EX-HN 5)

[**Locatioin**] This acupoint is located between the lateral end of the eyebrow and the outer canthus and in the depression about one finger-breadth posterior. (Fig. 2 – 4 – 92)

[**Indications**] Migraine, headache, eye disorders and trigeminal neuralgia.

〔**Needling method**〕Perpendicular or ablique insertion 0. 3 ~ 0. 5 *cun* , or prick to cause bleeding.

15. 1. 4 Erjian(Ex-HN 6)

〔**Locatioin**〕On the top region of the auricle, fold the auricle forward, the point is at the apex of the auricle. (Fig. 2 – 4 – 92)

〔**Indications**〕Redness, swelling and pain of the eye, hordeolum, headache , sore throat.

〔**Needling method**〕Prick to cause bleeding.

15. 1. 5 Qiuhou(EX-HN 7)

〔**Locatioin**〕This acupoint is located on the region of the face, at the junction of the lateral one-fourth and the medial three-fourths of the infraorbital margin. (Fig. 2 – 4 – 91)

〔**Indications**〕Eye diseases such as optic neuritis, optic atrophy, glaucoma, early stage of cataract, myopia.

〔**Needling method**〕Pushing the eyeball upward gently, perpendicular insertion the needle slowly 0. 5 ~ 1. 5 *cun* along the orbital margin. do not lift and thrust or rotate the needle. Mosibustion is contraindicated.

15. 1. 6 Jinjin(EX-HN 12) ,Yuye(EX-HN 13)

〔**Locatioin**〕This acupoint is located on the veins on both sides of the frenulum of the tongue. (Fig. 2 – 4 – 93)

〔**Indications**〕(1)Canker sore ,tongue swelling. (2)Vomiting and diabetes.

〔**Needling method**〕Stab the tongue ,then prick to cause bleeding.

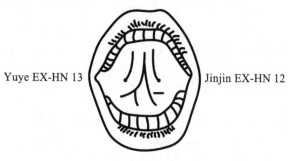

Yuye EX-HN 13　　　　　　　　　Jinjin EX-HN 12

Fig. 2 – 4 –93

15. 1. 7 Yiming(EX-HN 14)

[**Locatioin**]This acupoint is located 1 *cun* posterior to Yifeng (TE 17). (Fig. 2 – 4 – 92)

[**Indications**]Headache, vertigo, insomnia and eye diseases.

[**Needling method**]Perpendicular insertion 0. 5 ~ 1 *cun.*

15. 2 Acupoint on the chest and abdomen

Zigong(EX-CA 1)

[**Locatioin**]This acupoint is located on the lower abdomen, 4 *cun* directly below the umbilicus and 3 *cun* lateral to Zhongji (CV 3). (Fig. 2 –4 –94)

[**Indications**] Prolapse of uterus, irregular menstruation dismenorrhea, amenorrhea, hernia and sterility.

[**Needling method**]Perpendicular insertion 0. 8 ~ 1. 2 *cun.*

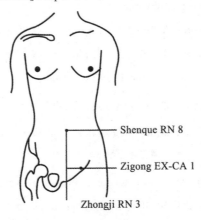

Shenque RN 8

Zigong EX-CA 1

Zhongji RN 3

Fig. 2 – 4 – 94

15. 3 Acupoints on the back

15. 3. 1 Dingchuan(EX-B 1)

[**Locatioin**]This acupoint is located below the spinous process of the seventh cervical vertebra and 0. 5 lateral to the posterior midline. (Fig. 2 – 4 – 95)

[**Indications**] Asthma and cough.

[**Needling method**] Perpendicular insertion 0. 3 ~ 0. 5 *cun*.

15. 3. 2 Jiaji(EX-B 2)

[**Locatioin**] A group of 34 acupoints on both sides of the spinal column, 0. 5 *cun* lateral to the lower border of each spinous process from the first thoracic vertebra to the fifth lumbar vertebra. (Fig. 2 – 4 – 95)

[**Indications**] (1) The acupoints on the upper portion of the thorax vertebrae on both sides mainly are used to treat diseases of the heart, lung, and upper extremities. (2) The acupoints on the lower portion of the thorax vertebrae on both sides mainly are used to treat diseases of the liver, gallbladder, spleen and stomach. (3) The acupoints on the lumbar vertebrae on both sides mainly are used to treat diseases of the urogenital system, the intestinal tract, the lumbasacral region and lower extremities.

[**Needling method**] Perpendicular insertion 0. 3 ~ 0. 5 *cun*, or use plum blossom needle for tapping.

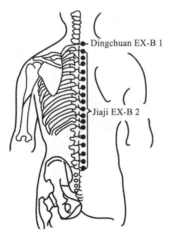

Dingchuan EX-B 1

Jiaji EX-B 2

Fig. 2 – 4 – 95

15. 3. 3 Weiwanxiashu(EX-B 3)

[**Locatioin**] This acupoint is located 1. 5 *cun* lateral to the lower border of the spinous process of the eighth thoracic vertebra. (Fig. 2 – 4 – 96)

[**Indications**] Stomachache, abdominal pain, diabetes and dry throat.

[**Needling method**] Oblique insertion 0. 3 ~0. 5 *cun*.

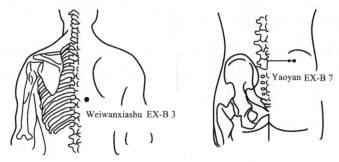

Weiwanxiashu EX-B 3

Yaoyan EX-B 7

Fig. 2 –4 –96   Fig. 2 –4 –97

15. 3. 4 Yaoyan(EX-B 7)

[**Locatioin**] This acupoint is located below the spinous process of the fourth lumbar vertebra and in the depression 3. 5 *cun* lateral to the spinous process of the fourth lumbar vertebra. (Fig. 2 –4 –97)

[**Indications**] Lumbago, irregular menstruation and leukorrhagia.

[**Needling method**] perpendicular insertion 0. 5 ~1 *cun*.

15. 3. 5 Shiqizhui(EX-B 8)

[**Locatioin**] This acupoint is located on the posterior midline and below the spinous process of the fifth lumbar vertebra. (Fig. 2 –4 –98)

[**Indications**] (1) Lumbosacral pain, metrorrhagia and metrostaxis. (2) Irregular menstruation and dysmenorrheal.

[**Needling method**] Perpendicular insertion 0. 5 ~1 *cun*.

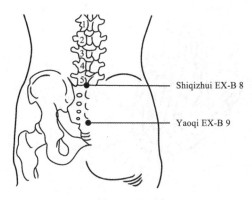

Fig. 2 – 4 – 98

15. 3. 6 Yaoqi(EX-B9)

[**Locatioin**] This acupoint is located 2 *cun* directly above the coccyx.
(Fig. 2 – 4 – 98)

[**Indications**] Epilepsy, insomnia, constipation and haemorrhoids.

[**Needling method**] Subcutenous insertion upward 1 ~ 1. 5 *cun*.

15. 4 Acupoints on the upper limbs

15. 4. 1 Yaotongdian(EX-UE 7)

[**Locatioin**] This acupoint is located on the dorsum of the hand, midway
between the transverse wrist crease and metacarpophalangeal joint, between
the second and third metacarpal bones, and between the fourth and fifth metacarpal bones, four acupoints in all on both hands. (Fig. 2 – 4 – 99)

[**Indications**] Acute sprain of waist.

[**Needling method**] Perpendicular insertion 0. 3 ~ 0. 5 *cun*.

15. 4. 2 Wailaogong(EX-UE 8)

[**Locatioin**] On the dorsum of the hand, between the second and third
metacarpal bones, 0. 5 *cun* posterior to the metacarpophalangeal joint. (Fig.
2 – 4 – 99)

[**Indications**] Stiff neck, pain of the hand and arm.

[**Needling method**] Perpendicular insertion 0. 3 ~ 0. 5 *cun*.

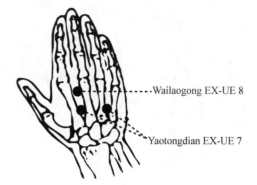

····Wailaogong EX-UE 8

····Yaotongdian EX-UE 7

Fig. 2 – 4 – 99

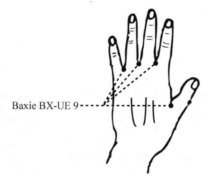

Baxie BX-UE 9····

Fig. 2 – 4 – 100

15. 4. 3 Baxie(EX-UE 9)

[**Locatioin**]This acupoint is located on the dorsum of the hand, at the junction of the white and red skin of the hands webs, eight in all, making a loose fist to locate the acupoints. (Fig. 2 – 4 – 100)

[**Indications**]Dysphoria, numbness of fingers, pain of eyes, swelling and pain of arms due to snake bite.

[**Needling method**]Ablique insertion upward 0. 3 ~ 0. 5 *cun*.

15. 4. 4 Sifeng(EX-UE 10)

[**Locatioin**]This acupoint is located on the palmar surface, in the midpoint of the transverse creases of the proximal interphalangeal joints. There are four acupoints on each hand. (Fig. 2 – 4 – 101)

[**Indications**]Infantile malnutrition and whooping cough.

[**Needling method**] Prick to cause bleeding or squeezing some yellow liquid out.

15. 4. 5 Shixuan(EX-UE 11)

[**Locatioin**] This acupoint is located on the tips of the ten fingers, about 0. 1 *cun* distal to the nails. (Fig. 2 – 4 – 101)

[**Indications**] Coma, epilepsy, high fever and sore throat.

[**Needling method**] Subcutenous insertion 0. 1 ~ 0. 2 *cun*, or prick to cause bleeding.

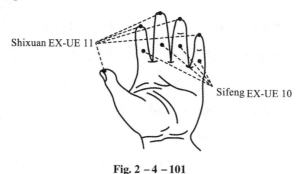

Shixuan EX-UE 11

Sifeng EX-UE 10

Fig. 2 – 4 – 101

15. 5 Acupoints on the lower limbs

15. 5. 1 Heding(EX-LE 2)

[**Locatioin**] This acupoint is located on the knee and in the depression of the midpoint of the superior patellar border. (Fig. 2 – 4 – 102)

[**Indications**] Knee joint pain, weakness of the foot and leg, and paralysis.

[**Needling method**] Perpendicular insertion 0. 8 ~ 1 *cun*.

15. 5. 2 Xiyan(EX-LE 5)

[**Locatioin**] This acupoint is located in the two depressions medial and lateral to the patellar ligament when the knee is flexed. These two acupoints are also called medial Xiyan(EX-LE 5) and lateral Xiyan respectively. (Fig. 2 – 4 – 102)

[**Indications**] Knee pain, heaviness and pain of the leg and beriberi.

[**Needling method**] Oblique insertion 0. 5 ~ 1 *cun*.

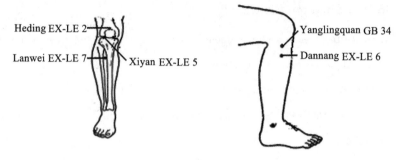

Heding EX-LE 2

Lanwei EX-LE 7

Xiyan EX-LE 5

Yanglingquan GB 34

Dannang EX-LE 6

Fig. 2 – 4 – 102   Fig. 2 – 4 – 103

15. 5. 3 Dannang(EX-LE 6)

[**Locatioin**] This acupoint is located superior and lateral to the shank in the depression 2 *cun* directly below the small head of the fibia. (Fig. 2 – 4 – 103)

[**Indications**] Acute and chronic cholecystitis, cholelithiasis, biliary ascariasis and flaccidity and obstruction syndromes of the lower limbs.

[**Needling method**] Perpendicular insertion 1. 5 ~ 2 *cun*.

15. 5. 4 Lanwei(EX-LE 7)

[**Locatioin**] This acupoint is located anterior and superior to the shank, 5 *cun* below Dubi and one finger breadth lateral to the anterior border of the tibia. (Fig. 2 – 4 – 102)

[**Indications**] Acute and chronic appendicitis, dyspepsia and paralysis of lower limbs.

[**Needling method**] perpendicular insertion 1. 5 ~ 2 *cun*.

15. 5. 5 Bafeng(EX-LE 10)

[**Locatioin**] This acupoint is located on the dorsum of foot, in the depressions on the webs between toes, proximal to the margins of the webs, four acupoints on each foot. (Fig. 2 – 4 – 104)

〔**Indications**〕Beriberi, pain of toe, swelling and pain of foot due to snake bite.

〔**Needling method**〕Oblique insertion 0. 5 ~ 0. 8 *cun* or prick to cause bleeding.

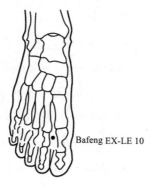

Bafeng EX-LE 10

Fig. 2 – 4 – 104

Knowledge point 5   Acupuncture and
Moxibustion techniques

Acupuncture and moxibustion are two different therapeutic methods. Acupuncture also known as needling is a procedure by which diseases can be prevented and treated through proper insertion of needles into points accompanied by different manipulation. In clinic, the needles of common use are the filiform needle, the cutaneous needle, the intradermal needle, the three edged needle, among which, the filiform needle is the commonest.

Moxibustion treats and prevents diseases by applying heat to points or certain place of the human body. The material used is chiefly "moxa wool" in the form of a cone or stick. Since ancient time moxibustion and acupuncture have been used together very often in clinical practice.

1. Manipulation of filiform needles

1. 1 The structure and specification

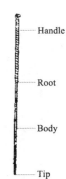

Fig. 2 –5 –1

The filiform needles are widely adopted at present in clinic. It is mainly made of stainless steel. A filiform needle may be divided into five parts: the handle, the tail, the tip, the body and the root. The filiform needles vary in length and diameter. (Fig. 2 –5 –1, Table 2 –5 –1, Table 2 –5 –2)

Table 2 –5 –1 Length of the needle

cun	0. 5	1	1. 5	2	2. 5	3	3. 5	4	4. 5	5
mm	15	25	40	50	65	75	90	100	115	125

Table 2 – 5 – 2 Gauge of the needle diameter

Gauge	26	28	30	32	34
Dia(cm)	0. 45	0. 38	0. 32	0. 26	0. 22

1. 2 Filiform needle practice

As the filiform needle is fine and pliable, it is difficult to insert it into the skin without some strength exerted by the fingers and conduct manipulations. An appropriate finger force is the guarantee to minimize the pain and raise the therapeutic effects.

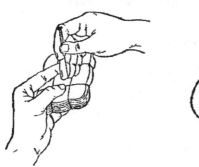
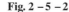
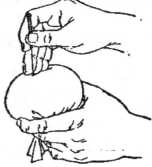

Fig. 2 – 5 – 2   Fig. 2 – 5 – 3

1. 2. 1 Practice with sheets of paper

Fold fine and soft tissue into a small packet 5 ~ 8 cm in size and 2 cm in thickness, then bind the packet with gause thread. Hold the paper packet in the left hand and the needle handle in the right hand. Rotate the needle into the packet and turn it out. Repeat the practice until you feel it is easy to do, then practice the rotating clockwise and counter-clockwise exercise as well as the lifting and thrusting manipulation. (Fig. 2 – 5 – 2)

1. 2. 2 Practice with a cotton cushion

Make a cotton cushion of about 6 ~ 7cm in diameter wrapped in gauze. The practice made on the paper packet can be also done on the cotton cushion. As the cushion is softer than the paper packet, more basic techniques of reinforcement and reduction, such as the manipulation of combining lifting, thrusting and rotating, can be practiced on it.

1. 2. 3 Practice on your own body

This may follow the practice on the paper and cushion so as to have the personal experience of the needling sensation, this practice requires pain free no bent of the needle and good needling sensation radiating to certain direction. Treatment can not be conducted on the patient unless you are able to insert the needle properly and skillfully.

1. 3 Preparation prior to acupuncture treatment

1. 3. 1 Inspection of the instruments

Needles of various sizes, trays, forceps, moxa wool, jars, sterilized cotton balls, 75% alcohol, or 1. 5% tincture iodine, or 2% gentian violet, should be carefully inspected and prepared before use.

1. 3. 2 Posture of the patient

An appropriate posture of the patient is significant for correct location of points, manipulation for acupuncture and moxibustion, retention of needle, and in prevention of fainting, bent, stucking and breaking of the needle, generally, the proper posture of the patient should be convenient for manipulation and comfortable to the patient. The common posture in the practices are as follow.

(1) Supination.

Suitable for the points on the head and face, chest and abdomen and the four limbs. (Fig. 2 – 5 – 4)

(2) Pronation.

Suitable for the points on the head, neck, back, lumbus, buttocks and the posterior aspects of the lower limbs. (Fig. 2 – 5 – 5)

(3)Lateral recumbent posture.

Suitable for the points at the lateral side of the body. (Fig. 2 – 5 – 6)

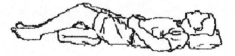

Fig. 2 – 5 – 4

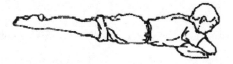

Fig. 2 – 5 – 5

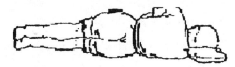

Fig. 2 – 5 – 6

(4)Sitting in supination.

Suitable for the points on the head and face, chest and abdomen and the four limbs. (Fig. 2 – 5 – 7)

(5)Sitting in pronation.

Suitable for the points on the head, neck, and back. (Fig. 2 – 5 – 7)

(6)Sitting with inclining position.

Suitable for points on the vertex, the temple, the auricular place and the cheek. (Fig. 2 – 5 – 7)

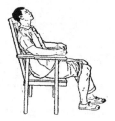
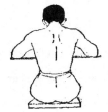
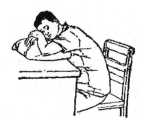

Sitting in supination   Sitting in pronation   Sitting with inclining position

Fig. 2 – 5 – 7

1. 3. 3 Sterilization

(1) Needle sterilization.

Autoclave sterilization: Needle should be sterilized in an autoclave at 1. 5 atmospheric pressure and 125 degree for 30 minutes.

Boiling sterilization: Needles and other instruments are boiled in water for 30 minutes. This methods is easy and effective without need of special equipment.

Medicinal sterilization: Soak the needles in 75% alcohol from 30 to 60 minutes. Then take them out and wipe off the liquid from the needles with a piece of sterile dry cloth. The needle tray and forceps which have directly contacted with the filiform needles should also be sterilized. Besides, needles used on infectious disease should be sterilized and stored in separately.

(2) Disinfection of the acupuncturist's fingers.

Before needling, the acupuncturist should wash his or her hands with soapsuds or 75% alcohol cotton balls.

(3) Disinfection of the region selected for needling.

The area selected for needling must be disinfected with 75% alcohol cotton ball or first with 2% tincture iodine and then by an 75% alcohol cotton ball to remove the iodine. The later is suitable for blood-letting with three-edged needle, or for plum blossom needle tapping.

1. 4 Puncture of filiform needle

1. 4. 1 Insertion

The needles should be inserted by coordination of both hands. While conduting the insertion, the thumb and index finger of the right hand hold the handle of the needle with the middle finger of the same hand being against the body of the needle, the tip of the needle is punctured rapidly into the point with a certain finger force, and then the needle is rotated to deep layer. The right hand is called "the puncturing hand". The left hand is known as the "pressing hand". In clinic, the common methods of insertion are as follows.

(1) Nailing insertion of the needle.

Inserting the needle aided by the pressure of the finger of the pressing hand. (Fig. 2 – 5 – 8)

Press beside the acupuncture point with the nail of the thumb or the index finger of the left hand and keep the needle tip closely to the nail and then insert the needle into the point. This method is suitable for short needles.

(2) Holding insertion of the needle.

Inserting the needle with the help of puncturing and pressing hands. (Fig. 2 – 5 – 9)

Wrap the needle body with a cotton ball by the thumb and the index finger of the left hand, leaving 0.2 ~ 0.3 cm of its tip exposed and hold the needle handle with the thumb and index finger of the right hand. As the needle tip is directly over the selected point, insert the needle swiftly into the skin with the right hand. This method is suitable for long needles.

(3) Relaxed insertion of the needle.

Inserting the needle with the fingers stretching the skin. (Fig. 2 – 5 – 10)

Stretch the skin where the point is located with the thumb and the index finger of the left hand, hold the needle with the right hand and insert it into the point rapidly to a required depth. This method is suitable for the points on the abdomen where the skin is loose.

(4) Lifting and pinching insertion of the needle.

Inserting the needle by pinching the skin. (Fig. 2 – 5 – 11)

Pinch the skin up around the point with the thumb and index finger of the left hand, insert the needle rapidly into the point with the right hand. This method is suitable for puncturing the points on the face, where the muscle and skin are thinnish.

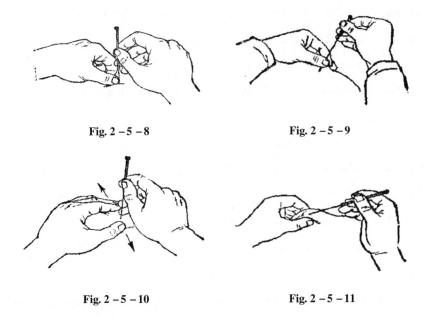

Fig. 2 – 5 – 8   Fig. 2 – 5 – 9

Fig. 2 – 5 – 10   Fig. 2 – 5 – 11

1. 4. 2 Angle and depth of insertion

An appropriate angle and depth of insertion depend on the location of the points, the therapeutic purpose and the shape of the patient, fat or thin.

(1) The angle between the needle and the skin.

The angle refers to one formed by the needle and the skin surface as the needle is inserted. Generally, there are three kinds: perpendicular, oblique and horizontal. (Fig. 2 – 5 – 12)

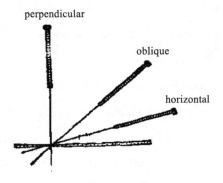

perpendicular

oblique

horizontal

Fig. 2 – 5 – 12

Perpendicular insertion: in this method, the needle is inserted perpendicularly, forming a 90 degree angle with the skin. Most points on the body can be punctured in this way.

Oblique insertion: the needle is inserted obliquely to form an angle of approximately 45 degree with the skin, suitable for the points where the muscle is thin or close to the important viscera. Points on the chest and back are often needled in this way.

Horizontal insertion (also known as transverse insertion): The needle is inserted horizontally to form a 15 ~ 25 degree angle with skin. This method is commonly used in the places where the muscle is thinnish.

(2) Depth of needle insertion.

Depth of needle insertion refers to the depth of the needle body within the skin.

Clinically, the depth of insertion mostly depends on the constitution of the patient, the location of the points and the pathological condition. (Table 2 - 5 - 3)

Table 2 - 5 - 3 The selection of acupuncture depth

depth	constitution	age	pathological condition	location
deep insertion	strong or fat	youth	yin syndrome or severe disease	limbs, buttocks, abdomen
shallow insertion	weak or thin	old or child	yang syndrome or new disease	head, face, chest, back

1. 4. 3 The fundamental manipulation techniques

(1) Needling manipulation.

Lifting and thrusting: the so-called lifting and thrusting is conducted by lifting the needle to superficial layer after the needle is inserted to a desired depth, then, thrust the needle to a deep layer. (Fig. 2 - 5 - 13)

Twirling or rotating: after the needle is inserted to a desired depth, twirl and rotate the needle clockwise and counter-clockwise continuously. (Fig. 2 – 5 – 14)

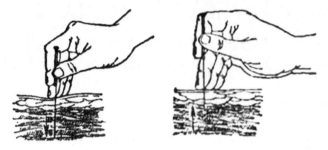

Fig. 2 – 5 – 13

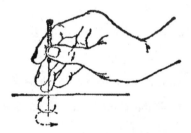

Fig. 2 – 5 – 14

(2) The supplementary manipulation technique.

Under certain conditions the supplementary manipulation techniques are employed after insertion. In clinic, the following six kinds of technique are commonly applied.

Pressing: slightly press the skin along the course of the meridian or around the point to pomote the flow of qi and blood. This method is used promote the arrival of qi. (Fig. 2 – 5 – 15)

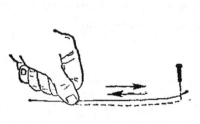

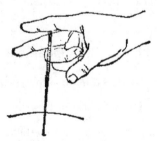

Fig. 2 – 5 – 15   Fig. 2 – 5 – 16

Flying: twirl the needle several times and then suddenly separate the thumb and the index finger from it (the movement of the fingers looks like the birds' wing waving). This method is used to strengthen the needling sensation. (Fig. 2 – 5 – 16)

Scraping: the thumb (the index finger or the middle finger) of the right hand is placed on the tail end to keep the needle steady, scrape the handle with the nail of the index finger (the middle finger or the thumb) of the right hand upward or downward. This methods is used to strengthen the needling sensation and promote the dispersion of the sensation. (Fig. 2 – 5 – 17)

Plucking: pluck the handle of the needles lightly, causing it to tremble. This methods is often used to strengthen the stimulation in order to get needling sensation. (Fig. 2 – 5 – 18)

Shaking: if the needle is inserted perpendicularly, shaking the needle handle as the movement of a scull can strengthen the needling sensation. If the needle is inserted obliquely or horizontally, shaking the needle handle can make the needling sensation transmit toward a certain direction. (Fig. 2 – 5 – 19)

Trembling: hold the needle with the fingers of the right hand and apply quick lift-thrust or twirl movement in small amplitude to cause vibration. This method is used to promote the arrival of *qi* or strengthen the needing sensation.

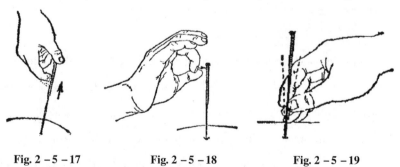

| Fig. 2 – 5 – 17 | Fig. 2 – 5 – 18 | Fig. 2 – 5 – 19 |

1. 4. 4 Manipulations and arrival of *qi* (Needling sensation)

Manipulation here refers to the methods of needling to induce needling sensation. The arrival of *qi* refers to the sensation of soreness, numbness or a distention feeling around the point when the needle is inserted to a certain depth. At the same time, the operator may feel tightness around the needle.

In the process of acupuncture, if the arrival of *qi* is delayed, or no sensation is obtained, the factors influencing the arrival of *qi* should be found out. It may be due to the inaccurate location of the points, improper depth, angle or direction of the needle insertion, readjustment of the point location, depth, angle or direction of the insertion is necessary. If the weakness with *qi* deficiency or other causes leads to the delayed arrival of *qi*, manipulations can be applied for promoting the *qi*. It is also possible to arrive by adding moxibustion or retaining the needles.

1. 4. 5 Reinforcing and reducing methods

Reinforcing and reducing methods refer to specific needling manipulations used to treat asthenia and sthenia syndromes. The method which is applied to strengthen healthy *qi* and invigorate the body resistance as well as improve the weakened physiological functions is called reinforcing, while the other one which is able to eliminate the pathogenic factors is known as reducing.

(1) Commonly used reinforcing and reducing methods in clinic treatment.

Reinforcing and reducing by twirling and rotating the needle: when the *qi* is obtained after insertion of the needle, rotating the needle gently and slowly with small amplitude is called reinforcing, while rotating the needle rapidly and heavily with large amplitude is known as reducing. It is also considered that rotating the needle with the thumb forward forceful and backward with the index finger means reinforcing, while rotating the needle with the index finger forward forcefully backward with the thumb means reducing.

Reinforcing and reducing by lifting and thrusting the needle: after needling sensation appears, the reinforcing is obtained by lifting the needle gently and slowly, while thrusting the needle heavily and rapidly. The reducing is achieved by lifting the needle forcefully and rapidly, while thrusting the needle gently and slowly.

The reinforcing and reducing achieved by rapid and slow insertion and withdrawal of the needle: during manipulations, the reinforcing method is conducted by inserting the needle slowly and withdrawing it rapidly. The reducing is performed by inserting the needle rapidly and withdrawing it slowly.

The reinforcing and reducing achieved by keeping the hole open or close: on withdrawing of the needle, pressing the needling hole quickly to close it and prevent the healthy *qi* from escaping is called reinforcing. Shaking the needle to enlarge the hole while withdrawing it and keeping the hole open is known as reducing.

The reinforcing and reducing achieved by the direction the needle tip pointing to: the needle tip pointing to the direction of the meridian is known as reinforcing while the needle tip pointing against the meridian direction is considered as reducing.

The reinforcing and reducing achieved by means of respiration: in the method, the reinforcing is achieved by inserting the needle when the patient breathes out and withdrawing the needle when the patient breathes in. The opposite way of practice means reducing.

Mild reinforcing and reducing when the needle is inserted into the acupoint and the needling sensation appears, lift and thrust as well as twirl and rotate the needle evenly and gently at moderate speed, then withdraw the needle.

(2) The influence factors of the effects of reinforcing or reducing.

The functional conditions of the patient: under different pathological conditions, acupuncture may produce different regulating functions, either reinforcing or reducing. If an individual is in a collapse condition, acupuncture functions to rescue *yang* from collapse. When an individual is under a condition of internal pathogenic heat, acupuncture functions to expel the heat. This dual regulating function is closely related to the defensive ability of human body.

Therapeutic properties of the acupoints: acupoints have relative specifi city as far as the therapeutic properties are concerned, some points tend to reinforce the body resistance, such as, Guanyuan(CV 4), Mingmen(GV 4), Qihai(CV 6), Zusanli(ST 36), Gaohuang(UB 43), which are mainly applied for deficiency syndromes. And some points such as Shaoshang (LU 11) and Shixuan(EX-UE 11), which have the propertity of clearing away heat and promoting the resuscitation are employed often for excessive heat syndromes.

Needling methods: needling methods are important for reinforcing or reducing. in order to achieve reinforcing or reducing effects, ancient acupuncturists did create a considerable number of reinforcing and reducing methods of needling. The common reinforcing and reducing methods in clinic are introduced above.

1. 4. 6 Retention and withdrawal the needle

(1) Retention.

Retention means to keep the needle in place after the use of needling manipulations. The purpose of it is to prolong the needling sensation and for further manipulation. Whether the needles should be retained or not and the duration of retention depend on the patients' condition. In general, the needle is retained for ten to thirty minutes after the application of needling manipulations. But for some chronic, intractable, painful and spastic cases, the time of retention may be appropriately prolonged. For some diseases, the duration may be as long as several hours. Meanwhile, manipulation may be given at intervals in order to strengthen the therapeutic effects.

(2) Withdrawal.

For the withdrawal of the needle, press the skin around the acupoint slightly with sterilized dry cotton ball held by the pressing hand, rotate the needle gently and lift it slowly to the subcutaneous level with puncturing hand, then withdraw it quickly and press the punctured point with sterilized dry cotton ball for a while to prevent bleeding.

1. 4. 7 Management of possible accidents

Although acupuncture is safe, some accidents may take place due to negligence of contraindications, imperfect manipulations or lack of the knowledge of anatomy. The possible accidents are seen as follows:

(1) Fainting during acupuncture.

Cause: this is often due to nervousness, delicate constitution, hunger, over-fatigue, improper position or forceful manipulation.

Manifestations: during acupuncture treatment, there may appear dizziness, vertigo, nausea, pallor, palpitation, chest distress, cold sweating and weak pulse. In severe cases, there may be cold extremities, drop of blood pressure, incontinence of urine and stool, and loss of consciousness.

Management: acupuncturist should stop needling immediately and withdraw all the needles, then soothe the patient and help the patient to lie down as well as offer some warm or hot water to the patient. The symptoms will disappear after a short rest. In severe cases, press hard with the finger-nail or needle Renzhong (GV 26), Suliao (GV 25), Neiguan (PC 6) and Zusanli (ST 36), apply moxibustion to Baihui (GV 20), Qihai (CV 6) and Guanyuan (CV 4). Generally, For patients will usually recover, if not, other emergency measures should be taken.

Prevention: for patients being treated by acupuncture for the first time or those of sensitive individuals, a brief account of needling should be given to them prior to the treatment to relieve their nervousness and supination is adopted. The manipulation should not be too forceful. needles are not retained for long time. During the treatment, if there appear some prodromal symptoms such as pallor, sweating or dizziness, management should be taken promptly.

(2) Stuck needle.

Cause: this may result from nervousness, strong spasm of the local muscle after the insertion of the needle, twirling the needle with too large amplitude or in one direction only causing muscle fibers to bind, or from a change of the position of the patient after the insertion of the needles.

Manifestations: when stuck needle happens, the acupuncturist may find difficult or impossible to rotate, lift and thrust the needles. The patient feels unbearably painful.

Management: the methods used to cope with such accidents vary according to the conditions of the patients. If the needle is stuck due to excessive rotation in one direction, the condition will release when the needle is twirled in the opposite direction. If stuck needle is caused by temporary muscle spasm, leave the needle in place for a while, then withdraw it by ritating, or by inserting another needle nearby to disperse the *qi* and blood, and to relieve the spasm. If the stuck needle is caused by changing of the position of the patient, the original posture should be resumed and then withdraw the needle.

Prevention: nervous patients should be encouraged to relax their tension. Manipulation should not be too forceful. Avoid puncturing the muscular tendon during insertion. Twirling the needle in only one direction shall not be allowed. During retention of the needles, the posture of the patient should remain unchanged.

(3) Bent needle.

Cause: this may arise from unskillful manipulation or too forceful manifestation, or the needle striking on the hard tissue or a sudden change of the patient's position or the handle of needle being touched or pressed by something or from an improper management of the stuck needle.

Manifestation:for the acupuncturist, it is difficult to lift, thrust, rotate and withdraw the needle. At the same time, the patient feels painful.

Management:when the needle is bent, lifting, thrusting and rotating shall be no longer conducted. The needle may be removed slowly and withdrawn by following the course of bend. If the bent needle is caused by the change of the patient's posture, help him to resume the original position, relax the local muscle and remove the needle. Never try to withdraw the needle with force so as not to break the needle inside the body.

Prevention:during the retention of the needle, the patient should not change the position; the acupuncturist should manipulate the needle gently, avoiding forceful manipulation. And during the retention period, the needle handle shall in no case be impacted or pressed by an external force.

(4) Broken needle.

Cause:result from the poor quality of the needle or eroded base of the needle, from too manipulation of the needle, from strong muscle spasm or a sudden movement of the patient when the needle is in place or from withdrawing a stuck needle.

Manifestations:the needle body is broken during manipulation and the broken part is below the skin surface or a little bit out of the skin surface.

Management:when the needle is broken, the acupuncturist should kep calm, ask the patient not to change the position to prevent the broken needle from going deeper into the body. If the broken part protrudes from the skin, remove it with forceps or fingers. If the broken part is at the same level of the skin, press the tissue around the site until the broken end is exposed, then remove it with forceps. If it is completely under the skin, surgery should be resorted with the help of x-ray to find out the exact location of the broken needle.

Prevention:the quality of the needle should be inspected carefully prior to the treatment. The patient is advised not to change the position. The needle body should not be inserted into the body completely and a little part should be exposed outside the skin. manipulatin should be performed gently, avoiding forceful manipulation lest the needle be broken. Inserting needle, if it is bent, the needle should be withdrawn immediately.

When the needle body is broken, the patient should be told to keep calm to prevent broken needle from going deeper into the body. If the broken part protrudes from the skin, remove it with forceps or fingers. If the broken part is at the same level of the skin, press the tissue around the site until the broken end is exposed, and then removes it with forceps. If it is completely under the skin, surgery should be resorted with the help of x-ray to find out the exact location of the broken needle.

(5) Hematoma.

Cause: this may arise from injury of the blood vessels during insertion or from no pressing of the point after withdrawing the needle.

Manifestation: local swelling, distension and pain after the withdrawal of the needle. The skin of the local place is blue and purplish.

Management: generally, a slight hematoma may disappear automatically. If the local swelling, distension and pain are serious, cold compression can be used to stop immediate bleeding. After bleeding is stopped, hot compress can be applied to help disperse the hematoma.

Prevention: avoid injuring the blood vessels and points are pressed with sterilized cotton ball as soon as the needle is withdrawn.

(6) Pneumatothorax.

Cause: on puncturing the acupoints located on the supraclavicular fossa, chest, back, axilla and hypochondriac region, injury the pleura and lung due to deep insertion.

Manifestation: sudden chest distress, pectoralgia, and short breath. In severe cases, there may exhibit dyspnea, cyanosis of the lips and nails, sweating and drop of blood pressure. Physical examination may find hyperresonance in percussing the chest, attenuation or disappearance of vesicular respiration, or shift of the trachea to the healthy side.

Management: if it is mild, the patient rest in half-lying position and take some antitussive and antiseptic. The patient should be treated under careful inspection. In severe cases, emergency measures should be employed at once.

Prevention: to avoid an accident, the acupuncturist should be careful on the angle direction and depth of needling where the points located on the chest, the back and the hypochondriac places.

1. 4. 8 Precautions in acupuncture treatment

(1) It is inadvisable to give acupuncture treatment to the patients who are either hungry, overeaten, drunk or exhausted. For patients with weak constitutions, or those with severe or chronic illness and deficiencies of *qi* and blood, strong needle manipulation should be avoided, and it is better to choose the supination position.

(2) It is contraindicated to puncture acupoints on the abdomen of women who are up to three months pregnant. For those who have been pregnant for more than three months, acupoints of the abdomen or the lumbo-sacral area is contraindicated. Acupuncture is also contraindicated on the following acupoints during pregnancy, Hegu (LI 4) , Sanyinjiao (SP 6) , Kunlun (UB 60) , and Zhiyin (UB 67).

(3) Acupoints on the vertex of infants should not be needled when the fontanel is not closed. Acupoints on the places with infection, ulcer, scars or tumor should not be needled.

(4) Patients with disturbance of blood coagulation and hemorrhagic tendency should not be punctured.

(5) Acupoints on the ocular area, napex, or close to the vital organs or large blood vessels should be carefully needled. It is inadvisable to do deep needling on the acupoints of the chest, ribs, lumbar region or upper back, especially for patients with swelling and enlargement of liver or spleen.

(6) To prevent accidentally puncturing the urinary bladder, the direction, angles and depths of needle insertions should be carefully controlled when needling patients with urine retention.

2. Manipulations of moxibustion

Moxibustion is a therapy which treats and prevents diseases with heat stimulation on the acupoints or certain locations of human body. Through there are quite a few materials used for moxibustion, the leaf of moxa remains the chief ingredient.

2. 1 The functions of moxibustion

2. 1. 1 Warm the meridians to dispel cold

Moxibustion can give heat stimulation to the acupoints or the part of body, and thus moxibustion can warm the meridians to dispel cold. Clinically, it is used for all diseases caused by cold obstruction, blood stagnation and blockages of the meridians.

2. 1. 2 Suppoting *yang* to strengthen the original *qi*

Moxibustion can warming *yang* and strengthen *qi* and recuperate depleted *yang*, and thus moxibustion can be widely applied to many serious diseases due to insufficiency, sinking or depletion of *yang qi*.

2. 1. 3 Remove blood stasis and dissipate pathological accumulation

Moxibustion, with its heat, has the effect of keeping *qi* activity free, *ying qi* and *wei qi* in balance, and in turn, it dispels blood stasis and dissipates pathological accumulation. In the clinical, it is commonly used to treat diseases related to *qi* and blood stagnation.

2. 1. 4 Prevent disease and maintain health

Applying moxibustion frequently at Guanyuan (CV 4) , Qihai(CV 6)Zusanli (ST 36)etc. May prevent and treat diseases as the body resistance invigorated and the immunity stregthened.

2. 2 Classification of moxibustion

2. 2. 1 Moxibustion with moxa

(1)Moxibustion with moxa cone.

Moxa cone is a cone-shaped wool, the size of which varies from the sizes of wheat grain to the size of a Chinese date. (Fig. 2 – 5 – 20)

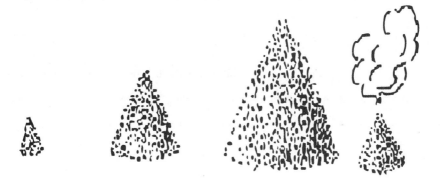

Fig. 2 – 5 – 20

The measurement unit of moxibustion is called "Zhuang". The burning out of one moxa cone is called one Zhuang. The moxibustion with moxa cones is classified into direct and indirect moxibustion.

①Direct moxibustion.

A moxa cone placed directly on the point and ignited is called direct moxibustion. it is subdivided into scarring moxibustion, and no scarring moxibustion. (Fig. 2 – 5 – 21)

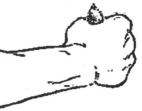

Fig. 2 – 5 – 21

Scarring moxibustion (also known as blistering moxibustion):

Prior to moxibustion, apply some garlic juice to the site in order to increase the adhesion and stimulation of the moxa cone to the skin, then put the moxa cone of the required size on the point, when the moxa cone completely burns out, it is replaced by a new one. Repeat this procedure untill blisters are formed. Normally about one week after the moxibustion, suppuration is formed at the local region. About five to six weeks later, the wound heals automatically, the scab exfoliates and scar is formed. During the combustion when a patient painful, the surrounding place of the moxibustion site can be gently tapped with hand so as to reduce pain. This method is indicated for certain chronic diseases, such as asthma, the pulmonary tuberculosis, and intractable pain.

No scarring moxibustion.

A moxa cone is placed on a point and ignited. When about two thirds of a moxa cone burnt or the patient feels a burning pain, remove the cone and place another one. The moxibustion continues until the local skin becomes reddish but without blister. Usually each point can be moxibusted for 3 ~ 7 cones without suppuration and scar formation. So this method is easy to be accepted by the patients and is used widely, often for cold and deficient disorders such as asthma, chronic diarrhea, indigestion, etc.

②Indirect moxibustion (also known as moxibustion with material isolation):

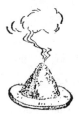

Fig. 2 −5 −22

The ignited moxa cone is isolated from the skin by some materials, sush

as ginger, salt, garlic and monkshood cake in order to avoid burning the skin.
(Fig. 2 – 5 – 22)

Moxibustion with ginger.

Cut a slice of ginger about 2 ~ 3 cm wide and 0. 2 ~ 0. 3 cm thick, punch numerous holes on it and place it on the point selected. On top of this piece of ginger, a moxa cone is placed and ignited. When the patient feels scorching, remove it and ignite another. Repeat this till the skin becomes reddish. This method is always used to treat obstructive syndrome due to pathogenic wind-cold, vomiting, abdominal pain and diarrhea due to weakness and cold of spleen and stomach.

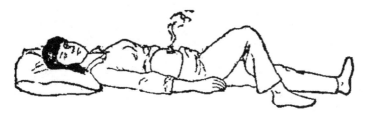

Fig. 2 – 5 – 23

Moxibustion with garlic.

Cut a slice of garlic 0. 2 ~ 0. 3 cm thick (a large single clove of garlic is desirable), punch several holes on it, put it on the acupoint with the ignited moxa cone above. Every 3 ~ 4 units of moxa cones are burnt out, renew a slice of garlic and continue moxibustion therapy. Repeat this till the skin becomes reddish. This method is often used for scrofula, pulmonary tuberculosis and the early stage of carbuncle and furuncle.

Moxibustion with salt.

This method is usually applied at the umbilicus. Fill umbilicus with salt to the level of the skin, place a moxa cone on the top of the salt and then ignite it. (Fig. 2 – 5 – 23)When it burns out, renew another one. Generally,3 ~ 9 units are used each time. For cases with acute diseases,more units may be used with no limit to the number of units. This method is often used for the symptoms of excessive sweating, cold limbs and impalpable pulse resulted from acute vomiting and diarrhea, or flaccid type of wind stoke and postpartum fainting.

Moxibustion with monkshood cake.

A cake 3 cm in diameter and 0.3 cm in thickness, made of monkshood powder mixed with alcohol, is punched with holes in it, and placed on the site for moxibustion with moxa cone, which is ignited and burnt on the top of it. This method is good for warming and strengthening kidney *yang* and thus adopted to treat impotence, seminal emission, premature ejaculation, infertility and ruptured abscess resistant to healing.

(2) Moxibustion with moxa stick.

Moxa stick is prepared by wrapping mugwort wool with a piece of paper. It is cylinder-shaped, 1.5cm in diameter and 20cm in length. There are three kinds of method: mild-warm moxibustion, circling moxibustion and sparrow-pecking moxibustion.

①Mild-warm moxibustion.

Ignite a moxa stick at its one end and place it two to three centimeters away over the site to bring a mild warmth to the local place, but not burning pain, for some fifteen minutes until the skin becomes slightly red. This method is suitable for to treat various diseases. (Fig. 2 – 5 – 24)

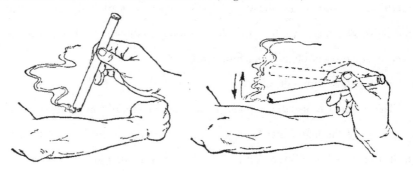

Fig. 2 – 5 – 24   Fig. 2 – 5 – 25

② "Sparrow-pecking" moxibustion.

Put an ignited moxa stick near the patient's skin, move it up and down like a bird pecking so as to give strong heat to the applied spot. This method is more often used as emergency treatment. (Fig. 2 – 5 – 25)

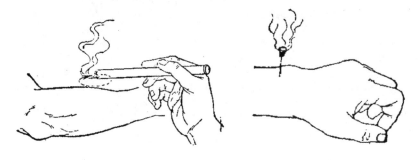

Fig. 2 – 5 – 26   Fig. 2 – 5 – 27

③Circling moxibustion.

Keep an ignited moxa stick at a fixed distance from the patient's skin, 3cm or so away the skin around the acupoint, move moxa stick in a circular direction or left and right. This method is suitable to treat rheumatic pain. (Fig. 2 – 5 – 26)

(3) Moxibustion with warmed needle.

Moxibustion with warmed needle is a method of acupuncture combined with moxibustion. This method has the function of warming the meridians and promoting the flow of *qi* and blood so as to treat *Bi*-syndromes caused by cold-damp and paralysis. (Fig. 2 – 5 – 27)

(4) Moxibustion with mild moxibustioner.

Mild moxibustioner, also known as container for moxibustion, is a metal cylindrical container made of 2 shells. The inside one being a small cylinder with cross-openings on its wall to hold the moxa wool, the outside one is cylindrical, also with cross-openings on its wall, it is attached with handle and support. Clinically, there may be other types of mild moxibustioner, however, the basic structure is similar. (Fig. 2 – 5 – 28)

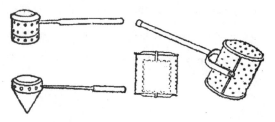

Fig. 2 – 5 – 28

On applying, ignite the moxa wool or moxa stick placed inside the container, and move the container forward and backward over the acupoint or the affected area to let heat radiate from the bottom, or keep the container on certain distance away from the acupoint until the local area becomes red. This method is suiable for the disorder over large area, particularly, for women and children, and those who fear to be treated by other ways of moxibustion.

2. 3 Cautions of moxibustion

2. 3. 1 Order for moxibustion

Moxibustion is generally applied to the upper part first, and then to the lower part. Treat the back first, the abdominal region second. The head first and the four extremities secod. It is applied to *yang* meridians first, then *yin* meridians. First less units used, then more units.

2. 3. 2 Reinforcing and reducing with moxibustion

For reinforcement, do not assist combustion by blowing, let the moxa burn naturally till it burns out. For reduction, blow air to it time after time to make the combustion vigorous. In practice, moxibustion can be conducted according to the patient's condition and the properties of the acupoints.

2. 3. 3 Moxibustion contraindication

(1) In principle, excess heat syndrome or the syndrome of *yin* deficiency with heat signs are contraindicated to moxibustion.

(2) Scarring moxibustion should not be applied to the face and head,

and the place close to the large blood vessels and the regions of tendons.

(3) The abdomen and lumbosacral region are not allowed to use moxibustion in pregnancy.

(4) For the patient with coma, numbness of the extremities or dysesthesia, excessive dose of moxibustion is not advisable, so that burning may be avoided.

(5) After scarring moxibustion, the patient should not do heavy physical labour and must keep the local skin clean to avoid infection during suppuration of the post-moxibustion sore. If the post-moxibustion sore is infected, apply antiphlogistic plaster to it.

3. Cupping therapy

Cupping, also termed as "horn method" in the ancient China, is a therapy in which a jar is attached to the skin surface to cause local congestion and blood stasis through the negative pressure created by consuming the air inside the cup with fire or other methods.

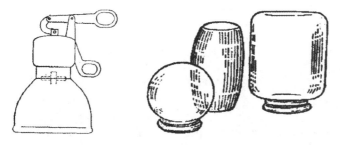

Fig. 2 – 5 – 29

3. 1 Types of cups

There are four types commonly used in the clinic: glass cup, bamboo jar, ceramic (pottery) cup and suction cup. (Fig. 2 – 5 – 29)

3. 2 Methods of creating suction inside the cup

3. 2. 1 Fire cupping method

With this method, negative pressure is created by introducing an ignited material inside the cup to consume the air thereby making the cup suck itself onto the skin. In the clinic, there are four kinds method can be used.

(1) Fire-twinkling (flashing) method.

Clamp a cotton ball soaked with 95% alcohol with a forceps or nipper, ignite it and insert it into the cup, make the ignited cotton for one circle inside the cup and immediately take it out and press the cup on the selected location. It is commonly applied in the clinic. (Fig. 2 −5 −30)

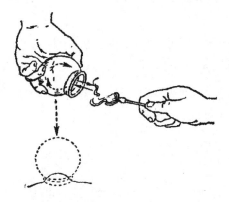

Fig. 2 −5 −30

(2) Fire-throwing method.

Throw a piece of ignited paper or an alcohol cotton ball into the cup, then rapidly put the mouth of the cup firmly against the skin on the desired position. This method is applied to the lateral side of the body.

(3) Alcohol firing method.

Place one to three drops of alcohol into a cup (not much so as to prevent it from dripping out of the cup to burn the skin), distribute evenly the alcohol on the wall by turning the cup. Then the alcohol is ignited and the cup is immediately pressed on to the place to be treated.

(4) Cotton-sticking method.

Stick a piece of proper sized alcohol cotton on the lower one third of the inner wall of the cup, ignite the cotton and the cup is then placed on the selected location.

3. 2. 2 Water-suction method

With this method, the negative pressure is created when boiling water draws the iar out of the cup so that it can attach to the skin. generally, a bamboo cup is chosen to put in the boiling water or herbal liquid for several minutes; then the cup is grasped with clamped, with the mouth firmly pressed against a cold towel. The cup is immediately placed on the selected location and attached to the body surface.

3. 2. 3 Suction cup method

A suction cup is placed firming on the chosen area, where a device is used to withdraw the air. When a sufficient amount of negative pressure is produced, the cup will attacl itself to the skin. The negative pressure can be adjusted according to the quantity of air withdrawn, to regulate the suction force.

3. 3 Application of cupping

Clinically in different pathological conditions, following options of cupping may be applied.

3. 3. 1 Mobile (walking) cupping

Prior to the treatment, apply lubricant oil, such as vaseline, on the skin, the cup then is sucked to the skin in the way as explained in the previous methods. Hold the cup with the right hand and slide it around and back to the affected area until the skin becomes congested. It is suitable for treatment of a large area, such as the back, the lumbus, the buttocks and the thigh. (Fig. 2 – 5 – 31)

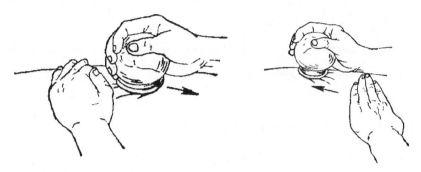

Fig. 2 – 5 – 31

3. 3. 2 Successive flash cupping

In this method, apply repeatedly and swiftly the cup cover the same place until the skin becomes flush and congested. (Fig. 2 – 5 – 32) It's extensively used to treat a variety of diseases, especially in situations where it is inadvisable to use retention cupping, such as with kids and on the cheeks of young ladies.

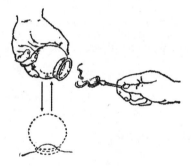

Fig. 2 – 5 – 32

3. 3. 3 cupping with blood-letting

This is also referred to as cupping with collateral-pricking. After disinfecting the treatment area, it is punctured with three-edged needle to causing bleeding, or tapped with plum-blossom needle, then apply cupping to induce more bleeding. This method may be used to treat acute sprain and contusion with blood stasis as well as skin and external diseases, including carbuncle, furuncle, erysipelas, neurodermatitis and psoriasis.

3. 3. 4 Retaining needle and cupping

During the retention of the needle, a cup is sucked over the needling are-

a. The needle is withdrawn when the cup is removed.

3. 4 Removal of the cup

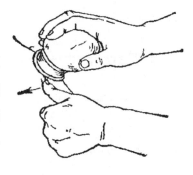

Generally, the cup is retained in the location for 10 ~ 15 minutes, in this period the local place would become congested with violet colored blood stasis formation. The cup is then removed. On removal, hold the cup with the right hand and press

Fig. 2 – 5 – 33

the skin beside the edge of the cup with the left hand to let the air come into the cup, and release cup. (Fig. 2 – 5 – 33)

3. 5 Indications

Cupping therapy has the action of warming the meridians, invigorating *qi* and blood and blood circulation, relieving blood stagnation, alleviating pain and swelling and dispelling damp and cold. It is commonly applied in *bi*-syndromes (such as lumbago, lower limb pain, shoulder and back pain), gastrointestinal tract disorders (such as gastralgia, abdominal pain) and pulmonary diseases (such as cough and asthma), and as well as some external diseases, including carbuncle, erysipelas, neurodermatitis.

3. 6 Precautions

(1) It should not be used in patients with high fever and convulsion, edema as well as areas with large blood vessels, allergic skin or skin ulcer and the abdominal and sacral location of the pregnant woman.

(2) Cares should be taken to avoid burning or scorching the skin. retention of the cup should not be too long lest impairment of the skin be caused.

(3) If the local congestion is severe after the removal of the cup, it is forbidden to perform cupping on the region again. Blister for the small blister, no

treatment is needed. the big one, drainage of liquid with a sterilize syringe, application of gentian violet and gauze to prevent infection are indicated.

4. Three eged needle

The three-edged needle, a needle for bloodletting, presently made of stainless steel, being 2 *cun* long, is shaped in a round handle, a triangular head and a sharp tip.

4. 1 Manipulation methods

Hold the handle of the three-edged needle with the thumb and the index finger of the right hand, the middle finger supporting against the lower part of the needle with 0. 1 ~ 0. 2 *cun* of the tip exposed. On pricking, the left hand holds the finger, the toe, or pinches, stretches the skin of the selected point. There are four commonly applied methods.

4. 1. 1 Point Pricking

First, push and press the skin around the point to gather the blood, hold the handle of the three-edged needle with the right hand, prick the disinfected point swiftly about 2 ~ 3 mm deep for bloodletting and withdraw the needle immediately, gently squeeze the skin around the pricked spot to lot a few drops of blood, afterwards press the punctured point with a sterilized cotton ball to stop bleeding, for instance, prickly Shaoshang (LU 11) to treat sore throat, pricking the apex of the auricle for conjunctivitis.

4. 1. 2 Scattered Pricking

Prick a number of spots at the affected location, or around a small place of a red swelling, then press the skin or apply cupping to let the stagnated blood escape to alleviate swelling and pain. In case of intractable tinea, carbuncles, erysipelas, sprain and contusion, the local place can be pricked by this method.

4. 1. 3 Collateral Pricking

After disinfection of the skin, prick the selected superficial vein to let a little blood, afterwards, press the punctured hole with a sterilized dry cotton ball to stop bleeding, e. g. pricking the superficial vein at the popliteal space and the medial side of the elbow for sun stoke and pricking several spots on the red threads of the affected location for acute lymphangitis.

4. 1. 4 Prinking

In the operation, the left hand press or pinches up the disinfected skin, prick superficially the point or the reactionary spot with a three-edged needle to let blood or fluid, or further prick 0. 5 cm deep to break the tissue fiber, afterwards, cover the punctured site with gauze. This method is applied for multiple folliculitis, neck scrofula which are treated by pricking the reactionary spots at the both sides of the vertebra. For hemorrhoids, prick the reactionary spots at the lumbar sacral place.

4. 2 Indications

The three-edged needling has the function of dispelling blood stasis and heat and assisting resuscitation, promoting the flow of qi and blood in meridians. It is advisable to treat excess syndrome and heat syndrome as well as cold syndrome of excess type, e. g. high fever, syncope, apoplexy with spasticity, sore throat, red, swelling and pain of the eyes, ringworm, early stage of carbuncles or furuncle, sprains or bruises, malnutrition, hemorrhoids, obstinate Bi-syndromes, erysipelasand numbness of fingers or toes.

4. 3 Precautions

Puncturing the skin with three-edged needle is strong stimulation, thus, fainting should be prevented.

Strict sterilization must be applied to the area to be pricked to prevent infection.

The operation should be slightly, superficial and rapid to avoid excessive bleeding, injuring the deep large artery. The quantity of bleeding depend on the patient's condition, generally, no more than 3 ml is necessary.

It is inadvisable to apply this method to the treatment of the patients with poor constitution, pregnancy and bleeding tendency.

Treatment is applied once daily or once every other day, three to five treatments constitute one course, for acute case, it may be given twice daily. If a large amount of bloodletting is made, it is advisable to apply the treatment once or twice a week; to apply the pricking method, it is performed once for 3 ~ 7 days and one course consisting 3 ~ 5 treatments, and 10 ~ 14 days-off between two courses.

5. Cutaneous needle

The cutaneous needle is also termed as the plum-blossom needle and seven-star needle. The pinhead of the cutaneous needle is like a small hammer. The length of its handle is about 15 ~ 19 cm. One of its ends is assembled with a lotus pod-shaped base, on which stainless steel needles are embedded. The names are given according to different numbers of needles inlaid, e. g. Plum-blossom needle (5 needles), seven-star needle (7 needles) or arhat needle (18 needles).

5. 1 Manipulation

After routine sterilization on needles and the tapping area with a 75% of alcohol, hold the handle of the needle with the thumb, middle and ring fingers and the index finger against the middle section of the handle and tap vertically on the skin with a gentle movement of the wrist. While tapping, the needle tips should be held perpendicularly over the skin, the places should be exact and strength should be even. Different places and strength may be used according to different treatment requirments.

5. 1. 1 Tapping places

The places to be tapped may be along the course of meridian, or on the points selected, or local areas.

(1)Tapping along the meridians.

Tapping along the meridians, is mostly used on the governor vessel and bladder meridians of foot-*taiyang*, which are located from the nape of the neck to the lumbo-sacral area. This method is also used on the meridians below the elbow or knee joints, on which the *yuan*-source acupoints, *luo*-connecting acupoints, *xi*-cleft acupoints and other specifice acupoints are dispersed.

(2)Tapping on the acupoints.

Tapping on the acupoints, is most commonly used acupoints of various specific acupoints, Huatuojiaji and *Ashi* acupoints.

(3)Tapping on the local areas.

Tapping on the local areas, is used on the affected areas.

5. 1. 2 The intensity of stimulation and course of treatment

The tapping may be light, moderate or heavy in accordance with the constitution, the age, the pathological condition of the patients and the location of the acupoints.

(1)Gentle tapping.

Light tapping is done until the skin becomes flush and congested. This is used on on the head and face, also on the places with thin muscles. It is applied for the kids, the women, the weak and the elderly, as well as patiens with deficiency syndromes or those with requiring extensive treatments.

(2)Heavy tapping.

Heavy tapping is conducted by exerting a relatively strong force until the skin becomes apparently flush and a slight bleeding with a little pain. This method is commonly applied to tender points on the back and buttocks area of strong, young patients, and those excessive syndromes, or acute outbreaks.

(3) Moderate tapping.

Moderate-strength tapping is done between light and heavy stimulation, until the skin becomes congestion and with slight pain, but no bleeding, suitable for the majority of the patients, ordinary diseases and general locations.

In general, treatments with tapping are done once a day or every other day, 10 treatments constitute a complete course, with an interval of 3 ~ 5 days between each course.

5. 1. 3 Indications

The cutaneous needling is used to treat disorders of the nervous system and dermatosis, e. g. headache, hypochondriac pain, dizziness and vertigo, insomnia, myopia, painful joints and paralysis, gastro-intestinal disease, dysmenorrhea and various kinds of skin disease.

5. 1. 4 Precautions

(1) The tips of the needles should be sharp, smooth and free from any hooks. On tapping, the tips of the needles should strike the skin at a right angle to the surface to reduce pain.

(2) Sterilize the needles, and the location of treatment should be disinfected. After heavy tapping, the local skin surface should be cleaned and disinfected to prevent infection.

(3) Tapping is not allowed to apply to the location of trauma and ulcers.

6. Ear acupuncture

Ear acupuncture treats and prevents diseases by stimulating certain points in the auricle with needles or other tools. Diagnosis can be made by observing, pressing and measuring the electrical resistance on the auricular points. It is commonly used therapy in clinical acupuncture treatment.

6. 1 Terminology for the anatomical regions of the auricular surface（Fig. 2 – 5 – 34）

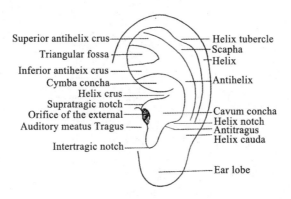

Superior antihelix crus
Triangular fossa
Inferior antiheix crus
Cymba concha
Helix crus
Supratragic notch
Orifice of the external
Auditory meatus Tragus
Intertragic notch

Helix tubercle
Scapha
Helix
Antihelix
Cavum concha
Helix notch
Antitragus
Helix cauda
Ear lobe

Fig. 2 – 5 – 34

6. 2 Distribution of auricular acupoints

The distribution of auricular points on the auricle is just like a inverted fetus with the head downwards and the buttocks upwards. (Fig. 2 – 5 – 35) The acupoints located on the ear lobe and around it are related to the head and face, those in the scapha to the upper arm, those on the antihelix and its two crura to the trunk and the lower limbs, those in the middle part of the ear (including cymba conchae and cavum con-

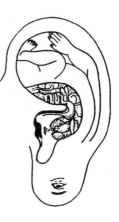

Fig. 2 – 5 – 35

chae) to the internal organs, and those mainly in the middle of the ear (the principal part of antihelix) to the trunk. Those arranged as a ring around helix crus to the digestive tract.

6. 3 Location and indication of the commonly used auricular acupoints (Fig. 2 – 5 – 36)

In order to measure the points exactly, according to its anatomy, the auricle is divided into zones in every portion in the national standard of nomenclature and location of auricular points. There are 91 points in all.

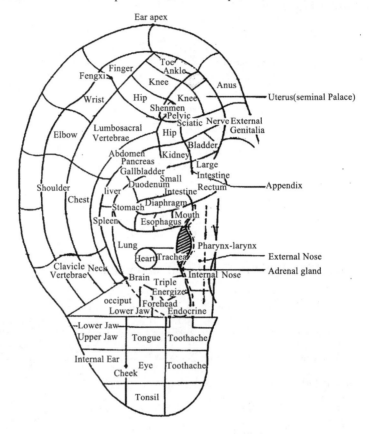

Fig. 2 – 5 – 36

6. 3. 1 Ear acupoints on the helix

The helix is divided into 12 zones. The helix crus is Zone 1. The area from the notch of the helix crus to the upper bodder of inferior antihelix crus is divided into 3 equal portions. They are from bottom to top, Zones 2, 3 and 4. The portion of the helix from the upper border of the inferior antihelix crus to anterior border of superior antihelix crus is Zone 5. Zone 6 of helix is from the anterior border of the superior antihelix crus to the apex of ear. The upper border of helix tubercle is Zone 7, and from the upper to the lower border of helix tubercle is Zone 8. There are 4 equal portion from the lower border of helix tubercle to the notch between the helix and the lobe. They are, from top to bottom, Zone 9, 10, 11 and 12. (Table 2 – 5 – 4)

Table 2 – 4 Ear acupoints on the helix

name	location	Indication
hX$_1$. Centerof ear (diaphragm)	the helix crus	hiccup, urticaria, dermatosis, infantile enuresis, hemoptysis
HX$_2$. Rectum	on the end of the helix approximate to the superior tragic notch	constipation, diarrhea, prolapse of the rectum, hemorrhoids
HX$_3$. Urethra	on the helix at the level with the lower border of the inferior antihelix crus	enuresis, frequency, urgency and pain of urination, retention of urine
HX$_4$. External genitalia	on the helix at the level with the upper border of the inferior antihelix crus	testitis, pruritus of vulva
HX$_5$. Anus	anterior to the triangular fossa	hemorrhoids. and fissure
HX$_{6.7}$. Ear apex	at the tip of the helix	fever, hypertension, acute conjuntivetis, insomnia
HX$_8$. Tubercle (liver *yang*)	on the helix tubercle	dizziness, headache, hypertension
HX$_{9\text{-}12}$. Lun$_{1\text{-}4}$	on the helix, that isHX$_9$-HX$_{12}$	fever, tonsilitis, upper respiratory tract infection

6. 3. 2 Ear acupoints on the scapha

The scahha is separated into 6 equal section, which are listed in descending order as Zone1, 2, 3, 4, 5and 6. (Table 2 – 5 – 5)

Table 2 – 5 – 5

name	location	indication
SF$_1$. Finger	at the top of the scapha	disorders of the fingers such as pain, numbness, etc
SF$_{1,2i}$ Fengxi (Allergic Point)	midpoint between Finger and wrist	urticaria, pruritus of skin, asthma, allergic rhinitis

Continued

name	location	indication
SF$_2$. Wrist	inferior to finger	pain of the wrist
SF$_3$. Elbow	inferior to wrist	external humeral epicondylitis and pain of the elbow
SF$_{4,5}$. Shoulder	inferior to the Elbow	scapulohumeral periarthritis
SF$_6$. Clavicle	at level with the helix-tragic notch	peripheral arthritis of the shoulder

6. 3. 3 Ear acupoints on the antihelix

The antihelix is separated into 13 sections.

The superior crus of the antihelix is separated into 3 equal sections: The lower third is Zone 5. he middle, Zone 4 and the upper is divided into 2 equal sections. The inferior section is Zone 3 of antihelix. The superior section is separated into two equal parts; The posterior half is Zone 2 and anterior half is Zone 1.

The inferior crus of the antihelix is also separated into 3 equal sections: The middle and anterior 2/3 are Zone 6 and the posterior 1/3 is Zone 7.

The body of antihelix is separated into 5 equal sections. Then divided into two segments along the concha border: an anterior 1/4 and a posterior 3/4. The anterior -superior 2/5 is Zone 8. The posterior- superior 2/5 is Zone 9. The anterior-middle 2/5 is Zone 10. The posterior-middle 2/5 is Zone 11. Anterior inferior 1/5 section is Zone 12 and the posterior-inferior 1/5 section is Zone 13. (Table 2 − 5 − 6,2 − 5 − 7,2 − 5 − 8)

Table 2 − 5 − 6 Ear acupoints on the the superior antihelix crus

name	location	indication
Ah$_1$. Heel	medial and superior angle of the superior antihelix crus	heel pain

Continued

name	location	indication
AH$_2$. Toe	lateral and superior angle of the superior antihelix crus	paronychia, pain of the toe
AH$_3$. Ankle	inferior to the toes and heel	ankle sprain
Ah$_4$. Knee	middle third of the superior antihelix crus	swelling and pain of the knee joint, sciatica
AH$_5$. Hip joint	lower third of the superior antihelix curs	pain of the hip joint, sciatica

Table 2 −5 −7 Ear acupoints on the inferior antihelix crus

name	location	indication
Ah$_6$. Sciatic Nerve	anterior 2/3 of the inferior antihelix crus	sciatica, paralysis of lower extremities
Ah$_{6a}$. Sympathetic (end of inferior antihelix crus)	the terminal of the inferior antihelix crus	palpitation, angina pectoris, spontaneous sweating, functional disorders of the automatic nervous system, gastrointestinal pain and spasm, biliary colic, ureteral colic
AH$_7$. Buttocks	the posterior 1/3 of the inferior antihelix curs	sciatica, gluteal fascitis

Table 2 −5 −8 Ear acupoints on the antihelix body

name	location	indication
AH$_8$. Abdomen	superior 2/5 of the anterior part of the antihelix body	Abdominal pain and distension, diarrhea, acute lumbar sprain, dysmenorrhea

Continued

name	location	indication
AH$_9$. Lumbosacral Vertebrae	posterior to the abdomen	pain of the Lumbosacral region
AH$_{10}$. Chest	the middle 2/5 of the anterior part of the antihelix body	chest and hypochondriac pain, intercostals neuralgia, mastitis
AH$_{11}$. Thoracic Vertebrae	posterior to the chest	chest pain, premenstrual pain of the breast, mastitis, insufficient lactation
AH$_{12}$. Neck	inferior 1/5 of the anterior part of the antihelix body	stiffneck, swelling and pain of the neck
AH$_{13}$. Cervical Vertebrae	posterior to the neck	stiffneck and cervical vertebrae syndrome

6. 3. 4 Ear acupoints on the triangular fossa

The triangular fossa is separated into three sections: the middle 1/3 is Zone 3. The anterior 1/3 is devided into three equal parts: superior, middle and inferior. The superior 1/3 is Zone 1, and the middle and inferior 2/3 are Zone 2. The posterior 1/3 has two equal sections: the superior 1/2 is Zone 4 and the inferior 1/2 is Zone 5.

Table 2 – 5 – 9 Ear acupoints on the triangular fossa

name	location	indication
TF$_1$. Upper triangular fossa	superior anterior 1/3 of the triangular fossa	hypertension
TF$_2$. Internal Genitalia	the inferior part of the anterior 1/3 of the triangular fossa.	irregular menstruation, dysmenorrhea, leukorrhagia, dysfunctional uterine bleeding, impotence, seminal emission, prospermia, prostatitis
TF$_3$. Middle triangular fossa	the middle 1/3 of the triangular fossa	asthma

Continued

name	location	indication
TF_4. Shenmen	the superior part of the posterior 1/3 of the triangular fossa	insomnia, dream-disturbed sleep, epilepsy, hypertension, neurasthenia
TF_5. Pelvis	the inferior part of the posterior 1/3 of the triangular fossa	pelvic inflammation, appendagitis, irregular menstruatin, pain in the lower abdomen

6. 3. 5 Ear acupoints on the tragus

The tragus is separated into 4 zones. The lateral suface is separated into 2 e-qual parts. The superior part is Zone 1 of the tragus, and the inferior part is zone 2of the tragus. The same separation is done on the medial surface of the trague: the superior and inferior parts are zone 3 and 4 respectively. (Table 2 −5 −10)

Table 2 −5 −10 Ear acupoints on the tragus

name	location	indication
TG_1. Upper tragus	superior 1/2 of the lateral surface	obesity, pharyngitis, rhinitis
TG_2. Lower tragus	inferior 1/2 of the lateral surface	obesity, rhinitis, nasal obstruction
$TG1_0$. External Ear	supratragic notch close to the helix	external otitis, tympanitis, tinnitus, dizziness
$TG_{1.2i}$. External Nose	center of the lateral surface of tragus between Zone1 and Zone2	nasal obstruction, rhinitis, simple obesity
TG_{1p}. Tragic Apex	top of the upper eminence of the tragus	fever, toothache
TG_{2p}. Adrenal Gland	top of the lower eminence of the tragus	hypotension, dizziness, rheumatic arthritis, parotitis, asthma, circulatory collapse pruritus, pain syndrome

Continued

name	location	indication
TG_3. Throat	upper half of the medial aspect of the tragus	hoarseness, acute and chronic pharyngitis, tonsillitis
TG_4. Internal Nose	lower half of the medial aspect of the tragus	rhinitis, paranasal sinusitis, epistaxis

6. 3. 6 Ear acupoints of the antitragus

The antitragus is separated into 4 zones. From the apex of the antitragus and the midpoint between the antitragus and the helix notch, 2 vertical lines are drawn to the upper line of the ear lobe separating the lateral surface of the antitragus and its posterior aspect into 3 parts: the anterior part is Zone 1, the middle, Zone 2 and the posterior part is Zone 3. The medial surface of the antitragus is Zone 4. (Table 2 – 5 – 11)

Table 2 – 5 – 11 Ear acupoints of the antitragus

name	location	indication
AT_1. Forehead	anterior part of the lateral aspect of the antitragus	headache, dizziness, insomnia, dream-disturbed sleep
AT_2. Temple	middle portion of the lateral aspect of the antitragus	migraine, dizziness
AT_3. Occiput	posterior portion of the lateral aspect of the antitragus	dizziness, headache, insomnia, asthma, epilepsy, neurasthenia
AT_4. Subcortex	medial aspect of the antitragus	pain syndrome, insomnia, tertian malaria, neurosism, pseudomyopia
$AT_{1.2.4i}$. Antitragic Apex	top of the antitragus	asthma, bronchitis, parotitis, neurodermatitis, testitis and epididymitis

Continued

name	location	indication
$AT_{2,3,4i}$. Midpoint of the rim	midpoint between the antitragic apex and helix-tragic notch	enuresis, auditory vertigo, functional uterine bleeding
$AT_{3,4}$, AH_{12i} Brain stem	helix-tragic notch between the antitragus and the antihelix	vertigo, occipital headache, and pseudomyopia

6. 3. 7 Ear acupoints of the concha

The concha is separated into 18 zones by labeling points and lines. Given that the junction of the middle and upper 1/3 of the inner margin, between the helix crus notch and the inferior crus of the antihelix, is point A. Within the concha, a horizontal line is drawn posteriorly from the end of the helix crus to the antihelix, whose intersection at the concha margin of the antihelix is point D. The junction of the middle and posterior 1/3 of the above line, from the end of the helix crus to point D, is point B. The junction of the upper 1/4, and the lower 3/4 of the posterior edge of the orifice of the external auditory meatus is point C. A curve which is similar to the edge of the cymba concha on the antihelix, is drawn from point A to B. Then another curve whose arc is similar to the inferior border of the helix crus is drawn from point B to C.

Bwtween the anterior segment of line BC and the inferior border, the helix crus is separated into three equal portions: the anterior 1/3 is Zone 1 of the concha, the middle 1/3, Zone 2 and the posterior 1/3 is Zone 3. The portion at the end of the helix crus, anterior to line ABC is Zone 4. The area within the anterior segment of line AB, the superior border of the helix crus, and the inner border of the helix, is separated into 3 equal portions: the posterior 1/3 is Zone 5, the middle is Zone 6 and the anterior 1/3 is Zone 7.

The junction of the anterior and middle 1/3 of the inferior border of the inferior antihelix crus connects with point A to become a line. The area on the cymba concha, anterior to that line is Zone 8. The part behind the anterior segment of line AB and Zone 8 is divided into 2 equal anterior and posterior portions that form Zones 9 and 10 respectively. Within the cymba concha, above the posterior segment of line AB, the area between the posterior border of Zone 10 and line BD is separated into two equal portions: the upper 1/2 is Zone 11, and the lower is Zone 12. The helix notch is connected with point B to become a line. The area on the cavum concha posterior to and below line BD is Zone 13. Given that the center of the cavum concha is the center of a circle, draw a circle with the diameter equal to the distance between that center and line BC, the circle is Zone 15. Two tangent lines crossing the apogee and perigee of Zone 15 are drawn respectively to the posterior wall of the external auditory foramen. The area between the two tangent lines is Zone 16. The area around Zone 15 and 16 is Zone 14. Connect the perigee of the external auditory foramen with the midpoint of the concha border of the antihelix to form a line. Then separate the area on the cavum concha below that line into two equal portions: the upper half is Zone 17, the lower Zone 18. (Table 2 - 5 - 12)

Table 2 - 5 - 12 Ear acupoints of the conchae

name	location	indication
CO_1. Mouth	anterior third of the area inferior to the helix crus	facial paralysis, stomatitis, cholecystitis, cholelithiasis, withdrawal syndrome
CO_2. Esophagus	middle 1/3 of the area inferior to the helix crus	esophagitis, esophagismus
CO_3. Cardia	lateral 1/3 of the area inferior to the helix crus	cardiospasm, nervous vomiting
CO_4. Stomach	end of he helix crus	gastrospasm, gastritis, gastric ulcer, insomnia, toothache, indigestion

Continued

name	location	indication
CO_5. Duodenum	posterior 1/3 of the area within the helix crus, part of the helix and line AB	duodenal ulcer, pylorospasm, cholecystitis, cholelithiasis
CO_6. Small Intestine	middle 1/3 of the area within the helix crus, part of the helix and line AB	indigestion, bellyaches, abdominal distention, tachycardia
CO_7. Large Intestine	anterior 1/3 of the area within the helix crus, part of the helix and line AB	diarrhea, constipation, cough, acne
$CO_{6.7i}$. Appendix	between small and large intestine	appendicitis, diarrhea
CO_8 Angle of Cymba Conchae	at the medial superior angle of cymba conchae	prostitutes, urethritis
CO_9. Bladder	middle inferior part of inferior antihelix crus	cystitis, enuresis, anuresis, lumbago, sciatica, occipital headache
CO_{10}. Kidney	posterior inferior part of inferior antihelix crus, directly above small intestine	lumbago, tinnitus, dizziness, insomnia, gynecopathy, enuresis, impotence, seminal emission
$CO_{9,10i}$. Ureter	between kidney and bladder	colic pain of the ureter calculus
CO_{11}. Pancrease & Gallbladder	between liver and kidney	pancreatitis, cholecystitis, cholelithiasis, migraine, herpes zoster, tympanitis, tinnitus
CO_{12}. Liver	posterior inferior part of the cymba conchae	hypochondriac pain, dizziness, hypertension, eye diseases, irregular enstruation, premenstrual syndrome, menopausal syndrome
middle of the cymba conchae	between the small intestine and kidney	abdominal pain and distention, ascariasis of the biliary tract

Continued

name	location	indication
CO_{13}. Spleen	posterior and superior part of the cavum conchae	abdominal distention, diarrhea, constipation, poor appetite, indigestion, irregular menstruation, leukorrhagia
CO_{15}. Heart	central depression of the cavum conchae	palpitation, insomnia, hysteria, angina pectoris, arrhythmia, neurosism
CO_{16}. Trachea	midpoint heart and orifice of external auditory meatus	cough and asthma
CO_{14}. Lung	around theheart and trachea	cough, asthma, chest distress, cutaneous pruritus, constipation, withdrawal syndrome, simple obesity
CO_{17}. Triple energizer	posterior and inferior to the orifice of external auditory meatus and between lung and endocrine	constipation, edema, abdominal distention, simple obesity
CO_{18}. Endocrine	anterior and inferior part of cavum conchae medial to the intertragic notch	dysmenorrhea, impotence, irreular menstruation, menopause syndrome, dysfunction of endocrine

6. 3. 8 Ear acupoints of the ear lobe

The ear lobe is separated into 9 zones. From the lower border of the cartilage of the intertragic notch to the lower border of the ear lobe, three equidistant horizontal and two equidistant vertical lines are drawn, dividing the area is vertically and equally into 9 zones. These zones are numbered anterior to posterior and from top to bottom: Zone 1,2 and 3 of the lobe are located in the upper area. Zone 4, 5 and 6 in the middle and Zone 7,8 and 9 in the lower area. (Table 2 −5 − 13)

Table 2 – 5 – 13 Ear acupoints of the ear lobe

name	location	indication
LO_1. Tooth	anterior and superior part of the frontal surface	toothache, paradontitis, hypo-tension
LO_2. Tongue	middle and superior part of the frontal surface	glossitis, stomatitis
LO_3. Jaw	posterior and superior part of the frontal surface	toothache, disorder of the temporo-mandibular joint
LO_4. Frontal Ear lobe	anterior and medial part of frontal surface	neurosism, toothache
LO_5. Eye	center of the frontal surface	acute conjunctivitis, hordeolum, pseudomyopia
LO_6. Internal ear	posterior and medial part of the frontal surface	auditory vertigo, tinnitus, impaired hearing
$LO_{5,6i}$. Cheek	between the eye and internal ear	facial paralysis, trigeminal neuralgia, acne, facial spasm, mumps
$LO_{7,8,9}$. Tonsil	inferior part of the frontal surface	tonsilitis, pharyngitis

6. 3. 9 Ear acupoints of the back auricle

The dorsal surface of ear is separated into 5 zones. Two horizontal lines are drawn through the locations on the dorsal surface corresponding to the beginning of the trunk of the two branches of the helix and the helix notch respectively, which divide the dorsal surface of ear into 3 parts: the upper area is Zone 1, the lower area Zone 5 and the middle area is separated into 3 equal portions. The medial 1/3 is Zone 2, the central 1/3 is Zone 3, and the lateral 1/3 is Zone 4. (Table 2 – 5 – 14)

Table 2 - 5 - 14

name	location	indication
P₁. Heart	upper part of the dorsal surface	palpitation, insomnia, excess dreaming
P₂. Lung	inner and middle part	asthma, pruritus
P₃. Spleen	center	stomachache, indigestion, poor appetite
P₅. Kidney	lower part of the dorsal surface	headache, dizziness, neurasthenia
GP₅. Groove of back auricle	the groove formed by the two branches of the antihelix	hypertension, cutaneous pruritus

6. 3. 10 Ear acupoints of the ear root

The location and indications of the acupoints on the ear root are shown in Table 2 - 5 - 15.

Table 2 - 5 - 15

name	location	indication
R₁. Upper ear root	highest portion of ear root	epistaxis
R₃. Root of the ear vagus	junction of the dorsal surface of the auricle and mastoid	cholecystitis, cholelithiasis, ascariasis of the bilary tract, abdominal pain, diarrhea, nasal obstruction, tachycardia
R₂. Lower ear root	lower portion of ear root	hypotension, lower limb paralysis, sequelae to infantile paralyssis

6. 4 Clinical application of auricular acupoints

6. 4. 1 Pain diseases

Various sprains and bruises, headache, neuropathic pain.

6. 4. 2 Inflammatory and infectious diseases

For example, acute and chronic colitis, parodontitis, mumps.

6. 4. 3 Dyfunctional diseases

Functional disturbances of the gastrointestinal tract, cardiac neurosis, irregular menstruation and neurasthenia.

6. 4. 4 Hypersensitivity an allergies

Urticaria, asthma, allergic rhinitis, and allergic colitis.

6. 4. 5 Endocrine diseases and metabolic disorders

Hyperthyroidism and/or hypothyroidism, diabetes, and menopausal syndromes.

6. 4. 6 Miscellaneous

Auricular acupuncture is effective for inducing lactation and labor and for preventing and treating transfusion and infusion reactions. In addition, it is also widely used for cosmetology, smoke cessation, drug withdrawal, age retardation and for the prevention of diseases and health care maintenance.

6. 5 Manipulation

6. 5. 1 Auricular acupoints selection principles

(1) Acupoints selection according to the affected area.

When the patients are ill, there are specific points on the corresponding area of the auricle that will be pressure sensitive, this is the basis for the selection of points to be treated, such as the Stomach point for the gastrointestinal diseases, etc.

(2) Acupoints selection according to the differentiation of syndromes based on the theory of the *zang-fu* organs.

Examples: lung and large intestine for skin diseases, kidney for cavities, etc.

(3) Acupoints selection according to the differentiation of syndromes based on the meridian theory.

(4)Acupoints are selected according to the routes and manifestations of the twelve meridians. Corresponding auricular acupoints are selected on their physiological function and pathological reactions. Examples: the bladder, pancreas and gallbladder acupoints for sciatica, the large intestine point for toothache, etc.

(4) Acupoints selection according to the physiology and pathology of modern medicine: some auricular acupoints are named according to the theories of western medicine examples: points endocrine, adrenal gland, sympathetic, etc. Their functions coincide with western medical theory, so the points can be selected based on their functions. Example: point adrenal gland for inflammatory diseases.

(5)Acupoints selection according to the clinical experience.

Some acupoints have been identified in clinic to be useful for treating other diseases besides local disorders. Example: acupoint Middle Ear for blood and skin diseases. Acupoint Shenmen for pain and tranquilizing, etc.

6. 5. 2 Manipulation methods

There are various methods to stimulate auricular acupoints. Some of the commonly used techniques are as follows.

(1)Filiform needling.

It refers to use the filiform needle to insert in the auricular acupoints. It is common way to treat diseases. The following procedures are observed when needling the auricular acpoints with filiform needles.

Acupoints selection and sterilization: following the selection of auricular acupoints for needling (include he sensitive spots detected by a needle probe or auricular acupoint detected). Strict disinfection should be done before acupuncture with a 2. 5% tincture iodine, followed by removing the iodine with a 75% alcohol cotton ball. Manipulations should begin after the alcohol on the auricle dries.

Body position and insertion: generally, patients are allowed to sit, however-er, but the elderly and weak, or severe conditions or nervous, it is advisable to let them down. Select No. 28 ~ 30, 0. 3 ~ 0. 5 *cun* needles made of stainless steel, stablize the auricle with the thumb and index fingers, and support the back of the ear with the middle finger of the left hand to control the depth of insertion and relieve pain. Then hold the filiform needle with the right hand and insert it into the point, either with the swift thrust or the slow twisting method. The insertion depth will depend on the thickness of the auricle, which will vary from patient to patient. Generally, penetrate the cartilage 0. 2 ~ 0. 3 *cun*, deep enough for the needle to stand erect without hanging.

Retention and removal of needle: the needles are usually retained for 20 ~ 30 minutes. The needles should be retained longer for chronic diseases, painful diseases, shorter and mild stimulation in children and elders. While the needles are retained, it is advisable to manipulate them at 10 minutes in-tervals. Removal of the needles is the last manipulation of a treatment. Hold the auricle with one hand, withdraw the needle quickly and perpendicularly, then immediately press the puncture hole with a dry sterilized cotton ball for a while to prevent bleeding.

(2) Electrotherapy.

After the needling sensation is obtained, connect the two electrodes to the handles of the needles in accordance with the electrotherapy technique. The current time is usually 10 ~ 20 minutes. This method is advisable for diseases of the nervous system, spasm and pain of the internal organs, and asthma.

(3) Needle embedding therapy.

Treating auricular acupoints by embedding intradermal needles is suitable for chronic and pain diseases. First, stabilize the ear with one hand, after route disinfection, clamp the handle of an intradermal needle with forceps in the oth-er hand, gently insert the needle into the selected point and stabilize it with adhesive tape. In general, the needle is embedded in the auricle on the same side as the affected area, or both if necessary. Each point should be pressed 3 times each day by the patient. The needle should be retained for 3 ~ 5 days after each treatment. A therapeutic course consists of 5 treatments.

(4) Auricular-seed-pressing therapy.

It is a simple stimulating method by pressing and adhering seeds on the auricular point. This method is safe, painless and fewer side-effects. It will not cause auricular perichondritis. It is suitable for the elderly people and children or the patient who is afraid of acupuncture. The material, such as rape seed, a mung bean, radish seed, a seed of vaccaria segetalis, magnetic bead, etc. can be used. When applying, first put the vaccaria segetalis on a piece of adhesive tape 0. 6cm × 0. 6cm, clamp it with forceps and tape it over the selected points; instruct the patients to press the seeds 30 ~ 30 seconds, 3 ~ 5 times a day. The adhesive tape should be replaced every 3 ~ 7 days. Both ears can be used alternately. The stimulation intensity depends on the patient's condition. In general, slight stimulation is advisable for children, pregnant women, and elderly patients or those with weakness or neurasthenia. Strong stimulation is advisable for acute pain.

(5) Acupoint injection therapy.

This therapy involves the injection of micro-amounts of medication into the auricular acupoints. A tuberculin syringe with a NO. 26 needle is usually selected. The appropriate medication is drawn according to the patient's condition. The auricle is stabilized with one hand, following the administration of a route skin test, the opposite hand slowly injects 0. 1 ~ 0. 3ml of medication into the auricular acupoints, creating a small hillock. Possible reactions might include pain, distension, redness and the sensation of heat. After the injection, the puncture hole is gently pressed with a sterilized, dry, cotton ball. This therapy may be administered once every other day.

6. 5. 3 Precautions

(1) Strict disinfection is necessary to prevent infection. If redness and

swelling occur on the puncture point, swab 2. 5% tincture of iodine, or apply an ignited moxa stick to the area.

(2) When treating sprains and motor disabilities, ask patients to move their affected extremities after insertion to enhance the therapeutic effects.

(3) Needling is contraindicated with pregnant women or those with history of habitual abortion.

(4) It is necessary for elderly or weak patients to take proper rest before and after needling, also gentle manipulation to guarantee safety is needed.

(5) Auricular acupuncture is inadvivisable for cases with severe structural diseases or serious anemia. Also, strong stimulation is not suitable for those with severe cardiac diseases or hypertension.

(6) Precautions should be taken to prevent needle fainting during auri cular acupuncture treatment. As per usual, appropriate measures should be taken in the event that is done occur.

7. Scalp Acupuncture

Scalp acupuncture therapy involves needling specific stimulation areas of the scalp for the prevention and treatment of disease. It originated from two theories, the theory of traditional *zang-fu* organs and meridians and the projection area of cortical functional localization on the scalp. Corresponding scalp lines were then defined based on these theories.

7. 1 Standard scalp acupuncture locations and indications

All the standard, basic lines of scalp acupuncture are located on the scalp. There are 4 areas corresponding to their anatomic names on the skull: frontal, parietal, temporal and occipital, and 14 basic lines on each hemisphere, plus the midline (25 lines in all comprise the left side, right side and the center). Their nomenclature, locations and indications are as following. (Fig. 2 –5 –37) (Table 2 –5 –16, 2 –5 –17,2 –5 –18)

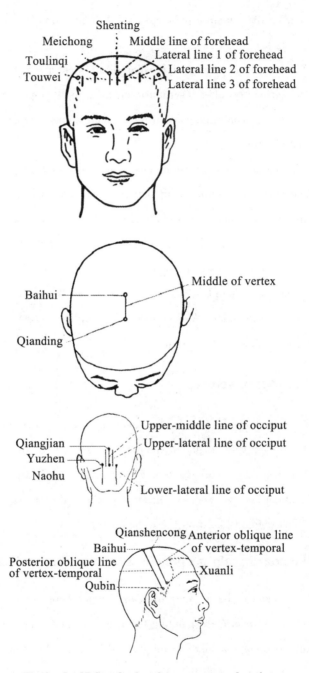

Shenting
Meichong Middle line of forehead
Toulinqi Lateral line 1 of forehead
Touwei Lateral line 2 of forehead
Lateral line 3 of forehead

Middle of vertex
Baihui
Qianding

Upper-middle line of occiput
Qiangjian Upper-lateral line of occiput
Yuzhen
Naohu
Lower-lateral line of occiput

Qianshencong Anterior oblique line
Baihui of vertex-temporal
Posterior oblique line
of vertex-temporal
Qubin Xuanli

Fig. 2 – 5 – 37 Standard scalp acupuncture locations

Table 2 – 5 – 16 Frontal scalp acupuncture locations and indications

name	location	indication
Frontal Mid-Line (MS 1)	forehead area, 1 *cun* in length from Shenting(GV 24), straight down along the meridian (Fig. 2 – 5 – 37)	epilepsy, mental disorder, rhinopathy
Frontal Lateral Line 1(MS 2)	forehead area, 1 *cun* in length from Meichong (BL 3) straight down along the meridian (Fig. 2 – 5 – 37)	coronary heart disease, bronchial asthma, bronchitis, insomnia, nasal disorders
Frontal Lateral Line 2 (MS 3)	forehead area, 1 *cun* in length from Toulin *qi* (GB 15) straight down along the meridian (Fig. 2 – 5 – 37)	acute and chronic gastritis, gastric and duodenal ulcers, liver and gallbladder diseases
Frontal Lateral Line 3 (MS 4)	forehead area, 1 *cun* in length from the point 0. 75 *cun* medial to Touwei (ST 8) straight down (Fig. 2 – 5 – 37)	dysfunctional uterine bleeding, impotence, seminal emission, hysteroptosis

Table 2 – 5 – 17 Vertex and temporal scalp acupuncture locations and indications

name	Location	indication
Vertex Mid-Line (MS 5)	vertex area, from Baihui (GV 20) to Qianding (GV 21) along the midline of the head	disorders of waist and lower extremities, e. g. paralysis, pain and numbness. cortical diuresis, hysteroptosis and hypertension
Anterior Vertex-Temporal Oblique Line (MS 6)	vertex area and cephalic region. From Qianshencong (1 *cun* ante-rior to Baihui (GV 20) obliquely to Xuanli(GB 6)	this entire line is divided into 5 equal parts: The upper 1/5 is used for treating paralysisof the contralateral lower limb and trunk. The middle 2/5 are for paralysis of contralateral upper limb. The lower 2/5 are for central facial paralysis, motor aphasia, salivation, cerebral atherosclerosis
Posterior Vertex-Temporal Line (MS 7)	vertex area and cephalic region,1 *cun* posterior and parallel to the anterior oblique line of vertextemporal. From Baihui (GV 20) obliquely to Qubin(GB7)	this entire line is divided into 5 equal parts: the upper 1/5 is used to treat paraesthesia in the contralateral lower limb and trunk. The middle 2/5 are for paraesthesia in the upper limb. and the lower 2/5 are for paraesthesia on the head and face
Lateral Vertex Line 1(MS 8)	vertex area, 1. 5 *cun* lateral to GV, 1. 5 *cun* in length posterior from Tongtian (BL 7) along the meridian	disorders of waist and lower extremities, e. g. paralysis, pain and numbness

Continued

name	Location	indication
Lateral Vertex Line 2 (MS 9)	vertex area, 2. 25 *cun* lateral to GV, 1. 5 *cun* in length posterior from ZhengYing (GB 17) to Chengling (GB 18).	impairment of the shoulders, arms and hands, such as paralysis, numbness or pain
Anterior Temporal Line (MS 10)	temporal area, from Hanyan (GB 4) to Xuanli (GB 6).	migraine, motor aphasia, peripheral facial paralysis
Posterior Temporal Line (MS 11)	temporal area, from Shuaigu (GB 8) to Qubin (GB 7)	migraine, tinnitus, deafness, vertigo

Table 2 – 5 – 18 Occipital scalp acupuncture locations and indications

Name	Location	Indication
Upper Occipital Mid-Line (MS 12)	occipital area, from Qiangjian (GV 18) to Naohu (GV 17), 1. 5 *cun* in length	eye disease, foot ringworm
Upper Occipital Lateral Line (MS 13)	occipital area, 0. 5 *cun* lateral and parallel to the upper-mid-line of the occiput	cortical visual disorders, cataract, myopia
Lower Occipital Lateral Line (MS 14)	occipital area, 2 *cun* in length from Yuzhen (BL 9) straight down	ataxia due to cerebellar diseases and paraequilibrium

7. 2 Indications for scalp acupuncture therapy

Scalp acupuncture therapy is mainly used to treat cerebral disorders in clinic, e. g, hemiplegia as a sequelae of apoplexy, numbness of the extremities, aphasia, vertigo, tinnitus, chorea, epilepsy, cerebral palsy, etc. It is also applied for headache, low back and leg pain, trigeminal neuralgia, and diseases of nervous system.

7. 3 Manipulations methods

Sitting or lYing positions required. Scalp acupoints should be selected according to the diagnosis. The hair is separated and the acupoint is sterilized with the routine method.

7. 3. 1 Insertion of the needle

Generally, select a 1. 5 ~ 3 *cun* filiform needle, No. 28 ~ 30, at a 15 ~ 30 angle, rapidly insert the needle subcutaneously, when the needle reaches the subgaleal layer and the practitioner feels the insertion resistance becomes weak, further insert the needle by twirling method, which parallels with the scalp, insertion varies with the areas, generally 0. 5 ~ 1. 5 *cun*. After the needle being inserted to the required depth, conduct manipulation.

7. 3. 2 Manipulation

In scalp acupuncture, the needle is manipulated only by twirling method, no lifting or thrusting of the needle. The depth of insertion keeps constant, the needle handle is held with the palmar surface of the thumb and the radial aspect of the index finger. Twirl the needle by rapidly and continuously flexing and extending the metacarpophalangeal joint of the index finger(or use electro-acupuncture to replace twirling of the needle). The twirling speed should be approximately 200 times per minute. Twirl the needle continuously for 2 ~ 3 minutes after the needle has been inserted, and retain the needle for 20 ~ 30 minutes. Repeat this manipulation 2 ~ 3 times, then withdrawn the needle. The needle retention time may be extended depending on the patholo gical condition. For hemiplegia, during the manipulation and retention of the needle, the patient is encouraged to exercise the affected limbs so as to enhace the therapeutic effect. In severe case, passive movement of the limbs of the patient should be done.

7. 3. 3 Withdrawal needle

Press the scalp around the acupoint with the left hand, hold the needle handle and rotate it gently and slowly as you withdraw it with the right hand. Pressure should be applied to the puncture hole immediately to prevent bleeding.

7. 3. 4 Course of treatment

Scalp acupuncture is applied once daily or once every other day, one course consisting of ten sessions of treatment. Between two courses, there is five to seven days break.

7. 4 Precautions

Due to the presence of hair on the scalp, strict sterilization should be done to prevent infection.

Due to duration and strong stimulation of scalp acupuncture, the practitioner should keep a close eye on the complexion of the patient in order to decrease the incidence of needle fainting.

Scalp acupuncture therapy is inadvisable for infants when their fontanels have not yet closed.

Stroke due to cerebral hemorrhage with coma, fever, high blood pressure, etc. In the acute stage is not suggested to treat by scalp acupuncture. The treatment may be applied until the pathological state is stable. However, scalp acupuncture therapy should be used as early as possible for patients with hemiplegia due to cerebral infarction. Scalp acupuncture should be used cautiously for patients with acute inflammation, high fever and heart failure.

There is a high incidence of bleeding when doing scalp acupuncture, due to the abundance of blood vessels in the scalp. Therefore, it is important to press the acupuncture hole with dry, cotton ball for 12 minutes following the withdraw of the needles.

Knowledge point 6　Acupuncture and Moxibustion treatment

1. Therapeutic functions of acupuncture and moxibustion

Acupuncture and moxibustion treatment is completed by acupoints prescription and needling or moxibustion manipulations. According to the therapeutic properties of acupoints and needling or moxa mani by means of acupuncture methods herapeutic function of acupuncture and moxibustion can be classified as follows:

1.1 Dredging the meridians and collaterals

The meridians and collaterals are the pathways for *qi* and blood to circulate in the whole body. They pertain to the *zang-fu* organs interiorly and extend over the body exteriorly. Dredging the meridians and collaterals refers to regulate *qi* and blood, remove obstruction from the meridians and collaterals by means of acupuncture methods to stimulate acupoints or regions on the body so as to treat diseases.

1.2 Regulating *yin-yang*

Regulating *yin-yang* means to use acupuncture methods to adjusts the relative predomination of *yin* and *yang* and relative decline of *yin* and *yang*. The purpose of regulating *yin* and *yang* is to reduce the excess and supplementary deficiency. Regulating *yin-yang* by acupuncture and moxibustion treatment is completed by Acupoints prescription and needling or moxa manipulations.

1. 3 Strengthening healthy *qi* (body resistance) and eliminating the pathogenic factors

The occurrence of disease results from the struggle between pathogenic factors and healthy-*qi* (body resistance) which exists in the whole course of disease. Strengthening healthy *qi* usually refers to " nourishing therapy ". By means of strengthening healthy *qi*, deficiency can be improved, body resistance can be reinforced and pathogenic factors can be eliminated. Eliminating the pathogenic factors refers to " purgation therapy ". Eliminating the pathogenic factors is helpful for restoring and strengthening healthy. The acupuncture and moxibustion treatment is based on the function of strengthening healthy *qi* and eliminating the pathogenic factors.

2. General principles of acupuncture and moxibustion treatment

The general principles of acupuncture and moxibustion are worked out by practicing repeatedly under the guidance of the theories of TCM. They are of universal significance in decision of the treatment methods and selection of points and manipulations.

2. 1 Reinforcing deficiency and reducing excess

Reinforcing deficiency means deficiency syndrome treated with reinforcing method to strengthen the body resistance, and reducing excess just means excess syndrome treated with reducing method to eliminate the pathogenic factors. By different manipulations of acupuncture and moxibustion stir up the autoregulation mechanism of the human body, strengthen the body resistance and eliminating the pathogenic factors are achieved in clinic.

2. 2 Clearing away the heat and warming the cold

Clearing away the heat means using cold or cool method to treat heat syndrome, and warming the cold means using warm or hot method to treat cold syndrome.

2. 3 Concentrating treatment on the root cause

Concentrating treatment on the root cause means to find the root cause of a disease and focus the treatment on it because the root cause is responsible for the emergency of syndrome. The process of searching root cause is the same as that of syndrome differentiation. However, for the treatment of severe urgent diseases, expectant treatment is required. Normally treat the secondary syndromes first and then deal with the root cause in emergency. If the root cause and secondary syndromes are all in the same situation, they must be treated simultaneously.

2. 4 Treating diseases according to individuality, locality and seasons

The occurrence, development and changes of disease involve a number of factors, including individual difference, geographical environment and seasonal variations which may affect the nature, duration and treatment of disease. So in treating disease, apart from following the above principles, one has to make corresponding changes according to individual condition, local environment and seasonal variations.

2. 4. 1 Abidance by individuality

Abidance by individuality means to decide treatment according to the age, sex, constitution and living habits of the patients.

2. 4. 2 Abidance by locality

Abidance by locality means to decide treatment according to geographical difference.

2. 4. 3 Abidance by seasonal variation

Seasonal variation means deciding treatment according to seasonal changes of weather.

3. Selection of acupoints and combination of acupoints

3. 1 Methods for selecting acupoints

3. 1. 1 Selection of proximal acupoints

Selection of proximal acupoints means to select points in the affected area and near the affected area. All points selected can treat the diseases of the local area and the adjacent area. The points can be selected from one meridian or several meridians, or just from the area of tenderness which is called "take tenderness as a point".

3. 1. 2 Selection of distant acupoints

It means to select acupoints distal to the affected area. The acupoints selected in this case are usually located below the elbows and knees. This method for selecting acupoints is based on the distribution of meridians and collaterals.

(1) Selecting points from the effected meridian.

Select relative points from the effected meridian for a disorder of the meridian and its pertaining and connecting organs.

(2) Selecting points from the involved meridian.

This method is also called "Selecting points from the other meridians" when meridian or certain *zang-fu* organs is diseased. Points are selected from the meridians which are related to the affected meridian or the diseased organ. The points are often selected from the meridians external internal relation meridians or meridians with the same name or other related meridians.

3. 1. 3 Selection of acupoints according to the symptoms

This method is used to select acupoint for the treatment of syndromes involving the whole body, the clinical manifestation of which are not limited to a certain local area according to the indication of acuponts and the theory of syndrome differentiation.

3. 2 Methods for the combination of acupoints

The prescription used in acupuncture treatment is composed of over two acupoints which are combined in the light of the syndromes. The purpose of combing acupoints are to strengthen the essential and comprehensive therapeutic effect. Therefore there are two ways to combine acupoints: one is to combine the acupoints with the same or similar indication and the other is to combine the corresponding acupoints according to pathological conditions or differentiation of syndromes. The most commonly used method are as follow.

3. 2. 1 Combination of points according to meridians

(1) Combination of points on the same meridian.

This method means selecting acupoints from the affected meridian of pertaining viscera.

(2) Exterior-interior point combination.

This method is based on the exterior interior relationship of *zang-fu* organs and the meridians. Points can be selected both from affected meridian and exterior interior relationship meridian at the seam time. The combination of *yuan* (primary) and luo (connecting) points is also included in this method. The first diseased meridian's *yuan* point selected, second disease meridian's *luo* point connected.

(3) Combination of points on the meridians with the same name.

This method means to select acupoints on the meridians of foot and hand with the same name.

3. 2. 2 Combination of points according to location

(1) Combination of the upper and lower points.

Upper means upper limbs and the areas above the lumber region, and lower refers to the lower limbs and the areas below the lumber region. The method of combination upper and lower points widely applied clinically. the method of combination the eight convergent Points is also an example of it.

(2) Combination of the front and back points.

The front refers to the chest and abdomen which are considered as the *yin* aspect. And the back means back and lower back which are referred to as the *yang* aspect. This method combines points located on the front and back to make up a prescription. The combination of the back-*shu* and front-*mu* points is included in this method.

(3) Combination of the left and right points.

Left means left side of the body and right means right side of the body including truck and limbs. The twelve regular meridians run symmetrically on the whole body. Points are often selected bilaterally for the disorder of the internal organs to strengthen the coordination of the functions of the meridians. Besides, the meridians also across at certain places so the points on the right side can be selected for a disorder on the left side and vice versa.

4. Application of special points

Most of the special points are located below the elbow or knees with special names and theory. They are frequently used in clinical treatment with specific methods.

4. 1 The Five-*shu* acupoints

There are 5 acupoints located below the elbow and knee on each of the 12 regular meridians, namely *Jing* (well), *Ying* (spring), *Shu* (stream),

Jing (river) and *He* (sea). Altogether there are 60 such acupoints.

Clinically *Jing*-well points is used to treat mental diseases, febrile diseases and emergent cases. *Ying*-spring points for febrile diseases. *Shu-stream* points for heavy sensation of the body and painful joints. *Jing*-river points for cough and asthma due to pathogenic cold and heat. *He*-sea points mostly for the disorders of six-*fu* organs, such as diarrhea and vomiting.

In addition, the selection of the *Five-shu* points can be made according to the combination of the *Five-shu* points with the five elements for treatment of diseases in the light of the theory "reducing the Child-acupoints to treat excess syndrome and reinforcing mother-acupoints to treat deficiency syndrome". For examples, reduccing Xingjian (LR 2), a *xing* (spring) point as well as a fire point for the excessive syndrome of the liver. This is an example of "reducing the son for an excessive syndrome". Reinforcing Ququan (LR 8), a *he* (sea) point and a water point for the deficiency syndrome of the Liver is an example of "reinforcing the mother for a deficiency syndrome".

4. 2 Application of the Back-*shu* and Front-*mu* acupoints

The back-*shu* points are acupoints on the back where *qi* of the *zang-fu* organs are infused. The front-*mu* points are acupoints on the chest and abdomen where *qi* of the *zang-fu* organs are accumulated.

The back-*shu* and front-*mu* acupoints are closely related to diseases of the viscera. When there is the pathogenic change in the viscera, the tenderness can be found on the corresponding back-*shu* or front-*mu* acupoints in order to help for diagnosis. In addition, the back-*shu* and front-*mu* acupoints can be used to treat visceral diseases.

The back-*shu* acupoints are mainly used to treat the disorders of five-*zang* organs and the front-*mu* acupoints are mainly used to treat the disorders of six-*fu* organs. In addition, the back-*shu* acupoints of *five-zang* organs can be used to treat the disorders of the related tissues and organs.

4. 3 Application of the *Yuan*-source and *Luo*-connecting acu-points

The *yuan*-source acupoints are places where the *yuan qi* infuses and ac-cumulates. The *yuan*-source acupoints are closely related to the *zang-fu* or-gans. Therefore, the disorders of *zang-fu* organs can be manifested on the *yuan*-source acupoints and can be treated by needling *yuan*-source acupoints.

The *luo*-connecting acupoints refer to the points where the fifteen collat-erals stem from the twelve meridians, the governor and conception vessels as well as the major collateral of the spleen. All the *luo*-connecting acupoints of the twelve meridians are located below the elbows and knees. These acupoints are used to treat the disorders of the regions that the meridians and collaterals run through as well as the disorders to the meridians in external and internal relation. The *luo*-connecting acupoints on the conception and govern vessels as well as the major *luo*-connecting acupoints of spleen are mainly used to treat diseases of the trunk.

The *yuan*-source and *luo*-connecting points can be used not only inde-pendently but also in combination. The method for the combination of *yuan*-source and *luo*-connecting acupoints is to select the corresponding *yuan*-source acupoint of the viscus primarily involved and corresponding *luo*-connecting acupoint of the viscus secondly involved. Usually this method is to deal with the disorders involving the meridians externally and internally related to each other.

4. 4 Application of the *Xi*-cleft acupoints

The *xi*-cleft acupoints are the sites where *qi* and blood from the meridians are deeply converged. Each of the twelve meridians and the four extraordinary vessels (*yin* heel vessel, *yang* heel vessel, *yin* link vessel and *yang* link ves-sel) has a *xi*-cleft acupoint on the limbs, amounting to sixteen in all.

Clinically *xi*-cleft acupoints are used to treat severe acute disorders of the meridians. The *xi*-cleft acupoints on the *yin* meridians are usually used to treat various blood syndromes and the *xi*-cleft acupoints on the *yang* meridians are often used to treat various pain syndromes.

4. 5 Application of the eight convergent acupoints

The eight convergent acupoints refer to the eight acupoints on the twelve meridians that are connected with the eight extraordinary vessels.

Clinically, they are effective in treating disorder of the relative 8 extra meridians. These eight convergent acupoints are divided into four groups and each goup is the fixed combination of the two acupoints on the hand and foot.

4. 6 Application of the eight confluent acupoints

Eight confluent acupoints, located on the trunk and four limbs below the knees and elbows, are the regions where the essence of *qi*, blood, tendons, vessels, bones, marrow, *zang* organs and *fu* organs converge.

In clinical treatment, apart from treating diseases of the meridian proper, they are frequently selected to treat the disorders related to the essence of the corresponding organs or tissues.

4. 7 Application of the lower *He*-sea acupoints

The lower *he*-sea acupoints refer to six acupoints on the three *yang* meridians of the foot where *qi* from the six-*fu* organs converge.

The lower *he*-sea acupoints are closely related to the six-*fu* organs and are used to treat the disorders of the six-*fu* organs.

4. 8 Application of the crossing acupoints

Crossing acupoints are those at the intersections of two or more meridians. Crossing acupoints are clinically used to treat diseases related to the meridian proper and the meridians crossed with the meridian proper.

5. Acupuncture and moxibustion therapy of the common diseases

5. 1 Sequela of apoplexy

Sequela of apoplexy refers to paralysis of limbs, deviation of the mouth and difficult in speaking after the attack of acute cerebrovascular diseases, similar to wind stroke and paralysis in TCM. It is caused by non-restroration of the visceral functions, retention of phlegm and blood stasis in the meridians as well as abnormal flow of meridian *qi*.

5. 1. 1 Syndrome differentiation

Paralysis of limbs on one side, accompanied by numbness or pain, deviation of the mouth, slurred speech or aphasia.

5. 1. 2 Treatment

[**Mainpoints**] Neiguan(PC 6), Renzhong (DU 26), Sanyinjiao(SP 6), Jiquan(HT 1), Weizhong(BL 40), Chize(LU 5).

[**Supplementaryary points**] For difficulty of swallowing, Fengchi(GB 20), Yifeng(SJ 17) and Wangu(GB 12) are added. For failing to extend fingers with stiffness, Hegu (LI 4) is added. For slurred speech, Lianquan(RN 23) is added, and Jinjin(EX-HN 12) and Yuye(EX-HN 13) are used with blood-letting method. For strephenopodia, penetrating method from Qiuxu(GB 40) to Zhaohai(KI 6) is used.

[**Method**] First puncture bilateral Neiguan(PC 6) perpendicularly for 0. 5 ~ 1 *cun*, using combinative reducing method of lifting-thrusting and twirling-rotating the needle for 1 minutes. Secondly puncture Renzhong(DU 26) obliquely upwards to the nasal septum for 0. 3 ~ 0. 5 *cun* with heavy bird-pecking method until the patient's eyeballs are moistened or tears flow down.

Thirdly puncture Sanyinjiao(SP 6)obliquely for 1 ~ 1.5 *cun*, at the angle of 45 degrees with the skin surface along the posterior border of the medial aspect of the tibia, with reinforcing method of lifting and thrusting the needle to make the affected low limb have tic for three times.

Select Jiquan(HT 1)point at 1 *cun* below the original location along the heart meridian to keep away from the armpit hair, puncture perpendicularly for 1 ~ 1.5 *cun* with reducing method of lifting and thrusting the needle to make the affected upper limb have tic for three times. Perpendicularly puncture Chize(LU 5)for 1 *cun* depth while the forearm bends to form an angle of 120 degrees with reducing manipulation of lifting and thrusting the needle until the affected arm and fingers have tic for three times. Select Weizhong(BL 40)point with the supine position and the lower limb lifted, puncture perpendicularly for 0.5 ~ 1 *cun*, with reducing method of lifting and thrusting to make the lower limb have tic for 3 times.

Puncture Fengchi(GB 20), Wangu(GB 12)and Yifeng(SJ 17)in the direction of the laryngeal protuberance for 2 ~ 2.5 *cun*, with reinforcing manipulation of twirling and rotating the needle in high frequency and small amplitude for 1 minute to each acupoint.

Puncture Hegu(LI 4)1 ~ 1.5 *cun* in depth with the needle tip toward Sanjian(LI 3), with reducing method of lifting and thrusting to make the patient's second finger or five fingers extended freely.

Puncture lianquan(RN 23)for 1.5 ~ 2 *cun*, with the needle tip towards the root of the tongue and reducing method of lifting and thrusting the needle. Prick Jinjin(EX-HN 12)and Yuye(EX-HN 13)with the three-edged needle to cause bleeding for 1 ~ 2 ml.

Puncture Qiuxu (GB 40)1.5 ~ 2 *cun* in depth with the needle tip toward Zhaohai(KI 6), until soreness and distension occurred locally.

5. 2 Insomnia

Insomnia refers to inability to have normal sleep, marked by difficulty to sleep, or easiness to wake up, or inability to sleep after waking up, or shallow sleep, keeping awake all nights. It is usually caused by anxiety, overstrain, emotional upsets, weakness and prolonged duration of illness as well as improper diet that lead to dysfunction of the heart, liver, spleen, and kidney as well as insufficiency of blood. Insomnia is mainly seen in neurosis in modern medicine.

5. 2. 1 Syndrome differentiation

(1) Liver-*qi* depression: dreaminess and easiness to wake up, dysphoria and susceptibility to rage, dizziness, distension or pain in the head, distending pain in the chest and hypochondrium, pale tongue with thin and white coating, taut pulse.

(2) Disharmony between heart and kidney: dysphoria and insomnia, dizziness, tinnitus, feverish sensation in the palms, soles and chest, soreness and weakness of the loins and knees, seminal emission, red tongue with thin and white coating, thin and rapid pulse.

(3) Deficiency of heart and spleen: difficulty to sleep, dreaminess and easiness to wake up, palpitation, poor memory, lassitude and listlessness, anorexia, pale complexion, light-colored tongue with thin and white coating, thin and weak pulse.

5. 2. 2 Treatment

(1) Body acupuncture.

[**Main acupoints**] Shenmen(HT 7), Sanyinjiao (SP 6), Baihui(GV 20) and Sishencong (EX-HN 1).

[**Supplementaryary points**] For liver-*qi* depression, Yanglingquan(GB 34) and Taichong (LR 3) are added. For exuberance of heart and liver fire,

Laogong (PC 8) , Shaofu (HT 8) , Xingjian(LR 2) are added. For phleghm-fire disturbing the heart, Zhongwan (RN 12) , Fenglong (ST 40) and Neiting (ST 44) are added. For disharmony between heart and the kidney, Shenshu (BL 23) , Taixi (KI 3) , and Xinshu(BL 15) are added. For deficiency of heart and spleen, Xinshu (BL 15) and Pishu (BL 20) are added.

[**Method**] For exuberant liver-fire and heart-fire, phlegm-heat attacking the heart, reducing method are used. For deficiency of heart and spleen, reinforcing method should be used. For disharmony between heart and the kidney, reducing method is used for Shenmen(HT 7) , reinforcing methods are used for other acupoints.

(2) Ear acupuncture.

[**Selection of acupoints**] Shenmen (TF_4) , Heart (CO_{15}) , Spleen (CO_{13}) , Kidney(CO_{10}) and Subcortex(AT_4).

[**Method**] Select 2 ~ 3 points for each treatment. A moderate stimulation is given and retain the needles for 20 minutes. The auricular-seed-pressing therapy is also applicable.

5. 3 Common cold

Common cold is an exogenous disease with nasal obstruction, headache, aversion to cold, fever, soreness and pain of the trunk and limbs, etc. It may be occur around the year, but more often in winter and spring. According to the difference in pathogenic factors, constitution and clinical manifestations, this syndrome is manifested either as wind-cold or wind-heat with the complications of summer-heat and dampness. It may be caused by pathogenic wind, cold and dampness that block the pores, stagnate *yang-qi* and hinder the dispersion of the lung, or by pathogenic wind, heat, summer-heat and dryness that affect the conveyance of the muscular interstices, leading to pathogenic factor to scorch the lung and the lung can not to depurate.

5. 3. 1 Syndrome differentiation

(1) Wind-cold : aversion to cold, fever, no sweating, headache, heaviness and soreness of the limbs, nasal obstruction, running nose, thin and white tongue coating, floating and tense pulse.

(2) Wind-heat : severe fever and slight aversion to cold, or sweating, distending headache, sore throat, dry mouth, nasal obstruction with yellowish discharge, thin and yellowish tongue coating, floating and rapid pulse.

(3) Summer-heat with damp : aversion to cold, fever, dull fever, unsmooth sweating, aching and heaviness in the four limbs, heavy and distending sensation in the head, fullness and oppression in the chest and epigastrium, nausea, loose stool, scanty and brown urine, red tongue with yellow-greasy tongue coating, a slow or superficial rapid pulse.

5. 3. 2 Treatment

(1) Body acupuncture.

[**Main acupoints**] Fengchi (GB 20), Dazhui (GV 14), Lieque (LU 7) , and Hegu (LI 4) , *Taiyang* (EX-HN 5).

[**Supplementaryary points**] For wind-cold, Feishu (UB13) and Fengmen (UB 12) are added. For wind-heat, Quchi (LI 11) and Chize (LU 5) are added. For summer-heat with damp type, Zhongwan (CV 12), Zusanli (ST 36) are added. For nasal obstruction or running nose Shangxing (GV 24) and Yingxiang (LI 20) are added. For sore throat Shaoshang (LU 9) is added. For severe dampness : Yinlingquan (SP 9).

[**Method**] Reducing method is used. Shaoshang (LU 9) is pricked for bloodletting. Dazhui (GV 14) and Fengmen (UB12) are used with moxibustion for wind-cold. Dazhui (GV 14) is used to prick for bloodletting and then a cupping is sucked over the pricked area for wind-heat.

(2) Three edged needle.

Three edged needle is used for cause bleeding on Erjian (EX-HN 6),

Shaoshang (LU 9) and Shang*yang* (LI 1). It is effective for wind-heat.

(3) Cupping.

[**Selection of acupoints**] Feishu (UB 13), GVDazhui (GV 14), Fengmen (BL 12), Dazhu (UB 11), and Shenzhu (GV 12).

[**Method**] Cupping or moving cupping is applied to the back, from Dazhui (GV 14) to the lower back up and down. Finally stop at Feishu (BL 13) for 10 ~ 20 minutes before removing the cup. It is effective for wind-cold especial having soreness and pain of the trunk and limbs.

5. 4 Cough

Cough, a main symptom of the lung problems, may result either from attack by exogenous factors disturbing the dispersion of the lung, or from disorders of the lung itself or other diseased *zang-fu* organs affecting the lung. Exogenous cause refers to attack by wind, cold, heat and dryness that lead to failure of lung to descend, failure of body fluids to distribute and obstruction of the trachea by sputum. Endogenous cause refers to dysfunction of the lung, spleen and kidney. Lung asthenia results in failure of descending; dysfunction of spleen leads to accumulation of dampness into phlegm which attacks the lung. Kidney asthenia brings about dysfunction of qi and upward adverse flow of qi, or invasion of liver fire into the lung leads to consumption of body fluid by lung heat.

5. 4. 1 Syndrome differentiation

(1) Wind-cold encumbering lung: cough with white and thin sputum, nasal obstruction and running nose, aversion to cold, fever, headache and general aching, thin and white tongue coating, floating and tight pulse.

(2) Wind-heat attacking lung: cough with yellow, thick and sticky sputum, difficulty in expectoration, fever and headache, thin and yellow tongue coating, floating and rapid pulse.

(3) Retention of phlegm and dampness in lung: cough with profuse sputum, white and sticky sputum easy to expectation, heavy cough, fullness and oppression in the chest and epigastrium, anorexia and abdominal distension, white and greasy tongue coating, soft and slippery pulse.

(4) Liver fire scorching lung: paroxysmal cough involving the rib-side, scanty and sticky sputum difficult to expectorate, or even blood in sputum, dry and itching throat, red eyes and bitter taste in the mouth, constipation and brown urine, tongue with red tip and margin, thin and yellow tongue coating, taut and rapid pulse.

(5) *Yin*-deficiency of the lung and kidney: dry cough without sputum or with scanty sputum, stickyor bloody sputum, dry throat, dysphoria with feverish sensation in the chest, palms and soles, night sweating and tidal fever, red tongue with a little coating, thin and rapid pulse.

5. 4. 2 Treatment

(1) Body acupuncture.

[**Main acupoints**] Feishu (BL 13), Lieque (LU 7), Tiantu(RN 22).

[**Supplementary points**] For wind-cold encumbering lung, Fengchi (GB 20) and Hegu(LI 4) are added. For wind-heat attacking lung, Dazhui (GV 14) and Quchi (LI 11) are added. For retention of phlegm and dampness in lung, Zusanli(ST 36) and Fenglong(ST 40) are added. For liver fire scorching lung, Xingjian(LR 2) and Yuji(LU 10) are added. For *yin*-deficiency of the lung and kidney, Shenshu(BL 23), Taixi(KI 3) and Gaohuang (BL 43) are added.

[**Method**] Needling techniques are selected according to the nature of the syndromes. For the treatment of wind-cold encumbering lung and retention of phlegm and dampness in lung, back-*shu* points can be needled with the addition of moxibustion or cupping.

(2) Acupoints application.

[**Selection of acupoints**] Dingchuan (EX-B 1), Feishu (BL 13), Dazhui (GV 14), Fengmen (BL 12), Gaohuang (BL 43), Tiantu (RN 22), Danzhong (RN 17) are used.

[**Method**] Baijiezi (Semen Sinapis Albae), Gansui (Radix Euphordiae Kansui), Xixin (Herba Asari), Yanhusuo (Rhizoma Corydalis), Rougui (Cortex Cinnamomi) and Dananxing (Arisaema Cum Bil) are prepared into paste which is applied to 3 ~ 4 acupoints each time. The application is changed once every 3 days and 10 days make up one course of treatment.

5. 5 Stomachache

Stomachache refers to a syndrome manifested by frequent pain in the upper abdomen, reduced appetite, nausea and vomiting. It may be caused by exogenous pathogenic factors and improper diet that lead to dysfunction of the spleen and stomach, failure of gastric qi to descend and upward adverse flow of turbid qi, or by emotional upsets, overstrain and weakness due to prolonged diseases that lead to depression of liver and stagnation, asthenia-cold in middle energizer and insufficiency of stomach yin, or by involvement of the collaterals in prolonged disease and stagnation of blood in the collaterals.

5. 5. 1 Syndrome differentiation

(1) Cold in the stomach: sudden onset of stomachache, severe pain, alleviation with warmth, aversion to cold and preference for warmth, nausea and vomiting, a thin white tongue coating and taut and tight pulse.

(2) Retention of food: distention and fullness in the epigastrium, unpressure pain, belching, acid regurgitation, alleviation of pain after vomiting, thick and greasy tongue coating as well as taut and slippery pulse.

(3) Liver-qi invading the stomach: distention of the stomach, epigastralgia involving the rib-sides, acid regurgitation, frequent belching and sighing

thin and white tongue coating as well as taut pulse.

(4) Stagnancy of *qi* and blood stasis: stabbing epigastralgia with fixed and unpressured pain, hematemesis or hematochezia in a severe case, purplish tongue with ecchymosis and unsmooth pulse.

(5) Deficiency-cold in the spleen and stomach: dull stomachache, preference for warmth and pressure, emaciation and spiritual lassitude, loose stool, pale tongue with thin and white tongue coating, deeply weak and slow pulse.

(6) Insufficiency of stomach *yin*: dull pain in the stomach, heartburn like hunger without appetite, dry mouth with desire to drink, red tongue with scanty coating as well as thin and rapid pulse.

5. 5. 2　Treatment

(1) Body acupuncture.

[**Main acupoints**] Neiguan (PC 6), Zhongwan (CV 12) and Zusanli (ST 36).

[**Supplementary points**] For cold in the spleen and stomach, Weishu (BL 21) and Shenque (CV 8) are added and moxibustion. For attack of the stomach by the liver-*qi*, Yanglingquan (GB 34), Taichong (LI 3) and *qi*men (LI 14) are added. For stagnancy of *qi* and Blood stasis, Danzhong (CV 17) and Geshu (BL 17) are added. For retention of food, Liangmen (ST 21) and Yianshu (ST 25) are added. For *yang* deficiency of spleen and stomach. Pishu (BL 20), Weishu (BL 21) and Qihai (CV 3) are added. For *yin* deficiency of Stomach, Weishu (BL 21), Taixi (KI 3) and Sanyinjiao (SP 6) are added.

(2) Method.

[**Method**] For liver-*qi* invading the stomach and stagnancy of *qi* and blood stasis, the even movement or reducing method may be used. For deficiency-cold in the spleen and stomach and insufficiency of stomach *yin*, the reinforcing method is adopted.

5. 6 Constipation

Constipation refers to a condition in which hard stool is difficult to excrete and defecation occurs once every more than two to three days. The feces are hard and elimination from the bowels is difficult and infrequent, every two days or more.

5. 6. 1 Syndrome Differentiation

(1) Excess type: difficult and infrequent defecation, perhaps every 3 to 5 days.

①Accumulation of heat, there are fever, dire thirst, foul breath, preference for cold drinks and diet, yellow and dry tongue with greasy coating, slippery and full pulse.

②Stagnation of *qi*, there are fullness and distending pain in the abdomen and hypochondriac (flank) regions, frequent belching, loss of appetite, thin greasy tongue coating and wiry or taut pulse.

(2) Deficiency type: difficult defecation due to weakness and unformed stool even no defecation for several days, accompanied with pale and lustreless complexion, lips and nails, dizziness and palpitation, pale tongue with thin and white coating, weak and thin pulse.

①Deficiency of *qi* and blood.

A pale and lusterless complexion lips and nails, dizziness, palpitation, listlessness and lassitude, a pale tongue with thin coating, a thready pulse.

②Deficiency of *Yang*.

Abdominal cold pain, a preference for warmth and aversion to cold, a pale tongue with white coating, a thready pulse of the deficiency type.

Cold type: no defecation for several days, accompanied with cold sensation and pain in the abdomen, preference for warmth and aversion to cold, pale tongue with white and moist coating, deep and slow pulse.

5. 6. 2 Treatment

(1) Body acupuncture.

[**Main acupoints**] Dachangshu (BL 45), Tianshu (ST 25), Zhigou (TE 6) and Shangjuxu (ST 37)

Tianshu (ST 25) is a *Mu*-point of *yangming* large intestine meridian of hand and shangjuxu (ST 37) is a Lower-he point of *yangming* large intestine meridian of hand. They two mean *Shu-mu* combination. Dachangshu (BL 45) is Back-*shu* point of *yangming* large intestine meridian of hand, they three acupoint can regulate *Fu-qi* of Large Intestine. Zhigou (TE 6) is a very experiential acupoint for constipation and it can dredge *qi* of triple energizer.

[**Supplementary points**]

For accumulation of heat, Hegu (LI 4) and Quchi (LI 11) are added.

For stagnation of *qi*, Zhongwan (CV 12) and Xingjian (LR 2) are added. For deficiency type, Pishu (BL 20) and Weishu (BL 21) are added. For cold type, Shengque (CV 8) and Qihai (CV 6) to which moxibustion is applied. For deficiency of *qi* and blood, Zusanli (ST 36), Qihai (CV 6) are added. For deficiency of *Yang*, Shenshu (BL 23) and Mingmen (GV 4) are added. For deficiency of *Yin* and Blood, Taixi (KI 3), Sanyinjiao (SP 6) and Zhaohai (KI 6).

[**Method**] The reinforcing method is used for deficiency type, the reducing method for excess type, and moxibustion for cold type.

(2) Electroacupuncture.

Daheng (ST 27) and Xiajuxu (ST 38) for 10 ~ 20 minutes, once every other day.

(3) Ear acupuncture.

[**Prescription**] Pt. lower portion of rectum, Pt. large intestine, Pt. subcortex, Pt. diaphragm, Pt. liver and Pt. spleen.

[**Method**] Find out the sensitive spots. Knead them by the hand for three to five times of day, stick and press seeds of semen vaccariae on them. Give the treatment once every three days, 15 treatments constitute a course.

[**Notes**] ①puncture has a good therapeutic effect in treating constipation, if several treatments take out ineffective, it's necessary to find out the possible reasons. ②Tell the patients to keep up physical exercise, take more vegetates, and cultivate a good habit of timing bowel movement.

5. 7 Headache

Headache is a subjective symptom. It can occur in various acute or chronic diseases. The causes are either attack by exogenous pathogenic wind or dysfunction of the liver, spleen and kidney that lead to retention of pathogenic factors in the meridians, or hyperactivity of liver-*yang*, or obstruction by phlegm and stagnation, or failure of *qi* and blood to nourish the head.

5. 7. 1 Syndrome differentiation

Wind attacking meridians: frequent severe headache, onset with the attack of cold and wind, pain involving the neck and back, thin and white tongue coating, float pulse.

Hyperactivity of liver-*yang*: headache, dizziness, occurrence with mental upsets or nervousness, dysphoria and susceptibility to rage, insomnia, flushed cheeks and bitter taste in the mouth, red tongue with thin and yellow coating, taut and rapid pulse.

Deficiency of both *qi* and blood: lingering headache, dizziness, blurred vision, spiritual lassitude and fatigue, pale complexion, pale tongue with thin and white coating, thin and weak pulse.

Obstruction of phlegm and dampness: headache with heaviness sensation, chest oppression, nausea, vomiting of phlegm and drool, white and greasy tongue coating, slippery pulse.

Qi stagnation and blood stasis: prolonged duration, fixed location of pain, prickly pain, or history of traumatic injury of the head, purplish tongue or with ecchymoses, thin and unsmooth pulse.

5. 7. 2 Treatment

(1) Body acupuncture.

[**Main acupoints**] Fengchi (GB 20) , Baihui (GV 20) , Taiyang (EX-HN 5) .

[**Supplementary acupoints**] For wind attacking meridians, acupoints should be selected according to the location of headache. Shangxing (GV 18) , yangbai (GB 14) , Yintang (EX-HN 3) andHegu(LI 4) are added for pain in the forehead. Shuaigu (GB 8) , Waiguan (TE 5) and Zulinqi (GB 41) are added for pain in side of the head; Taichong (LR 3) and Yongquan (KI 1) are added for pain in the vertex of the head; Tianzhu (BL 10) , Houxi (SI 3) and Kunlun (BL 60) are added for pain in the back of the head. For hyperactivity of liver-yang, Taichong(LR 3) , Taixi(KI 3) and Xingjian(LR 2) are added. For deficiency of qi and blood, Qihai(RN 4) , Zusanli(ST 36) , Pishi(BL 20) are added. For obstruction of phlegm and dampness, Yin-lingquan(SP 9) and Fenglong(ST 40) are added. For qi stagnation and blood stasis, Hequ(LI 4) , Sanyinjiao(SP 6) and Geshu(BL 17) are added.

[**Method**] Each time 4 ~ 6 acupoints are selected according to the patho-logical conditions. For the treatment of deficiency of both qi and blood, reinfor-cing needling technique and moxibustion are used for rest syndrome are nee-dled with reducing or mild reinforcing and reducing needling technique. For the treatment of the blood stasis, Taiyang(EX-HN 5) is pricked for bleeding.

(2) Ear acupuncture.

[**Selection of acupoints**] Subcortex(AT_4) , Occipital(AT_3) , Forehead (AT_1) , Temple (AT_2) , Liver (CO_{12}) , Gallbladsder (CO_{11}) and Shenmen (TF_4) .

[**Method**] Each time 3 ~ 4 acupoints are selected and the needles are re-tained for 30 minutes. Or Wangbuliuxingzi (semen vaccariae) is used for ear pressure.

5. 8 Facial paralysis

This disease is peripheral facial paralysis caused by an acute non-suppu-rating inflammation of the facial nerve in the stylomastoid foramen. It is termed "deviation of mouth and eye" in traditional Chinese medicine. It is caused by wind-cold or wind-heat attacking the meridians in the face, leading to obstruction of meridian qi, malnutrition of tendons and flaccidity of muscles.

5. 8. 1 Syndrome differentiation

Key points for syndrome differentiation: sudden onset in the morning with the manifestations of stiffness, numbness and looseness of the face, enlarge-ment of palpebral fissure, deviation of the angle of the mouth to the healthy side, disappearance of wrinkles on the forehead, the nasolabial groove becom-ing shallow and inability to draw eyebrows, frown, close eyes, show teeth, bulge cheeks and pout lips. In some patients pain appears behind the ear and in the face in the early stage.

(1) Windcold: patients mostly have the experience of catching cold after sleeping windward, or wind blowing on one side of the face too long. Normally, there are not necessarily any external symptoms.

(2) Wind heat: occurs after cold fever, or otitis media accompanied with pain in the inner ear and mastoid process.

5. 8. 2 Treatment

(1) Body acupuncture.

[**Main acupoints**] Cuanzhu (BL 2), Yangbai (GB 14), Sibai (ST 2), Quanliao(SI 18), Dicang (ST 4), Jiache (ST 6), and Hegu (LI 4).

[**Supplementary points**] For windcold, Fengchi(GB 20) and Fengmen (BL 12) are added with the reducing method. For windheat, Dazhui(GV 14) and Quchi (LI 11) are added with the reducing method. For deficiency of qi and blood, Pishu (BL 20), Weishu (BL 21), Sanyinjiao (SP 6) and Zusanli (ST 36) are added with the reinforcing method. For mastoidalgia, Yifeng (TE

17) is added. For shallow nasolabial groove, Yingxiang (LI 20). For deviation of the philtrum: Shuigou (GV 26). For deviation of the mentolabial groove, Chengjiang (CV 24) is added.

[**Method**] Dicang (ST 4) and Jiache (ST 6) are needled horizontally toward each other, Yangbai (GB 14) is needled horizontally toward downward. The acupoints on the face are needled with mild reinforcing and reducing method. The needling method in the early stage should be mild.

(2) Cutaneous acupuncture.

[**Selection of acupoints**] Yangbai (GB 14), Quanliao (SI 18), Diceng (ST 4) and Jiache (ST 6).

[**Method**] Use the cautaneous acupuncture to stimulate the acupoints until the skin of the points selected become congested. The needling is done once a day or once every other day. It is suitable for recovery.

5.9 Lumbago

Lumbago, also called "pain in the lumbar and spinal regions". The pain can be located on the spine or one side or both sides of the spine. Lumbago is mainly caused by retention of pathological wind, cold and dampness in the meridians, or by malnutrition of the and tendons due to kidney deficiency, or by inhibited flow of *qi* and blood in the meridians due to overstrain and impairment.

5.9.1 Syndrome differentiation

(1) Obstruction by pathogenic cold and dampness, cold pain and heaviness sensation in the loins, or pain involving the buttocks and legs, inflexibility, aggravation with cold and rain, thin and white tongue coating and deep or slow pulse.

(2) Stagnation of *qi* and blood, pricking and fixed pain, stiffness of the waist, inflexibility, purplish tongue or with ecchymoses, taut or unsmooth

pulse.

(3) Deficiency of kidney essence, slow onset, vague aching and lingering pain in the loins, aggravation with overstrain, weakness of loins and kness, pale complexion, dizziness, tinnitus, spiritual lassitude, cold limbs, frequent and clear urine, pale tongue, deep and thin pulse in the case of *yang* deficiency. Flushed cheeks, dysphoria, insomnia, dry mouth and throat, feverish sensation over palms and soles, yellow urine and dry feces, red tongue, thin and rapid pulse in the case of *Yin* deficiency.

5. 9. 2 Treatment

(1) Body acupuncture.

[**Main acupoints**] Shenshu(BL 23), Dachangshu(BL 25) and *Ashi* acupoints.

[**Supplementary acupoints**] For the syndrome of obstruction due to cold-dampness. Yao *Yang*guan (GV 3), Huantiao (GB 30), Chengfu (BL 36), Weizhong(BL 40) and Kunlun(BL 60) are added. For the syndrome of stagation of *qi* and blood, Geshu (BL 17), Ciliao (BL 32), Weizhong (BL 40), Yanglingquan(GB 34) and Feiyang(BL 58) are added. For the syndrome of kidney asthenia and essence consumption, Mingmen (GV 4), Qihaishu (BL 24), Guangyuanshu(BL 26), Ciliao(BL 32), Zusanli(ST 36) and Dazhong(KI 4) are added.

[**Method**] Kidney deficiency syndrome is treated with reinforcing needling technique, other syndromes are treated with reducing needling techniques. All the acupoints of cupping. If there is blood stagnation, Weizhong (BL 40) is punctured to let blood.

(2) Ear acupuncture.

[**Selection of acupoints**] lumbosacral Vertebrae(AH$_9$), Kidney(CO$_{10}$), Ear Shenmen(TF$_4$) and Subcortex(AT$_4$).

[**Method**] Each time 2 ~ 3 acupoints are selected and needled with medium and strong stimulation. The needles are retained for 20 ~ 30 minutes. Or Wangbuliuxingzi(semen vaccariae) is used for ear perssure.

5. 10 Sciatica

Sciatica is marked by pain radiating to the foot from lumbar region, buttocks, posterior side of the thigh and lateral side of the shank. The pain is usually unilateral and will be aggravated when the waist is bent or the lower limbs are moved. The causes of sciatica are various. Clinically it is divided into primary and secondary types. The secondary type is further classified into root and trunk types. Sciatica pertains to the conceptions of obstructive syndrome, lumbago and pain of loins and legs in TCM. It is mainly caused by exogenous pathogenic wind, cold and dampness that obstruct meridians, or by deficiency of *kidney-qi* and malnutrition of meridians, or by trauma, sprain, contusion and stagnation of *qi* and blood in meridians.

5. 10. 1 Syndrome differentiation

(1) Obstruction by cold-dampness: frequent attack after invasion of cold-dampness, pain and heaviness of loins and legs, inflexibility, subjective cold sensation in the affected region, aggravation in rainy and cold weather, white or white and greasy tongue fur, deep pulse.

(2) Deficiency of *kidney-qi*: slow onset, lingering duration, recurrence, aching pain in the loins, aggravation after work, weakness of waist and legs, pale complexion, light-colored tongue, deep and thin pulse.

(3) Stagnation of *qi* and blood: traumatic injury history of waist, stabbing pain in the waist and legs, aggravation in movement, purplish tongue, taut or unsmooth pulse.

5. 10. 2 Treatment

(1) Body acupuncture.

[**Main acupoints**] 3 ~ 5 lumbar Jiaji(EX-B 2), Dachangshu(BL 25),

Huantiao(GB 30) , Weizhong(BL 40) , Yanglingquan(GB 34) , Xuanzhong (GB 39) and Qiuxu(GB 40).

[**Supplementary acupoints**]For obstruction by cold-dampness, Yaoyang- guan(GV 3) , Zhibian (BL 54) , Chengfu (BL 36) , Feiyang (BL 58) , and Kunlun(BL 60) are added. For deficiency of *kidney-qi*, Shenshu(BL 23) and Dazhong(KI 4) are added. For stagnation of *qi* and blood, Shuigou (GV 26) , Weizhong(BL 40) , Houxi(SI 3) are added.

[**Method**] Each time 4 ~ 5 acupoints are selected according to the path- ological conditions. For the treatment of cold-dampness, reducing needing technique, warmed needling or moxibustion are used with the addition of cup- ping. For the treatment of kidney deficiency, reinforcing needling technique, warmed needling or moxibustion are used. For the treatment of stagnation with moxa cone are used. For the treatment of stagnation, bloodleting is done Weizhong(BL 40) or the collaterals around.

(2) Electro-acupuncture.

[**Selection of acupoints**] Lumbar Jiaji (EX-B 2) , Yanglingquan (GB 34) and Weizhong(BL 40).

[**Method**] After needling sensation is felt, impulse current is attached to the needles for 10 ~ 15 minutes, once a day.

5. 11 Stiff neck

Stiffness of neck is a commonly encountered damage of cervical soft tis- sues due to an improper position of the neck during sleep or attack of wind- cold into the back that prevents the smooth circulation of *qi* and blood in the meridians. Its main clinical manifestations are unilateral or bilateral acute sim- ple stiffness and pain of the neck and its associated limitation of movement.

5. 11. 1 Syndrome differentiation

Stiffness and pain in the neck, aggravation in movement, restricted movement, deviation of the head to the affected side, pain involving the shoulder, back or head, and evident local tenderness.

5. 11. 2 Treatment

(1) Body acupuncture.

[**Main acupoints**] *Ashi* points, Jianjing(GB 21) Wailaogong (EX-UE 8) and Houxi(SI 3).

[**Method**] Reducing method is used. First puncture remote acupoints Wailaogong (EX-UE 8) and Houxi(SI 3), and the patient ia asked to move the neck during the treatment. Then puncture local acupoits. After withdrawal of the needle, cupping is applied to local acupoint.

(2) Ear acupuncture.

[**Selection of acupoits**] Neck (AH_{12}) , Cervical Vertebra (AH_{13}) and Tenderness points.

[**Method**] Strong stimulation is used and the patient is asked to move the neck during the treatment. The needles are retained for 15 ~ 20 minutes.

5. 12 Cervical spondylopathy

Cervical spondylopathy is a syndrome due to long-term sprain, hyperosteogeny of the cervical vertebra, protrusion of intervetebral disc and thickening of ligament that stimulates or oppresses the cervical nerve root, spinal cord, vertebral artery or sympathetic nerve, causing pain and other symptoms. The main clinical manifestations are soreness, distension or pain of the neck, shoulder or arm, numbness of the fingers, etc. This disease pertains to obstructive syndrome in TCM. It is usually caused by invasion of pathogenic wind, cold and dampness into meridians, blocking the flow of *qi* and blood, or by deficiency of liver and kidney as well as insufficiency of *qi* and blood in the aged, leading to malnutrition of the tendons, or by impairment of the tendons and vessels due to long-term strain.

5. 12. 1 Syndrome differentiation

(1) Exogenous windcold attack: stiffness and pain in the neck or involving the arm and shoulder, cold limbs and numbness of hands, or heaviness
sensation, aggravation with wind and cold, accompanied by general aching,
thin and white tongue fur, floating and tense pulse.

(2) Stagnation of *qi* and blood: aching, distending pain or prickly pain in
the neck, shoulder and arm, or swelling and distension, or pain radiating to the
arm, accompained by dizziness and headache, mental depression, aggravation
with nervousness, thin and white tongue coating, taut and unsmooth pulse.

(3) Insufficiency of the liver and kidney: slow onset, numbness and dull
pain in the neck, shoulder and back, prolonged duration, aggravation with
overstrain, accompanied by dizziness, blurred vision, tinnitus, deafness,
aching and weakness of loins and kness, weakness of lower limbs, tender
tongue with thin coating, deep, thin and weak pulse.

5. 12. 2 Treatment

(1) Body acupuncture.

[**Main acupoints**] 3 ~ 5 Cervial Jiaji, Fengchi(GB 20) , Wangu(GB 12) ,
Dazhui(BL 11) , Tianzhu(BL 10) , Hegu(LI 4) and Zhongzhu(SJ 3).

[**Supplementary acupoints**] For exogenous wind-cold attack: Waiguan
(SJ 5) , Fengmen(BL 12) and Jianjing(GB 21) are added. For stagnation of
qi and blood, Quchi (LI 11) , Jianyu (LI 15) , Geshu (BL 17) and Yan-
glingquan(GB 34) are added. For insufficiency of liver and kidney, Ganshu
(BL 18) , Shenshu(BL 23) and Xuanzhong(GB 39) are added.

[**Method**] Reinforcing method is used for the treatment of insufficiency
of the liver and kidney. The rest two syndromes are treated with the reducing
method. The acupoints on the neck and back are needled with rotating and
twirling manipulations. Moxibustion can be used with the addition of cupping.

(2) Ear acupuncture.

[**Selection of acupoins**] Neck (AH_{12}), Cervial Vertebra (AH_{13}), Shoulder, Kidney (CO_{10}) and Ear Shenmen (TF_4).

[**Method**] Each time 2 ~ 3 acupoints are selected and needled with filiform needles and moderate and strong stimulation. The needles are retained for 20 ~ 30 minutes. The treatment is given once a day or once every other day. Or Wangbuliuxingzi (semen vaccariae) is used for ear point pressing.

5. 13 Scapulohumeral periarthritis

Scapulohumeral periarthritis is a chronic, retrograde and inflammatory disease of the shoulder joint capsule and the soft tissues around it, mostly due to exposure to cold, trauma and chronic strain of the shoulder. The main clinical manifestations are soreness and dysfunction of the shoulder. In the early stage, pain is the main symptom, while in the late stage dysfunction is the main symptom. The diseases are usually seen in those at the age of 50 or over. This disease pertain to the conception of obstrctive syndrome in TCM. It is caused either by invasion of pathogenic wind, cold and dampness due to deficiency, or by weakness in the aged and malnutrition of tendons and vessels, or by stagnation of qi and blood that block the meridians, prevent the flow of qi and blood and lead to dysfunction of the tendons and vessels.

5. 13. 1 Syndrome differentiation

Pain in the shoulder radiating to the neck and back, aggravated at night or by movement of the shoulder, limitation of the active and passive movements of the shoulder joints in all directions, especially of the abduction, extorsion and backward extension.

5. 13. 2 Treatment

(1) Body acupuncture.

[**Main acupoints**] Jianyu (LI 15), Jianliao (TE 14), Jianzhen (SI 9),

Binao (LI 14) , *Ashi* acupoints and Tiaokou (ST 38) .

[**Supplementary acupoints**] For pain of the anterior aspect of the shoulder, Hegu (LI 4) , Quchi (LI 11) and Zusanli (ST 36) . For pain of the lateral aspect of the shoulder and over scapula, Houxi (SI 3) , Waiguan(SJ 5) ,Tianzong (SI 11) and Yanglingquan (GB 34) . For pain involving the back ,Quyuan (SI 13) and Tianzong(SI 11) are added.

[**Method**] Several acupoints are selected each time according to the pathological conditions. Reducing method can be used. First puncture Tiaokou (ST 38) localed on the contralateral side of affected side with the point of the needle pointing to the direction of Chengshan(BL 57) and the patient is asked to move the shoulder joint during the manipulation of the needle. Moxibustion can be used in addition and cupping may be applied for reinforcement of the curative effect.

(2) Electro-acupuncture.

[**Selection of acupoints**] Jianyu (LI 15) , Jianliao (TE 14) , Jianzhen (SI 9) , Quchi(LI 11) and *Ashi* acupoints.

[**Method**] Each time 1 ~ 2 acupoint are selected. When needling sensation is felt, impulse current is attached to the needles for 10 minutes. This treatment is given once a day.

5. 14 Herpes zoster

Herpes zoster is clinically marked by clusters of blisters in the form of a belt in the areas distributing with peripheral nerves or certain part of skin and local burning pain. It usually appears on one side of the chest, face, eye, abdomen and thigh. TCM holds that it is caused by exogenous virulent wind, dampness and heat ,or by stagnant liver and gallbladder fire that fumigates meridians and skin with damp-heat in the spleen meridian. Prolonged stagnation of pathogenic factors in the meridians, unsmooth circulation of *qi* and blood and retention of blood stasis in the meridians may lead to lingering local pain.

5. 14. 1 Syndrome differentiation

In the early period there is pricking pain in the affected part and redness of local skin, then followed by clusters of macules, sudden appearance of blisters in the form of belt and severe pain. It may be accompanied by mild fever, general discomfort and anorexia. After 2 ~ 3 weeks, scab is gradually formed and exfoliates without any scar. In a few cases pain may linger for a longer time.

5. 14. 2 Treatment

(1) Body acupuncture.

[**Main acupoints**] Local *Ashi* acupoints and corresponding Jiaji points.

[**Supplementary acupoints**] For the stagnated fire in liver meridian, Taichong(LR 3) , Xingjian(LR 2) and Xiaxi(GB 43) are added. For the accumulated dampness heat in spleen and stomach, Yinlingquan(SP 9) , Neiting (ST 44) and Xuehai(SP 10) are added. For fever, Dazhui(GV 14) is added. For herpes zoster on the chest and hypochondria, Zhigou(TE 6) , Qimen(LR 14) , Geshu(BL 17) and Ganshu(BL 18) are added.

[**Method**] Reducing method is required to apply. More needles can be used to perform surrounded needling in the local area of pathological changes. Moxibustion can also be used. The three-edged needle is used to thrust 4 or 5 times 0. 5 *cun* away from both ends and several times more on both sides of the eruption according to its extent, slightly bleeding is given, then cupping is used.

(2) Ear acupuncture.

[**Selection of acupoints**] Reaction points, Ear Shenmen (TF_4) , lung (CO_{14}) , Liver(CO_{12}) , Subcortex(AT_4) and Adrenal Gland(TG_{2p}).

[**Method**] 2 ~ 3 points are selected each time, strong stimulation with retaining needle for 20 ~ 30 minutes.

5. 15 Sprain of soft tissues of the limbs

Sprain of soft tissues of the limbs refers to the sprain of the muscles, tendons and ligaments around the shoulders, elbows, hip joints, knees and ankles due to twisting or pulling without fracture, dislocation and contusion of the skin. The clinical manifestations are swelling, pain and dysfunction of the joints. This problem pertains to the improper exertion or falling and contusion that impair tendons and joints and result in stagnation of *qi* and blood in the local region and obstruction of meridians and collaterals.

5. 15. 1 Syndrome differentiation

The main manifestations are swelling, pain, dysfunction of the joints and cyanotic color of local skin. If there are signs of protrusive swelling and unsmooth movement of the joints, the sprain is severe.

5. 15. 2 Treatment

(1) Body acupuncture.

[**Main acupoints**] Local *Ashi* acupoints.

[**Supplementary acupoints**] For the treatment of the shoulders, Jianyu (LI 15), Jianliao(TE 14), Jianjing(GB 21) are added. For the treatment of the elbows, Quchi(LI 11), Xiaohai(SI 8) and Tianjing(TE 10) are added. For the treatment the wrist, Yangchi(TE 4), Yangxi(LI 5), Yanggu(SI 5) and Waiguan(TE 15) are added. For the treatment of hip joints, Huantiao(GB 30), Zhibian(BL 54) and Chengfu(EX-LE 5), Liangqiu(ST 34), Xiyangguan(GB 33) and Yanglingquan(GB 34) are added. For the treatment the ankles, Jiexi(ST 41), Kunlun(BL 60) and Qiuxu(GB 40) are added.

[**Method**] Reducing needling technique is used. local acupoints can be moxibusted or applied with cupping.

(2) Ear acupuncture.

[**Selection of acupoints**] Reaction points and Ear Shenmen(TF$_4$).

[**Method**] Medium and strong stimulation is required, the needles are retainde for 20 ~ 30 minutes and the needling is done once a day. For the treatment of old wound, Wangbuliuxingzi(semen vaccariae) can be used for ear acupressure.

5. 16 Dysmenorrhea

Dysmenorrhea refers to abdominal pain during or before and after mensturuation, usually affecting normal work and daily life. It is either primary dysmenorrhea or functional dysmenorrhea marked by no evident changes of the genitalia or secondary dysmenorrhea due to organic pathological changes of the genitalia. The clinical manifestations are mainly lower abdominal pain or lumbago before and after or during menstruation, even unbearable pain and regular occurrence with menstrual cycle. This disease usually caused by stagnation of liver *qi*, inhibition of blood flow or attack by cold during menstruation and unsmooth circulation of *qi* and blood, or by malnutrition of the uterine meridian due to deficiency of *qi* and blood as well as liver and kindey.

5. 16. 1 Syndrome differentiation

(1) Coagulation of cold-dampness: cold pain in the lower abdomen before or during menstruation, rejection to pressure and preference for warmth, unsmooth and scanty menorrhea with purplish and blackish clot, accompanied by cold body and limbs, aching joints, whitish greasy tongue fur, deep and tense pulse.

(2) *Qi* stagnation and blood stasis: distending pain in the lower abdomen before or during menstruation, unsmooth and scanty menorrhea with purplish and blackish clot, accompanied by distension in the chest, hypochondria and brest, purplish tongue or with ecchymoses, deep and taut pulse.

(3) Insufficiency of *qi* and blood: vague pain in the lower abdomen during or after menstruation, preference for pressure, light-colored and thin menorrhea, accompanied by pale complexion, lassitude, dizziness, light-colored tongue and weak pulse.

(4) Deficiency of both the liver and kidney: vague pain in the lower ab-

domen after menstruation, irregular menstruation, profuse or scanty menorrhea with light-red color and no blood clot, accompanied by aching and weakness of the loins and knees, restlessed sleep in the night, dizziness and tinnitus, reddish tongue with scanty fur and thin pulse.

5. 16. 2 Treatment

(1) Body acupuncture.

[**Main acupoints**] Zhongji(CV 3) , Ciliao(BL 32) and Sanyinjiao(SP 6).

[**Supplementary acupoints**] For coagulation of cold-dampness,
Guanyuan(CV 4) and Shuidao (ST 28) are added with heavy and frequent
moxibustion. For *qi* stagnation and blood stasis, Taichong(LR 3) and Xuehai
(SP 10) are added. For insufficiency of *qi* and blood, Pishu(BL 20) and Zu-
sanli(ST 36) are added. For deficiency of both the liver and kidney, Ganshu
(BL 18) , Shenshu(BL 23) and Taixi(KI 3) are added.

[**Method**] The teratment begins 3 ~ 5 days before menstruation. Ciliao
(BL 32) is needle 1. 5 *cun* into the posterior sacral foramen obliquely toward
the spinal column with reducing method and repeated manipulation to enable
warm sensation to transmit to the lower abdomen. Zhongji(CV 3) is needled
(urination is done first) obliquely downward to enable needling sensation to
transmit to the lower region. Sanyinjiao(SP 6) is needled obliquely upward to
enable needling sensation to transmit to the upper region. For the treatment of
coagulation of cold-dampness, reducing method can be used and local acupoints are dealt with needle-warming moxibustion or moxa-roll moxibustion.
For *qi* stagnation and blood stasis, reducing method is used and no moxibustion is applied. For insufficiency of *qi* and blood as well as deficiency of the
liver and kidney, reinforcing method is used with the addition of moxibustion.

(2) Ear acupuncture.

[**Selection of acupoints**] Internal Genitalia (TF_2) , Subcortex (AT_4) ,
Sympathetic Nerve (AG_{6a}) , Endocrine (CO_{18}) , Liver (CO_{12}) and Kidney

(CO_{10}).

［**Method**］Each time 2 ~ 4 acupoints are needled with medium and strong stimulation. Or Wangbuliuxingzi(senmen vaccariae)is used for ear acupressure alternatively on both ears, 3 ~4 times a day. The treatment begins 3 days before menstruation to prevent relapse.

5. 17 Insufficiency of lactation

Lactation starts in the gravida 2 or 3 days after the delivery. If there is insufficient lactation or even total absence of lactation, it is known as hypogalactia. It is caused by deficiency of *qi* and blood which results from weak constitution with deficiency of spleen and stomach or from large amounts of bleeding during delivery the baby, or due to mental upsets and stagnation of liver *qi* that lead to obstruction of milk collaterals and blockage of *qi* and blood as well as little milk to be secreted.

5. 17. 1 Syndrome differentiation

(1)Deficiency of *qi* and blood.

Little milk or no milk, no distention of the breast, pale face, poor appetite, short of breath, loose stool, pale lip and nails, pale tongue, thready pulse.

(2)Liver *qi* stagnation.

It is difficult to secrete milk with distention and pain in the breast, unstaube emotionally, fullness in the chest, constipation, scanty and yellow urine.

5. 17. 2 Treatment

［**Main acupoints**］Rugen (ST 18), Tanzhong (CV 17), Shaoze (SI 1).

［**Supplementary acupoints**］For liver *qi* stagnation, Qimen (L 14) and Taichong (LR 3) are added. For deficiency of *qi* and blood, Pishu (BL 20), Zusanli (ST 36)and sanyinjiao(SP 6)are added.

［**Method**］Shaoze(SI 1)is pricked to let blood. Reinforcing by needle and moxibustion is used for deficiency of *qi* and blood, and reducing method by needle for liver *qi* stagnation.

5. 18 Malposition of fetus

Malposition of fetus refers to the abnormal position of the fetus in uterus, such as occipitoposterior, breech presentation or transverse position, after thirty weeks of conception. It is made known by prenatal examination and usually seen in multiparas or those with lax abdominal wall. It commonly occurs to those women of multiple pregnancies and abdominal muscle weakness.

5. 18. 1 Treatment

[**Main acupoints**] Zhiyin (BL 67).

[**Method**] Moxibustion with moxa sticks is applied to Zhiyin (BL 67) bilaterally for 15 ~ 20 minutes while the pregnant woman sits in chair or lies supinely in bed with the belt loosened. Give the treatment once or twice every day till the fetal position is corrected.

5. 19 Infantile enuresis

Infantile enuresis refers to involuntary and recurrent urination during sleep among infants over there years old. Enuresis may occur once in several days in mild cases and every night in serious cases, accompanied by lassitude and emaciation. According to TCM, infantile enuresis is caused by insufficiency of *kidney-qi* which fails to consolidate the bladder, or by deficiency of lung and spleen-*qi* that fails to govern the lower energizer, or by stagnation of dampness heat in the liver meridian and disorder of the bladder in transforming *qi*.

5. 19. 1 Syndrome differentiation

(1) Insufficiency of kidney *yang*: the symptoms are enuresis during sleep even several times a night, clear and profuse urine, dispiritedness and lassitude, whitish complexion and cold limbs, aching and weakness of the loins

and knees, hypomnesis or poor mentality, light-colors tongue and thin pulse.

(2) Deficiency of spleen and *lung-qi*: the symptoms are enuresis during sleep, aggravation after fatigue, profuse and frequent urination, frequent spontaneous sweating, poor appetite, shortness of breath and no desire to speak, weakness of limbs loose stool, light-colored tongue and thin pulse.

5. 19. 2 Treatment

[**Main acupoints**] Guanyuan(CV 4), Zhongji(CV 3), Baihui (GV 20), Sanyinjiao(SP 6) and Pangguangshu(BL 28).

[**Supplementary acupoints**] For insufficiency of kidney *yang*, Shenshu (BL 23) and Mingmen(GV 4) are added. For deficiency of spleen and lung-*qi*, Pishu(BL 20), Feishu(BL 13), *qi*hai(CV 6) and Zusanli(ST 36) are added.

[**Method**] The acupoints are needle with filiform needles and reinforcing method or warmed needle or moxibustion with moxa-roll. Guanyuan (CV 4) and Zhongji(CV 3) are needled, after urination, obliquely downward with rotation of the needle for reinforcing purpose. Sanyinjiao(SP 6) is needled obliquely upward to direct the needling sensation to transmit upwards.

5. 20 Swelling and pain of eye

Swelling and pain of eye is an acute condition in various external eye disorders. The main symptoms are redness of the eye, swelling of the eyelids and pain of the eye. It is usually caused by retention of exogenous windheat in the meridians and stagnation of fire, or by exuberant liver and gallbladder fire attacking the eyes along the meridians.

5. 20. 1 Syndrome differentiation

(1) Exogenous pathogenic windheat: redness and swelling of eyes, photophobia and epiphora, excessive secretion of eyes, accompanied by headache, fever, red tongue with yellow coating and rapid pulse.

(2) Exuberance of liver and gallbladder fire: redness and swelling of eyes, photophobia and epiphora, excessive secretion of eyes, accompanied by bitter taste in the mouth, dry throat, dysphoria, constipation, red tongue with yellow coating, taut and rapid pulse.

5. 20. 2 Treatment

(1) Body acupuncture.

[**Main acupoints**] *Taiyang*(EX-HN 5), Jingming(BL 1), Fengchi(GB 20), Taichong(LR 3) and Hegu(LI 4).

[**Supplementary acupoints**] For exogenous pathogenic windheat, Shangxing(GV 23) and Quchi(LI 11) are added. For exuberance of liver and gallbladder fire, Xingjian(LR 2) and Xiaxi(GB 43) are added.

[**Method**] The acupoints are needled with filiform needles and reducing method. Moxibustion is not used. *Taiyang* (EX-HN 5) and Shangxing (GV 23) are pricked for bloodletting.

(2) Pricking Method.

This method can be on the tender point between two scapulars or on the points with 0. 5 *cun* lateral to Dazhui(GV 14). This method is used for acute conjunctivitis.

5. 21 Tinnitus and deafness

Tinnitus and deafness are two symptoms arising from auditory disturbance. Tinnitus is characterized by spontaneous ringing sound, and deafness is failing or less of hearing. Because of the similarities between these two conditions in etiology and treatment, they are discussed together. They are usually caused by upward rush of fire of the liver and gall bladder which obstructs *Shaoyang* meridians or by pathogenic wind evil blocking ear orifice, or by deficiency of kidney essence which fails to nourish the ears.

5. 21. 1 Syndrome differentiation

(1) Excess syndrome: sudden deafness, distended sensation and const-

sant ringing in the ear can not be eliminated by pressing the ear. In the case of excess fire of liver-gallbladder, there are distention in the head, flushed face, sore throat, irritability and bad temper and taut pulse. In the case of invasion of exogenous wind, there are adversion to cold and fever, superficial pulse.

(2) Deficiency syndrome: hard hearing afterchronic disease, intermittent tinnitus aggravated by strain and eliminated by pressing the ear, dizziness, soreness and aching of the loin, thin and rapid pulse.

5. 21. 2 Treatment

[**Main acupoints**] Yingfeng (TE 17), Tinghui (GB 2), Tinggong(SI 19), Zhongzhu (SJ 3).

[**Supplementary acupoints**] For excess fire of liver and gallbladder, Taichong (LR 3), Xiaxi(GB 43) are added. For invasion of exogenous wind, Waiguan (SJ 5), Hegu (LI 4) are added. For deficiency of kidney essence, Shenshu (BL 23) and Taixi(KI 3) are added.

[**Method**] Reducing method is used for excess syndrome. Reinforcing method is used for deficiency syndrome.

5. 22 Sore throat

Sore throat is a disease which is redness and sore in throat as well as discomfort swallowing. It is usually caused by sudden change of weather, weakness of defensive *qi*, invasion of pathogenic wind-heat into the lung meridian and retention of pathogenic wind-heat in the throat, or by deficiency of both the lung and kidney, failure of *yin* fluid to nurish the throat and hyperactivity of deficiency fire.

5. 22. 1 Syndrome differentiation

Pathogenic windheat: reddish swelling of the throat, difficult in swallowing, cough, accompanied by fever, headache, superficial and rapid pulse.

Excessive heat of lung and stomach: reddish swelling of the throat, difficult in swallowing, thirst, constipation, brown urine, red tongue, yellow tongue coating and full pulse.

Yin deficiency of lung and kidney: discomfort in the throat, dryness and mild pain in the throat, dry cough, feverish sensation in the palms and soles, reddish tongue with scanty coating and tihin and rapid pulse.

5. 22. 2 Treatment

(1) Excess syndrome.

[**Main acupoints**] Shaoshang(LU 11) and Lianquan(CV 23).

[**Supplementary acupoints**] For pathogenic wind-heat, Guanchong (SJ 1) and Hegu(LI 4) are added. For excessive heat of lung and stomach, Yuji(LU 10) and Neiting(ST 44) are added.

[**Method**] Shaoshang (LU 11) is pricked with three-edged needle for bloodletting. Other acupoints can be used reducing method.

(2) Deficiency syndrome.

[**Main acupoints**] Lianquan (CV 23), Yuji (LU 10), Taixi (KI 3) and Zhaohai(KI 6).

[**Supplementary acupoints**] For tidal fever and night sweating, Yinxi (HT 6) , Sanyinjiao(SP 6) and Fuliu(KI 7) are added.

[**Method**] The main acupoints are needled with mild reinforcing and reducing method while the compatible acupoints are needled with reinforcing technique. No moxibustion is applied.

5. 23 Simple obesity

Simple obesity refers to accumulation of fat in the body due to changes of the biochemical and physiological functions except those of endogenous and hereditary factors. Clinically body weight increase by 20% more than the standard lever is regarded as obesity, usually accompanied by abnormal changes of appetite and sleep, sweating, dry mouth and disorder of stool. TCM believes that obesity is mainly due to disorder of the spleen.

5. 23. 1 Syndrome differentiation

(1) Heat in the stomach and intestines: hyperorexia, polyphagia, dry mouth irritability and susceptibility to rage, constipation, brown urine, red tongue with yellow and greasy coating, slippery and powerful pulse.

(2) Deficiency of spleen and stomach-*qi*: pale complexion, poor appetite, abdominal distension after meal, spiritual lassitude, loose stool, light-colored tongue with tooth prints, thin and white tongue coating, thin and slow pulse.

(3) *Yang* deficiency of spleen and kidney: bright-white complexion, normal appetite or reduced appetite, dizziness and aching loins, aversion to cold and edema of limbs, often accompanied by irregual menstruation in women and impotence in men, light-colored tongue with tooth prints, scanty tongue coating, deep thin and weak pulse.

5. 23. 2 Treatment

(1) Body acupuncture.

[**Main acupoints**] Zhongwan(CV 12), Tianshu(ST 25), Quchi(LI 11), Yinlingquan(SP 9), Fenglong(ST 40) and Taichong(LR 3).

[**Supplementary acupoints**] For heat in the stomach and intestinse. Hegu(LI 4), Zusanli(ST 36) and Neiting(ST 44) are added. For deficiency of stomach and spleen-*qi*, Pishu(BL 20), Weishu(BL 21), Zusanli(ST 36) and Taibai(SP 3) are added. For *yang* deficiency of spleen and kidney, Qihai (CV 4), Guangyuan(CV 4), Shenshu (BL 23), Mingmen(GV 4) are added. For constipation, Tianshu (ST 25), Zhigou (TE 6) and Yanglingquan (GB 34) are added. For abdominal obesity, Guilai(ST 29), Xiawan(CV 10), Zhongji(CV 3) are added.

[**Method**] Heat in the stomach and intestines is treated with reducing method. Deficiency of spleen and stomach-*qi* or *yang* deficiency of spleen and kidney is treated with reinforcing or mild reinforcing and reducing method.

(2) Ear acupuncture.

[**Selection acupoints**] Hunger Point (External Nose) ($TG_{1,2i}$) , Mouth (CO_1) , Esophagus (CO_2) , Lung (CO_{14}) , Stomach (CO_4) , Endocrine (CO_{18}) and Pancreas and gallbladder(CO_{11}).

[**Method**] All the acupoints mentioned above are needled with filiform needles once every other day. For embedment of needles and ear pressure with Wangbuliuxingzi (semen vaccaria) , patients are advised to press themselves three times a day (in hunger, before meal and sleep) , each acupoint for 2 ~ 3 minutes. The two ears are pressed in alternation.

中国针灸

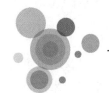

第一部分
中医学基础理论概要

学习掌握中医基础理论和中医诊断学的基本知识。

知识点目录

❖知识点 1　中医学理论体系的基本特点

❖知识点 2　阴阳学说

❖知识点 3　五行学说

❖知识点 4　脏象学说

❖知识点 5　气血理论

❖知识点 6　病因学说

❖知识点 7　中医四诊

❖知识点 8　辨证原则

知识点 1 中医学理论体系的基本特点

中医学是研究人体生理、病理、疾病的诊断与防治，以及摄生康复的一门传统医学科学，它有独具特色的理论体系。中医学理论体系的两大基本特点为整体观念和辨证论治。

1. 整体观念

中医学把人体内脏和体表各组织、器官看作一个有机的整体，同时认为四时气候、地土方宜、周围环境等因素对人体生理病理有不同程度的影响，既强调人体内部的统一性，又重视机体与外界环境的统一性。

1.1 人是一个有机整体

1.1.1 形体结构整体性——人体以五脏为中心，通过经络系统，把六腑、五体、五官、九窍、四肢百骸等全身组织器官有机地联系起来，构成一个表里相关、上下沟通、密切联系、协调共济、井然有序的统一整体。

1.1.2 生理机能的统一性——人体以五脏为中心，结构上不可分割，全身的组织器官在功能上相互为用。在五脏中，又以心为主宰，通过心与其他脏腑在功能上相互影响、配合。

1.1.3 病理变化的相关性——疾病变化的整体性是人有机整体性的另外一个表现和依据。脏腑病变既可相互影响，又可反映于体表，局部病理变化与整体病理反应密切相关。

1.1.4 疾病诊断的整体性——"四诊法"（望、闻、问、切）是中医诊病的基本方法。四诊是相互联系的，具体诊断疾病时需要"四诊合参"，这就是说，必须将四诊收集到的病情，进行综合分析，去粗取精，去伪存真，才能做出由表及里的全面的科学判断。

1.1.5 *疾病治疗的整体性*——人是一个有机的整体，临床治病必须从整体观念出发，不仅要重视局部，而且要重视全局。在方法上，既可通过治疗局部而影响全身，又可通过治疗全身而影响局部。

1.2 人与自然相统一

中医学认为，人是宇宙间的万物之一，与自然界息息相通，休戚相关。自然界的各种运动变化，如季节的更替、地域的差异等，都会直接或间接地影响到人体，而人体对这些影响，也必然相应地出现各种不同的生理活动或病理变化。人与自然有着统一的本原和属性，人产生于自然，人的生命活动必然受自然界规律的影响。人与自然的物质统一性决定生命和自然运动规律的统一性。

2. 辨证论治

辨证论治为辨证和论治的合称，既是中医学认识疾病和治疗疾病的基本原则，又是诊断和防治疾病的基本方法，是中医学术特点的集中表现，也是中医学理论体系的基本特点之一。

辨证即是认证、识证的过程。证是对机体在疾病发展过程中某一阶段病理反映的概括，包括病变的部位、原因、性质以及邪正关系，反映这一阶段病理变化的本质。所谓辨证，就是根据四诊所收集的资料，通过分析、综合，辨清疾病的病因、性质、部位，以及邪正之间的关系，概括、判断为某种性质的证。

论治又称施治，是根据辨证的结果，确定相应的治疗方法。辨证是决定治疗的前提和依据，论治是治疗的手段和方法。通过论治的效果可以检验辨证的正确与否。辨证论治是认识疾病和解决疾病的过程，是理论与实践相结合的体现，是理、法、方、药在临床上的具体运用，是指导中医临床工作的基本原则。

知识点 2　阴阳学说

中医学把阴阳学说应用于医学，形成了中医学的阴阳学说，促进了中医学理论体系的形成和发展。中医学的阴阳学说是中医学理论体系的基础之一和重要组成部分，是理解和掌握中医学理论体系的一把钥匙。中医学用阴阳学说阐明生命的起源和本质。人体的生理功能、病理变化、疾病的诊断和防治的根本规律，贯穿于中医的理、法、方、药。长期以来，阴阳学说一直有效地指导着临床实践。

1. 阴阳的医学含义

阴阳是相互关联的两种事物或是一个事物的两个方面。阴和阳的相对属性应用于医学，将人体中具有中空、外向、弥散、推动、温煦、兴奋、升举等特性的事物或现象统属于阳；具有实体、内守、凝聚、宁静、凉润、抑制、沉降等特性的事物或现象统属于阴。

中医学以水火为阴阳属性的标志，即水为阴，火为阳，称为阴阳之征兆。

2. 阴阳的相互作用

2.1 阴阳对立制约

对立是指处于一个统一体的矛盾双方的互相排斥、互相斗争。阴阳学说认为：阴阳双方的对立是绝对的，如天与地、上与下、内与外、动与静、升与降、出与入、昼与夜、明与暗、寒与热、虚与实、散与聚等等。阴阳两个方面的相互对立，主要表现于它们之间的相互制约、相互斗争。阴与阳相互制约和相互斗争的结果取得了统一，即取得了动态平衡。只有维持这种关系，事物才能正常发展变化，人体才能维持正常的生理状态；否则，事物的发展变化就会遭到破坏，人体就会发生疾病。

2.2 阴阳互根互用

互根指相互对立的事物之间的相互依存、相互依赖，任何一方都不能脱离另一方而单独存在。阴阳互根互用是阴阳之间的相互依存，互为根据和条件。阴阳双方均以对方的存在为自身存在的前提和条件。阳根于阴，阴根于阳，无阳则阴无以生，无阴则阳无以化。阳蕴含于阴之中，阴蕴含于阳之中。阴阳互根深刻地揭示了阴阳两个方面的不可分离性。阴阳互根是阴阳相互转化的内在根据。阴阳在一定条件下的相互转化，也是以它们的相互依存、相互为根的关系为基础的。

2.3 阴阳消长

消长乃增减、盛衰之谓。阴阳消长是阴阳对立双方的增减、盛衰、进退的运动变化。阴阳对立双方不是处于静止不变的状态，而是始终处于此盛彼衰、此增彼减、此进彼退的运动变化之中。其消长规律为阳消阴长，阴消阳长。阴阳双方在彼此消长的动态过程中保持相对的平衡，人体才得以保持正常的运动规律。

2.4 阴阳转化

转化即转换、变化，指矛盾的双方经过斗争，在一定条件下走向自己的反面。阴阳转化是指阴阳对立的双方，在一定条件下可以相互转化，阴可以转化为阳，阳可以转化为阴。阴阳转化是事物运动变化的基本规律。在阴阳消长过程中，事物由"化"至"极"，即发展到一定程度，超越了阴阳正常消长的阈值，事物必然向着相反的方面转化。阴阳的转化必须具备一定的条件，这种条件中医学称之为"重"或"极"。阴阳的消长（量变）和转化（质变）是事物发展变化全过程密不可分的两个阶段，阴阳消长是阴阳转化的前提，而阴阳转化则是阴阳消长的必然结果。

3. 阴阳学说在中医学中的应用

3.1 说明人体的组织结构

人体是一个有机整体，组成人体的所有脏腑、经络、形体、组织，既是有机联系的，又都可以根据其所在部位、功能特点划分为互相对立的阴阳两部分。

3.1.1 按解剖位置——人体的上半身为阳，下半身属阴；体表属阳，体内属阴；体表的背部属阳，腹部属阴；四肢外侧为阳，内侧为阴。

3.1.2 按脏腑功能——五脏为阴，六腑为阳。五脏之中，心肺为阳，肝脾肾为阴；心肺之中，心为阳，肺为阴；肝脾肾之间，肝为阳，脾肾为阴。而且每一脏之中又有阴阳之分，如心有心阴、心阳，肾有肾阴、肾阳，胃有胃阴、胃阳等。

3.1.3 经络分阴阳——在经络之中，也分为阴阳。经属阴，络属阳。而经之中有阴经与阳经，络之中又有阴络与阳络。

3.1.4 气血津液分阴阳——气为阳，血和津液为阴。

3.2 说明人体的生理功能

人体的生理功能是由贮藏和运行于脏腑、经络中的精和气为基础的。精藏于脏腑之中，主内守而属阴；气由精所化，运行于全身而属阳。精与气的相互产生、相互促进，维持了脏腑、经络、形体、官窍的功能活动稳定有序。人体维持正常的生理功能是体内阴阳动态平衡的结果。

3.3 说明人体的病理变化

疾病的发生发展过程就是邪正斗争的过程。邪正斗争导致阴阳失调,而出现各种各样的病理变化。无论外感病或内伤病,其病理变化的基本规律不外乎阴阳的偏盛或偏衰。

3.3.1 阴阳偏盛——阴盛和阳盛是属于阴阳任何一方高于正常水平的病变。

(1)阳盛则热:阳盛是病理变化中阳邪亢盛而表现出来的热的病变。阳邪致病,如暑热之邪侵入人体可造成人体阳气偏盛,出现高热、汗出、口渴、面赤、脉数等表现,其性质属热,所以称阳盛则热。

(2)阴盛则寒:阴盛是病理变化中阴邪亢盛而表现出来的寒的病变。阴邪致病,如纳凉饮冷,可以造成机体阴气偏盛,出现腹痛、泄泻、形寒肢冷、舌淡苔白、脉沉等表现,其性质属寒,所以称阴盛则寒。

3.3.2 阴阳偏衰——阴阳偏衰即阴虚、阳虚,是属于阴阳任何一方低于正常水平的病变。

(1)阳虚则寒:阳虚是人体阳气虚损,根据阴阳动态平衡的原理,阴或阳任何一方的不足,必然导致另一方相对的偏盛。阳虚不能制约阴,则阴相对偏盛而出现寒象。如机体阳气虚弱,可出现面色苍白、畏寒肢冷、神疲蜷卧、自汗、脉微等表现,其性质亦属寒,所以称阳虚则寒。

(2)阴虚则热:阴虚是人体的阴液不足。阴虚不能制约阳,则阳相对偏亢而出现热象。如久病耗阴或素体阴液亏损,可出现潮热、盗汗、五心烦热、口舌干燥、脉细数等表现,其性质亦属热,所以称阴虚则热。

临床上为了区别阳盛则热、阴盛则寒和阳虚则寒、阴虚则热,把阳盛则热称作实热,把阴虚则热称作虚热,把阴盛则寒称作实寒,把阳虚则寒称作虚寒。

3.4 用于指导辨证和临床诊断

由于阴阳偏盛偏衰是疾病过程中病理变化的基本规律,所以疾病的病理变化虽然错综复杂，千变万化，但其基本性质可以概括为阴和阳两大类。阴阳学说用于诊断学中，旨在分析通过四诊而收集来的临床资料和辨别证候。

四诊收集的色泽、声息、症状和脉象等临床信息经过区分，从而辨别证候的阴阳属性。阴阳是辨别证候的总纲，只有分清阴阳，才能抓住疾病的本质，对临床治疗具有重要的意义。

3.5 指导疾病治疗和用药

3.5.1 确定治疗原则

（1）阴阳偏盛的治疗原则：损其有余，实者泻之。阴阳偏盛，即阴或阳的过盛有余，为有余之证。阳盛则热属实热证，宜用寒凉药以制其阳，治热以寒，即"热者寒之"。阴盛则寒属寒实证，宜用温热药以制其阴，治寒以热，即"寒者热之"。因二者均为实证，所以称这种治疗原则为"损其有余"，即"实者泻之"。

（2）阴阳偏衰的治疗原则：补其不足，虚者补之。阴阳偏衰，即阴或阳的虚损不足，或为阴虚，或为阳虚。阴虚不能制阳而致阳亢者，属虚热证，治当滋阴以抑阳。若阳虚不能制阴而造成阴盛者，属虚寒证，治当扶阳以制阴。

3.5.2 归纳药物的性能

阴阳用于疾病的治疗，不仅用以确立治疗原则，而且也用来概括药物的性味功能，作为指导临床用药的依据。中药的性能是指药物具有四气、五味、升降浮沉的特性。四气（又称四性）有寒、热、温、凉。五味有酸、苦、甘、辛、咸。四气属阳，五味属阴。四气之中，温、热属阳；寒、凉属阴。五味之中，辛、甘属阳，酸、苦属阴。治疗疾病就是根据病情的阴阳偏盛偏衰，确定治疗原则，利用药物的阴阳偏性，选择相应的药物，从而达到纠正人体阴阳失衡，治疗疾病的目的。

知识点 3　五行学说

五行学说是中国古代的一种朴素的唯物主义哲学思想。五行学说认为宇宙间的一切事物都是由木、火、土、金、水五种物质元素所组成，自然界各种事物和现象的发展变化都是这五种物质不断运动和相互作用的结果。中医学把五行学说应用于医学领域，以系统结构观点来观察人体，阐述人体局部与局部、局部与整体之间的有机联系，以及人体与外界环境的统一，加强了中医学整体观念的论证。五行学说主要用于阐明五脏病机传变规律，揭示机体内部与外界环境的动态平衡的调节机制，揭示生理与疾病、疾病的诊断和防治的规律。

1. 五行的释义

"五"，是木、火、土、金、水五种物质；"行"，四通八达，流行和行用之谓，是行动、运动的古义，即运动变化，运行不息的意思。五行是指木、火、土、金、水五种物质的运动变化和相互作用。

2. 五行学说的含义

五行学说是以木、火、土、金、水五种物质的功能属性来归纳事物和现象的属性，并以五者之间相互促进、相互制约的关系来论述和推演事物之间的相互关系及复杂的运动变化规律的一种古代哲学思想。五行学说在中医学的应用主要是以五行的特性来分析归纳人体脏腑、经络、形体、官窍等组织器官和精神情志等各种功能活动，构建以五脏为中心的生理病理系统，进而与自然环境相联系，建立天人一体的五脏系统，并以五行的生克制化规律来分析五脏之间的生理联系，以五行的乘侮和母子相及规律来阐释五脏病机传变的相互影响，从而指导疾病的诊断和防治。

木曰曲直：曲直是指树木的枝条具有生长、柔和、能屈又能伸的特性——引申为凡具有生长、升发、条达、舒畅等性质或作用的事物和现象，归属于木；火曰炎上：炎上是指火具有炎热、上升、光明的特性——引申为凡具有温热、上升、光明等性质或作用的事物和现象，归属于火；土爰稼穑：稼穑泛指人类种植和收获谷物的农事活动——引申为凡具有养育、生化、承载、受纳性质或作用的事物和现象，归属于土；金曰从革：金有刚柔相济之性，金之质地虽刚硬，可作兵器以杀戮，但也有随人意而更改的柔和之性——引申为凡具有沉降、肃杀、收敛等性质或作用的事物和现象，归属于金；水曰润下：润下是指水具有滋润、下行的特性——引申为凡具有滋润、下行、寒凉、闭藏等性质或作用的事物和现象，归属于水。

由此可以看出，中医学上所说的五行不是指木、火、土、金、水这五种具体物质本身，而是五种物质不同属性的抽象概括。

3. 事物五行属性划分

五行学说根据五行特性，与自然界的各种事物或现象相类比，运用归类和推演等方法，将其最终分成五大类。

表 1 - 3 - 1　自然界事物的五行属性划分

自然界事物						五行属性
五音	五味	五色	五化	五气	五季	
角	酸	青	生	风	春	木
徵	苦	赤	长	暑	夏	火
宫	甘	黄	化	湿	长夏	土
商	辛	白	收	燥	秋	金
羽	咸	黑	藏	寒	冬	水

表 1 - 3 - 2 人体结构的五行属性划分

人体结构							五行属性
五脏	五腑	五官	五志	五体	五液	五脉	
肝	胆	目	怒	筋	泪	弦脉	木
心	小肠	舌	喜	脉	汗	洪脉	火
脾	胃	口	思	肉	涎	缓脉	土
肺	大肠	鼻	悲	皮	涕	浮脉	金
肾	膀胱	耳(二阴)	恐(惊)	骨	唾	沉脉	水

4. 五行的调节机制

五行正常的调节机制为相生相克，五行异常的调节机制是相侮相乘。

4.1 五行正常的调节机制 （生克制化）

4.1.1 相生规律：相生即递相产生、助长、促进之意。五行之间互相产生和促进的关系称作五行相生。五行相生的次序：木生火，火生土，土生金，金生水，水生木。

4.1.2 相克规律：相克即相互制约、克制、抑制之意。五行之间相互制约的关系称为五行相克。五行相克的次序：木克土，土克水，水克火，火克金，金克木。这种克制关系也是往复无穷的。

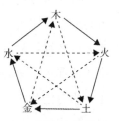

五行生克示意图
——▶代表相生
·····▶代表相克

在上述生克关系中，任何一行皆有"生我"和"我生"，"克我"和"我克"四个方面的关系。以木为例，"生我"者水，"我生"者火；"克我"者金，"我克"者土。

4.1.3 制化规律：五行中的制化关系是五行生克关系的结合。相生与相克是不可分割的两个方面。没有生，就没有事物的发生和成长；没有克，就不能维持正常协调关系下的变化与发展。因此，必须生中有克（化中有制），克中有生（制中有化），相反相成，才能维持和促进事物相对平衡协调和发展变化。五行之间这种生中有制、制中有生、相互生化、相互制约的生克关系，称为制化。其规律：木克土，土生金，金克木；火克金，金生水，水克火；土克水，水生木，木克土；金克木，木生火，火克金；水克火，火生土，土克水。

4.2 五行的异常调节机制 （乘侮胜复）

4.2.1 相乘规律：乘，即乘虚侵袭之意。相乘即相克太过，超过正常制约的程度，使事物之间失去了正常的协调关系。五行之间相乘的次序与相克同，但被克者更加虚弱。

4.2.2 相侮规律：侮，即欺侮，有恃强凌弱之意。相侮是指五行中的任何一行本身太过，使原来克它的一行，不仅不能去制约它，反而被它所克制，即反克，又称反侮。

4.3 五行学说在中医学中的应用

4.3.1 说明脏腑的生理功能及其相互关系

说明脏腑的生理功能：五行学说将人体的内脏分别归属于五行，以五行的特性来说明五脏的部分生理功能。木性可曲可直，条顺畅达，有生发的特性，故肝喜条达而恶抑郁，有疏泄的功能；火性温热，其性炎上，心属火，故心阳有温煦之功；土性敦厚，有生化万物的特性，脾属土，脾有消化水谷，运送精微，营养五脏、六腑、四肢百骸之功，为气血生化之源；金性清肃，收敛，肺属金，故肺具清肃之性，肺气有肃降之能；水性润下，有寒润、下行、闭藏的特性，肾属水，故肾主闭藏，有藏精、主水等功能。

说明脏腑之间的相互关系：中医五行学说对五脏五行的分属，不仅阐明了五脏的功能和特性，而且还运用五行生克制化的理论，来说明脏腑生理功能的内在联系。五脏之间既有相互产生的关系，又有相互制约的关系。用五行相生说明脏腑之间的联系：如木生火，即肝木济心火，肝藏血，心主血脉，肝藏血功能正常有助于心主血脉功能的正常发挥；用五行相克说明五脏间的相互制约关系：如心属火，肾属水，水克火，即肾水能制约心火，如肾水上济于心，可以防止心火之亢烈。

4.3.2 说明五脏病变的传变规律

由于人体是一个有机整体，内脏之间又是相互产生、相互制约的，因而在病理上必然相互影响。本脏之病可以传至他脏，他脏之病也可以传至本脏，这种病理上的相互影响称为传变。从五行学说来说明五脏病证的传变，可以分为相生关系传变和相克关系传变。

（1）相生关系传变：包括"母病及子"和"子病犯母"两个方面。

母病及子：系病邪从母脏传来，侵入属子之脏，先有母脏的病变，后有子脏的病变。如水不涵木，即肾阴虚不能滋养肝木，其临床表现在肾，则为肾阴不足，多见耳鸣、腰膝酸软、遗精等；临床表现在肝则为肝之阴血不足，多见眩晕、消瘦、乏力、肢体麻木，或手足蠕动，甚则震颤抽掣等。肾属水，肝属木，水能生木。若水不生木，其病由肾及肝，由母传子。由于相生的关系，病情虽有发展，但互相产生作用不绝，病情较轻。

子病犯母：系病邪从子脏传来，侵入属母之脏，即先有子脏的病变，后有母脏的病变。如心火亢盛而致肝火炽盛，有升无降，最终导致心肝火旺。心属火，肝属木，木能生火。肝为母，心为子，其病由心及肝，由于传母，病情较重。

（2）相克关系传变：包括"相乘"和"反侮"两个方面。

相乘是相克太过为病，如木旺乘土，又称木横克土。木旺乘土，即肝木克伐脾胃，先有肝的病变，后有脾胃的病变。由于肝气横逆，疏泄太过，影响脾胃，导致消化机能紊乱。木旺乘土，除了肝气横逆的病变外，往往是脾气虚弱和胃失和降的病变同时存在。肝属木，脾（胃）属土，木能克土，木气有余，相克太过，其病由肝传脾（胃）。病邪从相克方向传来，侵犯被克脏器。

相侮，又称反侮，是反克为害。如木火刑金，由于肝火偏旺，影响肺气清肃，临床表现既有胸胁疼痛、口苦、烦躁易怒、脉弦数等肝火过旺之证，又有咳嗽、咳痰，甚或痰中带血等肺失清肃之候。肝病在先，肺病在后。肝属木，肺属金，金能克木，今肝木太过，反侮肺金，其病由肝传肺。

4.3.3 用于指导疾病的诊断和治疗

（1）指导疾病的诊断

人体是一个有机整体，当内脏有病时，人体内脏功能活动及其相互关系的异常变化，可以反映到体表相应的组织器官，出现色泽、声音、形态、脉象等诸多方面的异常变化。由于五脏与五色、五音、五味等都以五行分类归属形成了一定的联系，这种五脏系统的层次结构，为诊断和治疗奠定了理论基础。因此，在临床诊断疾病时，就可以综合望、闻、问、切四诊所得的信息，根据五行的所属及其生克乘侮的变化规律来推断病情。

（2）指导疾病的治疗

五行学说不仅用以说明人体的生理活动和病理现象，综合四诊，推断病情，而且也可以根据五行生克规律确定治疗原则和治疗方法。如"补母和泻子法""滋水涵木法""培土生金法"等。

知识点 4　脏象学说

脏象学说的基本概念：脏象，原作臆象、藏象。脏，指隐藏于体内的脏器。象，其义有二，其一指脏腑的解剖形态；其二指脏腑的生理病理表现于外的征象。"象"是"脏"的外在反映，"脏"是"象"的内在本质，两者结合起来就叫作"脏象"。脏通"藏"。"藏象"今作"脏象"。脏象是人体系统现象与本质的统一体，是人体脏腑的生理活动及病理变化反映于外的征象。中医学据此作为判断人体健康和诊断、治疗疾病的依据。

根据生理功能特点，脏腑分为五脏、六腑和奇恒之腑三类。五脏：心、肺、脾、肝、肾；六腑：胆、胃、大肠、小肠、膀胱、三焦；奇恒之腑：脑、髓、骨、脉、胆、女子胞。

从形象上看，五脏属于实体性器官；从功能上看，五脏是主"藏精气"，即生化和贮藏气血、津液、精气等精微物质，主持复杂的生命活动。所以说："五脏者，藏精气而不泻也，故满而不能实。"（《素问·五脏别论》）满，指精气盈满；实，指水谷充实。满而不能实，就是说五脏贮藏的都是精气，而不是水谷或废料。从形象上看，六腑属于管腔性器官；从功能上看，六腑是主"传化物"，即受纳和腐熟水谷，传化和排泄糟粕，主要是对饮食物起消化、吸收、输送、排泄的作用。所以说："六腑，传化物而不藏，故实而不能满也。"（《素问·五脏别论》）六腑传导、消化饮食物，经常充盈水谷，而不贮藏精气。因传化不藏，故虽有积实而不能充满。奇恒之腑，形多中空，与腑相近，内藏精气，又类于脏，似脏非脏，似腑非腑，故称之为"奇恒之腑"。所以说："脑、髓、骨、脉、胆、女子胞，此六者，地气之所生也，皆藏于阴而象于地，故藏而不泻，名曰奇恒之腑。"（《素问·五脏别论》）脏象学说的内容主要为脏腑、形体和官窍等。其中，特别是以五脏为重点。五脏是生命活动的中心，六腑和奇恒之腑均隶属于五脏。因此，五脏理论是脏象学说中最重要的内容。

◆五脏系统

心、肺、脾、肝、肾称为五脏，加上心包络又称六脏。但习惯上把心包络附属于心，称五脏。五脏具有化生和贮藏精气的共同生理功能，同时又各有专司，且与躯体官窍有着特殊的联系，形成了以五脏为中心的特殊系统。其中，心的生理功能起着主宰生命活动的作用。

1. 心

心位于胸腔偏左，膈膜之上，肺之下，圆而下尖，形如莲蕊，外有心包卫护。心与小肠、脉、面、舌等构成心系统。心，在五行属火，为阳中之阳脏，主血脉，藏神志，为五脏六腑之大主，也为生命之主宰。心与四时之夏相通应。"心为君主之官，神明出焉。"（《素问·灵兰秘典论》）

1.1 心的生理功能

1.1.1 心主血脉

心主血脉，指心有主管血脉和推动血液循行于脉中的作用，包括主血和主脉两个方面。血就是血液。脉，既是脉管，又称经脉，为血之府，是血液运行的通道。心脏和脉管相连，形成一个密闭的系统，成为血液循环的枢纽。心脏不停地搏动，推动血液在全身脉管中循环无端，周流不息，成为血液循环的动力。

心主血脉的生理作用有二：一是行血以输送营养物质。心气推动血液在脉内循环运行，血液运载着营养物质以供养全身，使五脏六腑、四肢百骸、肌肉皮毛，甚至整个身体都获得充分的营养，以维持其正常的功能活动。二是生血，使血液不断地得到补充。胃肠消化吸收的水谷精微，通过脾主运化、升清散精的作用，上输给心肺，在肺部吐故纳新之后，贯注心脉变化而赤成为血液，故有"心生血"（《素问·阴阳应象大论》），"血生于心"（《质疑录》）之说。

心脏功能正常，则心脏搏动如常，脉象和缓有力，节律调匀，面色红润光泽。若心脏发生病变，则会通过心脏搏动、脉搏、面色等方面反映出来。如心气不足，血液亏虚，脉道不利，则血液不畅或血脉空虚，而见面色无华，脉象细弱无力等，甚则发生气血瘀滞，血脉受阻，而见面色灰暗，唇舌青紫，心前区憋闷和刺痛，脉象结、代、促、涩等。

1.1.2 心主神志

心主神志，即是心主神明，又称心藏神。心所主之神志，一般称之为狭义的神，是指人们的精神、意识、思维活动。

心藏神，为人体生命活动的中心。其生理作用有二：其一，主思维、意识、精神。在正常情况下，神明之心接受和反映客观外界事物，进行精神、意识、思维活动。其二，主宰生命活动。五脏六腑必须在心的统一指挥下，才能进行统一协调的生命活动。心为君主而脏腑百骸皆听命于心。心藏神而为神明之用。"心者，五脏六腑之大主也，精神之所舍也。"（《灵枢·邪客》）

1.2 心与五体、五官、九窍、情志的联系

1.2.1 在体合脉：脉是指血脉。心合脉是指全身的血脉都属于心，心有主管血脉和推动血液循行于脉中的作用。脉搏的形态可以反映心气的盛衰。

1.2.2 其华在面：华是光彩之义。其华在面指心的生理功能是否正常，可以显露于面部的面泽变化。心气旺盛，血脉充盈，面部红润有泽；心气不足，则可见面色白，晦滞；血虚则面色无华；血瘀则面色青紫。

1.2.3 开窍于舌：心开窍于舌指舌为心之外候，又称舌为"心之苗"。舌的功能是主司味觉和表达语言。舌的味觉功能和正确地表达语言有赖于心主血脉和心主神志的生理功能。心的阳气不足，则舌质淡白胖嫩；心的阴血不足，则舌质红绛瘦小；心火上炎则舌红，甚至生疮；若心血瘀阻，则舌质暗紫或有瘀斑；心主神志的功能异常，则出现舌

卷、舌强、语謇或失语。

1.2.4 在志为喜：心在志为喜指心的生理功能和精神情志的"喜"有关。喜，一般属于对外界刺激产生的良性反应，有益于心的生理功能。但喜乐过度，又可使心神涣散而不收，注意力难以集中，甚至可因为兴奋过度而诱发心疾，故有"喜伤心之说"。

2. 心包

心包是心脏外面的包膜，为心脏的外围组织。心包（络）与六腑中的三焦互为表里。由于心包（络）是心的外围组织，故有保护心脏，代心受邪的作用。脏象学说认为，心为君主之官，邪不能犯，所以外邪侵袭于心时，首先侵犯心包（络），故曰"诸邪之在于心者，皆在于心之包络"（《灵枢·邪客》）。实际上，心包受邪所出现的病变与心是一致的，故在辨证和治疗上也大体相同。

3. 肺

肺，位居胸中，左右各一，呈分叶状，质疏松。与心同居膈上，上连气管，通窍于鼻，与自然界之大气直接相通。与大肠、皮、毛、鼻等构成肺系统。在五行属金，为阳中之阴脏。主气司呼吸，助心行血，通调水道。肺与四时之秋相应。在五脏六腑中，位居最高，为五脏之长，故有"华盖"之称。肺脏娇嫩，不耐寒热燥湿诸气，称为"娇脏"。

3.1 肺的生理功能

3.1.1 肺主气

肺主气是肺主呼吸之气和肺主一身之气的总称。

（1）肺主呼吸之气

肺主呼吸之气是指肺通过呼吸运动，吸入自然界的清气，呼出体内的浊气，实现体内外气体交换的功能。肺为体内外气体交换的场所。肺吸入自然界的清气，呼出体内的浊气，实现了体内外气体的交换。通过不断地呼浊吸清，吐故纳新，促进气的生成，调节着气的升降出入运动，从而保证了人体新陈代谢的正常进行。

（2）肺主一身之气

肺主一身之气是指肺有主持、调节全身各脏腑之气的作用，即肺通过呼吸而参与气的生成和调节气机的作用。肺主一身之气的生理功能具体体现在两个方面：①气的生成作用：肺参与一身之气的生成，特别是宗气的生成。人体通过呼吸运动，把自然界的清气吸入于肺，又通过胃肠的消化吸收功能，把饮食物变成水谷精气，由脾气升清，上输于肺。自然界的清气和水谷精气在肺内结合，积聚于胸中的上气海（上气海，指膻中，位于胸中两乳之间，为宗气汇聚发源之处），便称之为宗气。②对全身气机的调节作用：所谓气机，泛指气的运动，升降出入为其基本形式。肺的呼吸功能是气的升降出入运动的具体体现。肺有节律地一呼一吸，对全身之气的升降出入运动起着重要的调节作用。

3.1.2 肺主宣肃

宣谓宣发，即宣通和发散之意。肃谓肃降，清肃下降之意。肺禀清虚之体，性主于降，以清肃下降为顺。肺宜清而宣降，其体清虚，其用宣降。宣发与肃降为肺气机升降出入运动的具体表现形式。肺位居上，既宣且降且以下降为主，方为其常。肺气必须在清肃宣降的情况下能保持其主气、司呼吸、助心行血、通调水道等正常的生理功能。

肺主宣发是指肺气向上升宣和向外布散的功能。其气机运动表现为升与出。其生理作用主要体现在三个方面：其一，吸清呼浊。经肺的呼吸，吸入自然界的清气，呼出体内的浊气；其二，输布津液精微。肺将脾所转输的津液和水谷精微，布散到全身，外达于皮毛，以温润、濡养五脏六腑、四肢百骸、肌腠皮毛；其三，宣发卫气。肺借宣发卫气，调节腠理之开阖，并将代谢后的津液化为汗液，由汗孔排出体外。因此，肺气失于宣散，则可出现呼吸困难、胸闷、咳嗽，以及鼻塞、喷嚏和无汗等症状。

肺主肃降是指肺气清肃、下降的功能，其气机运动形式为降与入。其生理作用除了利于肺的呼吸作用、输布津液精微之外，还有通调水道和清肃洁净的作用。肺主通调水道，肺为水之上源，肺气肃降则能通调水道，使水液代谢产物下输膀胱。肺司清肃洁净。肺的形质是"虚如蜂巢"，清轻肃净而不容异物。肺气肃降，则能肃清肺和呼吸道内的异物，以保持呼吸道的洁净。因此，肺气失于肃降，则可出现呼吸短促、喘促、咳痰等肺气上逆之候。

3.1.3 肺主行水

肺主行水是指肺的宣发和肃降对体内水液输布、运行和排泄的疏通与调节作用。由于肺为华盖，其位最高，参与调节体内水液代谢，所以说"肺为水之上源，肺气行则水行。"（《血证论·肿胀》）

人体内的水液代谢是由肺、脾、肾以及小肠、大肠、膀胱等脏腑共同完成的。肺主行水的生理功能是通过肺气的宣发和肃降来实现的。肺气宣发，一是使水液迅速向上向外输布，布散到全身，外达皮毛，"若雾露之溉"以充养、润泽、护卫各个组织器官；二是使经肺代谢后的水液，即被身体利用后的废水和剩余水分，通过呼吸、皮肤汗孔蒸发而排出体外。肺气肃降，使体内代谢后的水液不断地下行到肾，经肾和膀胱的气化作用，生成尿液而排出体外，保持小便的通利。

3.2 肺与五体、五官、九窍、情志的联系

3.2.1 在体合皮

皮指皮肤，是一身之表，具有防御外邪，调节体温和辅助呼吸的作用。肺气宣布卫气与体表皮肤，调节汗孔开阖，稳定体温，适应气候变化，抵御外邪，参与呼吸，排除浊气。肺气虚弱则汗孔开阖失司，出现多汗、少汗或者无汗的异常表现。肺气宣发卫气的功能异常则出现恶寒、发热等外感症状。

3.2.2 其华在毛

毛，也叫毫毛，常与皮肤统称为皮毛。肺气宣发肃降，输布精微物质以充养皮毛，则腠理固密，毫毛滋润有光泽。如果肺气虚弱，皮毛失于濡养则毫毛枯槁、稀疏。

3.2.3 开窍于鼻

鼻为呼吸之气出入的通道，鼻与喉相通而连于肺，故肺开窍于鼻，主司通气和嗅觉。喉为肺之门户，主司通气和发声。肺功能正常，则鼻窍通利，呼吸平稳，嗅觉灵敏。若肺失宣降，则可见鼻塞、流涕、喷嚏、咽痒、喑哑等。

3.2.4 在志为悲（忧）

悲忧为人体正常的情绪变化和情感反应。过度悲忧，则属于不良刺激，会造成肺气损伤，影响肺的宣发肃降功能，导致肺气不断虚耗，"悲则气消。"（《素问·举痛论》）

4. 脾

脾位于腹腔上部，膈膜之下，与胃以膜相连，"形如犬舌，状如鸡冠"，与胃、肉、唇、口等构成脾系统。主运化、统血、输布水谷精微，为气血生化之源，人体脏腑百骸皆赖以脾濡养，故有"后天之本"之称。在五行属土，为阴中之至阴。脾与四时之长夏相应。

4.1 脾的生理功能

4.1.1 脾主运化

运即转运输送；化即消化吸收。脾主运化，指脾具有将水谷化为精微，并将精微转输至全身各脏腑组织的功能。实际上，就是对营养物质的消化、吸收和运输的功能。脾主运化包括运化水谷和运化水湿两个方面。

脾运化水谷是指脾对饮食物的消化吸收作用。饮食物的消化和营养物质的吸收、转输，是在脾胃、肝胆、大小肠等多个脏腑共同参与下的一个复杂的生理活动，其中脾起主导作用。脾主运化水谷，包括了消化水谷、吸收转输精微并将精微转化为气血的重要生理作用。五脏六腑维持正常生理活动所需要的水谷精微，都有赖于脾的运化作用。由于饮食水谷是人出生之后维持生命活动所必需的营养物质的主要来源，也是生成气血的物质基础。饮食水谷的运化则是由脾所主，所以说脾为后天之本，气血生化之源。脾的运化功能强健，习惯上称作"脾气健运"。只有脾气健运，则机体的消化吸收功能才能健全，才能为化生气、血、津液等提供足够的养料，才能使全身脏腑组织得到充分的营养，以维持正常的生理活动。反之，若脾失健运，则机体的消化吸收功能便失常，就会出现腹胀、便溏、食欲不振以至倦怠、消瘦和气血不足等病证。

运化水湿又称运化水液，是指脾对水液的吸收和转输，调节人体水液代谢的作用，即脾配合肺、肾、三焦、膀胱等脏腑，调节、维持人体水液代谢平衡的作用。脾主运化水湿是调节人体水液代谢的关键环节。在人体水液代谢过程中，脾在运输水谷精微的同时，还把人体所需要的水液（津液）通过心肺而运送到全身各组织中去，以起到滋养濡润作用，又把各组织器官利用后的水液，及时地转输给肾，通过肾的气化作用形成尿液，送到膀胱，排泄于外，从而维持体内水液代谢的平衡。脾居中焦，为人体气机升降的枢纽，故在人体水液代谢过程中起着重要的调节作用。因此，脾运化水湿的功能健旺，既能使体内各组织得到水液的充分濡润，又不致使水湿过多而潴留。反之，如果脾运化水湿的功能失常，必然导致水液在体内的停滞，而产生水湿、痰饮等病理产物，甚则形成水肿。这也就是脾虚生湿、脾为生痰之源和脾虚水肿的发病机理。

4.1.2 脾主升清

升指上升和输布；清指精微物质。脾主升清是指脾具有将水谷精微等营养物质，吸收并上输于心、肺、头目，再通过心肺的作用化生气血，以营养全身，并维持人体内脏位置相对恒定的作用。如脾气不能升清，则水谷不能运化，气血生化无源，可出现神疲乏力、眩晕、泄泻等症状。脾气下陷（又称中气下陷）则可见久泄、脱肛甚或内脏下垂等。

4.1.3 脾主统血

统血，统是统摄、控制的意思。脾主统血指脾具有统摄血液，使之在经脉中运行而不溢于脉外的功能。脾统血是通过气摄血的作用来实现的。脾为气血生化之源，气为血帅，血随气行。脾的运化功能健旺，则气血充盈，气能摄血；气旺则固摄作用亦强，血液也不会溢出脉外而发生出血现象。反之，脾的运化功能减退，化源不足，则气血亏虚，气虚则统摄无权，血离脉道，从而导致出血。

4.2 脾与五体、五官、九窍、情志的联系

4.2.1 在体合肉，主四肢

肉，肌肉。脾气的运化功能与肌肉的壮实及其功能的发挥有密切的联系。脾气健运，则肌肉得以营养，肌肉发达有力，四肢灵活；脾气失运，则水谷精微化生无源，肌肉四肢失去濡养，则表现为肌肉四肢瘦削、软弱无力、倦怠，甚至痿废不用。

4.2.2 开窍于口

口是饮食物消化的开始。脾主运化，与饮食物消化密切相关，故开窍于口。饮食口味与脾的运化功能关系密切。脾气强健，脾胃经气通过经脉的联系，上输于口则口味正常，纳谷香甜；脾气虚弱，则食欲不振，口味异常，出现口淡无味、口黏、口甜等。

4.2.3 其华在唇

水谷精微上输于口，可以通过口唇的色泽反应脾气的强弱。脾气健运，则口唇色泽红润，感觉灵敏；如果脾气虚弱则口唇苍白、失润；如果脾胃湿热郁积，可以表现为口唇糜烂。

4.2.4 在志为思

思虑是正常的思维过程，脾气健运，气血充足，则思维活跃，记忆力强。但是，思虑过度则会耗气伤血，使得脾气郁滞，不思饮食，脘腹胀满。

5. 肝

肝位于腹部，横膈之下，右胁下而偏左。与胆、目、筋、爪等构成肝系统。主疏泄，喜条达而恶抑郁。在五行属木，为阴中之阳。肝与四时之春相应。肝脏的生理功能特点可以用"体阴而用阳"概括。肝为刚脏，以血为体，以气为用，体阴而用阳。肝为藏血之脏，血属阴，故肝体为阴；肝主疏泄，性喜条达，内寄相火，主升主动，故肝用为阳。

5.1 肝的生理功能

5.1.1 肝主疏泄

疏即疏通、疏导。泄即升发、发泄。肝主疏泄是指肝具有疏通、舒畅、条达以保持全身气机疏通畅达、通而不滞、散而不郁的作用。肝主疏泄是保证机体多种生理功能正常运转的重要条件。肝主疏泄在人体生理活动中的主要作用：

（1）调畅气机

肝主疏泄的生理功能，关系到人体全身的气机调畅。气机，即气的升降出入运动。升降出入是气化作用的基本形式。肝的疏泄功能，对全身各脏腑组织的气机升降出入之间的平衡协调，起着重要的疏通调节作用。

（2）促进消化吸收

肝主疏泄是保持脾胃正常消化吸收的重要条件。肝对脾胃消化吸收功能的促进作用是通过协调脾胃的气机升降和分泌、排泄胆汁而实现的。

　　胃气主降，受纳腐熟水谷以输送于脾；脾气主升，运化水谷精微以灌溉四旁。脾升胃降构成了脾胃的消化运动。肝的疏泄功能正常是保持脾胃升降枢纽能够协调不紊的重要条件。

　　胆附于肝，内藏胆汁，胆汁具有促进消化的作用。胆汁是肝之余气积聚而成。胆汁来源于肝，贮藏于胆，胆汁排泄到肠腔内，以助食物的消化吸收。肝的疏泄功能正常，则胆汁能正常地分泌和排泄，有助于脾胃的消化吸收功能。如果肝气郁结，影响胆汁的分泌和排泄，可导致脾胃的消化吸收障碍，出现胁痛、口苦、纳食不化，甚至黄疸等。

　　（3）调节精神情志

　　情感、情绪是指人类精神活动中以反映情感变化为主的一类心理过程。中医学的情志属狭义之神的范畴，包括喜、怒、忧、思、悲、恐、惊，亦称之为七情。肝通过其疏泄功能得以调畅气机，可调节人的精神情志活动。在正常生理情况下，肝的疏泄功能正常，肝气升发，既不亢奋，也不抑郁，舒畅条达，则人就能较好地协调自身的精神情志活动，表现为精神愉快，心情舒畅，理智清朗，思维灵敏，气和志达，血气和平。若肝失疏泄，则易于引起人的精神情志活动异常。疏泄不及，则表现为郁郁寡欢、多愁善感等；疏泄太过，则表现为烦躁易怒、头胀头痛、面红目赤等。

　　（4）调理冲任

　　妇女经、带、胎、产等特殊的生理活动，关系到许多脏腑的功能，其中肝脏的作用甚为重要，素有"女子以肝为先天"之说。妇女一生以血为重，由于行经耗血、妊娠血聚养胎、分娩出血等，无不涉及血，以致女子常有余于气而不足于血。冲为血海，任主胞胎，冲任二脉与女性生理机能休戚相关。肝为血海，冲任二脉与足厥阴肝经相通，而隶属于肝。肝主疏泄，可调节冲任二脉的生理活动。肝的疏泄功能正常，足厥阴经之气调畅，冲任二脉得其所助，则任脉通利，太冲脉盛，月经应时而下，带下分泌正常，妊娠孕育，分娩顺利。若肝失疏泄而致冲任失调，气血不和，从而引发月经、带下、胎产之疾，以及性功能异常和不孕等。

5.1.2 肝藏血生血

肝藏血是指肝脏具有贮藏血液、防止出血和调节血量的功能。肝有"血海"之称。

血液来源于水谷精微，生化于脾而藏受于肝。肝内贮存一定的血液，既可以濡养自身，以制约肝的阳气而维持肝的阴阳平衡、气血和调，又可以防止出血。因此，肝不藏血不仅可以出现肝血不足，阳气升腾太过，而且还可以导致出血。

调节血量。在正常生理情况下，人体各部分的血液量是相对恒定的。但是，人体各部分的血液，常随着不同的生理情况而改变。当机体活动剧烈或情绪激动时，人体各部分的血液需要量也就相应地增加，于是肝脏所贮藏的血液向机体的外周输布，以供机体活动的需要。当人们在安静休息及情绪稳定时，由于全身各部分的活动量减少，机体外周的血液需要量也相应减少，部分血液便归藏于肝。因肝脏具有贮藏血液和调节血量的作用，故肝有"血海"之称。

肝的疏泄与藏血之间的关系：肝主疏泄又主藏血。藏血是疏泄的物质基础，疏泄是藏血的功能表现。肝的疏泄全赖血之濡养作用，又赖肝之功能正常才能发挥其作用。所以肝的疏泄与藏血功能之间有着相辅相成的密切关系。就肝之疏泄对藏血而言，在生理上，肝主疏泄，气机调畅，则血能正常地归藏和调节。血液的运行不仅需要心肺之气的推动和脾气的统摄，而且还需要肝气的调节才能保证气机的调畅而使血行不致瘀滞。在病理上，肝失疏泄可以影响血液的归藏和运行。如肝郁气滞，气机不畅，则血亦随之而瘀滞，即由气滞而血瘀。若疏泄太过，肝气上逆，血随气逆，又可导致出血。就肝之藏血对疏泄而言，在生理上，肝主藏血，血能养肝，使肝阳勿亢，保证肝主疏泄的功能正常。在病理上，肝之藏血不足或肝不藏血而出血，终致肝血不足。肝血不足，血不养肝，疏泄失职，则夜寐多梦、女子月经不调等证相继出现。

5.2 肝与五体、五官、九窍、情志的联系

5.2.1 在体合筋

筋即筋膜，包括肌腱和韧带。肝血充足，筋得以濡养，则运动灵活有力，耐受疲劳，并能较快地解除疲劳，故肝又称为"罢极之本"。

5.2.2 其华在爪

爪即爪甲，包括指甲和趾甲，是筋的延续。爪甲有赖于肝血的濡养，其荣枯与肝气肝血的盛衰有密切关系。肝精肝血充足，则爪甲坚韧、红润有光泽；肝血亏虚，则爪甲痿软而薄，枯而色夭，甚至变形、脆裂。

5.2.3 开窍于目

目的视觉功能有赖于肝精肝血的濡养和肝气的疏泄。肝精、肝血充足，肝气调和则目能发挥其视物辨色的功能。肝血不足则出现视物不清、色盲；肝阴不足则两目干涩；肝阳上亢则头晕目眩；肝火上炎则目赤肿痛。

5.2.4 在志为怒

情志活动中，怒与肝的关系最密切。一定程度内的怒，对维持机体的生理平衡有重要意义。肝为刚脏，性喜条达而恶抑郁，故肝生怒志是肝的生理功能。情志不遂也会影响肝的功能：郁怒不解则肝气郁结；大怒暴怒则肝气上升太过、血随气逆，出现咳血、吐血等；肝血不足，不能濡养肝气则烦躁易怒。

6. 肾

肾位于腰部脊柱两侧，左右各一，右微下，左微上，外形椭圆弯曲，状如豇豆。肾与膀胱、骨髓、脑、发、耳等构成肾系统。主藏精，主水液，主纳气，为人体脏腑阴阳之本，生命之源，故称为先天之本；

在五行属水，为阴中之阳。四时与冬季相应。

6.1 肾的生理功能

6.1.1 肾藏精

肾藏精是指肾具有贮存、封藏人身精气的作用。精，有广义和狭义之分。广义之精是构成人体的维持人体生长发育、生殖和脏腑功能活动的有形的精微物质的统称，包括禀受于父母的生命物质，即先天之精，以及后天获得的水谷之精，即后天之精。狭义之精是禀受于父母而贮藏于肾的具有生殖繁衍作用的精微物质，又称生殖之精。

先天之精和后天之精的关系：先天之精和后天之精，其来源虽然不同，但却同藏于肾，二者相互依存，相互为用。先天之精为后天之精准备了物质基础，后天之精不断地供养先天之精。先天之精只有得到后天之精的补充滋养，才能充分发挥其生理效应；后天之精也只有得到先天之精的活力资助，才能源源不断地化生。即所谓"先天生后天，后天养先天"，二者相辅相成，在肾中密切结合而组成肾中所藏的精气。肾为先天之本，接受其他脏腑的精气而贮藏起来，当其他脏腑的精气充盛，肾精的生成、贮藏和排泄才能正常。

肾中所藏之精主要的功能有：促进生长发育，主司生殖和参与血液的生成。

（1）肾主生长发育

肾所藏之精气为生命的基础，在人的生、长、壮、老、已的过程中起主导作用。在整个生命过程中，由于肾中精气的盛衰变化，而呈现出生、长、壮、老、已的不同生理状态。人从幼年开始，肾精逐渐充盛，则有齿更发长等生理现象。到了青壮年，肾精进一步充盛，乃至达到极点，机体也随之发育到壮盛期，则真牙生，体壮实，筋骨强健。待到老年，肾精衰退，形体也逐渐衰老，全身筋骨运动不灵活，齿摇发脱，呈现出老态龙钟之象。由此可见，肾精决定着机体的生长发育，为人体生长发育之根。如果肾精亏少，影响到人体的生长发育，会出现生长发育障碍，如发育迟缓、筋骨痿软等；成年则出现未老先衰、齿摇发落等。

（2）肾主生殖

肾为先天之本，肾精的生成、贮藏和排泄，对人体的生殖能力有着重要的影响。人体生殖器官的发育及其生殖能力，均有赖于肾气的盛衰。人出生以后，由于先天之精和后天之精的相互滋养，从幼年开始，肾的精气逐渐充盛，发育到青春时期，随着肾精的不断充盛，便产生了一种促进生殖功能成熟的物质，称作天癸。于是，男子就能产生精液，女性则月经按时来潮，性功能逐渐成熟，具备了生殖能力。以后，随着人从中年进入老年，肾精也由充盛而逐渐趋向亏虚，天癸的生成亦随之减少，甚至逐渐耗竭，生殖能力亦随之而下降，以至消失。这充分说明肾精对生殖功能起着决定性的作用。如果肾藏精功能失常就会导致性功能异常，生殖功能下降。

（3）参与血液的生成

肾为先天之本，肾藏精，精能生髓，髓能化血。

6.1.2 肾主水液

肾主水液是指肾主持和调节人体水液代谢的功能。水液是体内正常液体的总称。肾主水的功能是靠肾阳对水液的气化来实现的。人体的水液代谢包括两个方面：一是将水谷精微中具有濡养滋润脏腑作用的津液输布周身；二是将各脏腑代谢利用后的浊液排出体外。人体的水液代谢与肺、脾、胃、小肠、大肠、膀胱、三焦等脏腑有密切关系，而肺的宣肃、脾的运化和转输、肾的气化共同构成调节水液代谢平衡的中心环节。其中，以肺为标，以肾为本，以脾为枢。肺、脾、膀胱等脏腑均有赖于肾的蒸腾气化功能，才能在水液代谢中发挥各自的生理作用。肾的气化作用贯穿于水液代谢的始终，居于极其重要的地位，所以有"肾主水""肾为水脏"之说。在病理上，肾主水功能失调，气化失职，开阖失度，就会引起水液代谢障碍。气化失常，关门不利，阖多开少，小便的生成和排泄发生障碍可引起尿少、水肿等病理现象；若开多阖少，又可见尿多、尿频等症状。

6.1.3 肾主纳气

纳，固摄、受纳的意思。肾主纳气是指肾具有摄纳肺吸入之气而调节呼吸的作用。人体的呼吸运动，虽为肺所主，但吸入之气，必须下归于肾，由肾气为之摄纳，呼吸才能通畅、调匀。如果肾的纳气功能减退，摄纳无权，吸入之气不能归纳于肾，就会出现呼多吸少、吸气困难、动则喘甚等肾不纳气的病理表现。肾主纳气是肾的封藏作用在呼吸运动中的体现。

6.1.4 滋养温煦其他脏腑

肾阴肾阳为脏腑阴阳之本：肾为五脏六腑之本，为水火之宅，寓真阴而涵真阳。五脏六腑之阴，非肾阴不能滋助；五脏六腑之阳，非肾阳不能温养。肾阴充则全身诸脏之阴亦充，肾阳旺则全身诸脏之阳亦旺盛。所以说，肾阴为全身诸阴之本，肾阳为全身诸阳之根。

6.2 肾与五体、五官、九窍、情志的联系

6.2.1 肾主骨

肾主骨，骨的生长发育有赖于肾精化生的骨髓的充养，肾中精和气促进机体生长发育。齿为骨之余，牙齿的生长、脱落和润泽、枯槁，反映了肾气的盛衰。

6.2.2 其华在发

发，指毛发、头发。发为血之余，肾精能生髓化血，血能养发。发质的疏密、色泽、质地也能反映肾气的盛衰。

6.2.3 肾开窍于耳及前后二阴

（1）开窍于耳

肾藏精生髓，填充骨髓、脊髓和脑髓。耳与脊髓相连。耳的听觉功能灵敏与否，与肾之精气的盛衰密切相关。

（2）开窍于前后二阴

前阴是指排尿和生殖的器官；后阴是指排泄粪便的通道。尿液的生成和排泄有赖于肾气的蒸化和固摄。粪便的排泄，本属于大肠传化糟粕的功能，但与肾气的推动和固摄也关系密切。

6.2.4 在志为恐（惊）

五志当中，恐（惊）属于肾。恐，是人们对事物惧怕的一种精神状态，是一种自知的恐惧，俗称"胆怯"。惊，惊吓，为不自知，事出意外而受到的惊吓。恐会伤肾，恐则气下。在恐惧的时候，往往会出现下肢酸软无力，甚至二便失禁的现象，这都是"恐而伤肾"的表现。

◆六腑系统

六腑是胆、胃、小肠、大肠、膀胱、三焦的总称。它们的共同生理功能是"传化物"，其生理特点是"泻而不藏""实而不能满"。六腑的生理特性是受盛和传化水谷，具有通降下行的特性。每一腑都必须适时排空其内容物，才能保持六腑通畅，功能协调，故有"六腑以通为用，以降为顺"之说。突出强调"通""降"二字，若"通"和"降"得太过与不及，均属于病态。

1. 胆

胆居六腑之首，又隶属于奇恒之腑，其形呈囊状，附于肝之短叶间。胆属阳属木，与肝相表里，肝为脏属阴木，胆为腑属阳木。胆贮藏排泄胆汁，主决断，调节脏腑气。

1.1 胆的生理功能

1.1.1 贮藏和排泄胆汁

胆汁，别称"精汁""清汁"，来源于肝脏。贮藏于胆腑的胆汁，由于肝的疏泄作用，使之排泄，注入肠中，以促进饮食物的消化。若肝胆的功能失常，胆的分泌与排泄受阻，就会影响脾胃的消化功能，而出现厌食、腹胀、腹泻等消化不良症状。若湿热蕴结肝胆，以致肝失疏泄，胆汁外溢，浸渍肌肤，则发为黄疸，以目黄、身黄、小便黄为特征。胆气以下降为顺，若胆气不利，气机上逆，则可出现口苦，呕吐黄绿苦水等。

1.1.2 主决断

胆主决断指胆在精神意识思维活动过程中，具有判断事物、做出决定的作用。胆主决断对于防御和消除某些精神刺激（如大惊大恐）的不良影响，以维持和控制气血的正常运行，确保脏器之间的协调关系有着重要的作用。胆能助肝之疏泄以调畅情志，肝胆相济则情志和调稳定。胆气豪壮者，剧烈的精神刺激对其所造成的影响不大，且恢复也较快；胆气虚弱的人，在受到精神刺激的不良影响时，易于形成疾病，表现为胆怯易惊、善恐、失眠、多梦等。

2. 胃

胃是腹腔中容纳食物的器官。其外形屈曲，分为上脘（包括贲门）、中脘和下脘（包括幽门）三部，上连食道，下通小肠。主受纳腐熟水谷，为水谷精微之仓、气血之海，胃以通降为顺，与脾相表里，脾胃常合称为后天之本。

2.1 胃的生理功能

胃主受纳和腐熟水谷

受纳是接受和容纳之意。胃主受纳是指胃接受和容纳水谷的作用。饮食入口，经过食道，容纳并暂存于胃腑，这一过程称之为受纳，故称胃为"太仓""水谷之海"。胃主受纳功能是胃主腐熟功能的基础，也是整个消化功能的基础。若胃有病变，就会影响胃的受纳功能，出现纳呆、厌食、胃脘胀闷等症状。

腐熟是饮食物经过胃的初步消化，形成食糜的过程。胃主腐熟指胃将食物消化为食糜的作用。胃接受由口摄入的饮食物并使其在胃中短暂停留，进行初步消化，依靠胃的腐熟作用，将水谷变成食糜，其精微物质由脾之运化而营养周身，未被消化的食糜则下行于小肠，不断更新，形成了胃的消化过程。如果胃的腐熟功能低下，会出现胃脘疼痛、嗳腐食臭等食滞胃脘之候。

胃主受纳和腐熟水谷的功能，必须和脾的运化功能相配合，才能顺利完成。脾胃密切合作，"胃司受纳，脾司运化，一纳一运"（《景岳全书·饮食》），才能使水谷化为精微，以化生气血津液，供养全身，故脾胃合称为"后天之本""气血生化之源"。

3. 大肠

大肠居腹中，其上口在阑门处接小肠，其下端紧接肛门，包括结肠和直肠。主传化糟粕和吸收津液。与肺相表里，属金，属阳。

大肠的生理功能

大肠主传导是指大肠接受小肠下移的饮食残渣，使之形成粪便，经肛门排出体外的功能。大肠接受由小肠下移的饮食残渣，再吸收其中剩余的水分和养料，使之形成粪便，经肛门而排出体外，是整个消化过程的最后阶段，故有"传导之腑""传导之官"之称。大肠重新吸收水分，参与调节体内水液代谢的功能，称之为"大肠主津"。大肠的主要功能是传导糟粕，排泄大便。大肠的传导功能，主要与胃之通降、脾之运化、肺之肃降以及肾之封藏有密切关系。

4. 小肠

小肠居腹中，上接幽门，与胃相通，下连大肠，包括回肠、空肠、十二指肠。主受盛化物和泌别清浊。与心相表里，属火属阳。

4.1 小肠的生理功能

4.1.1 受盛化物

受盛，接受，以器盛物之意。化物，变化、消化、化生之谓。小肠的受盛化物功能主要表现在两个方面：一是小肠受盛了由胃腑下移而来的初步消化的饮食物，起到容器的作用，即受盛作用；二指经胃初步消化的饮食物，在小肠内必须停留一定的时间，由小肠对其进一步消化和吸收，将水谷化为可以被机体利用的营养物质，精微由此而出，糟粕由此下输于大肠，即"化物"作用。在病理上，小肠受盛功能失调，传化停止，则气机失于通调，滞而为痛，表现为腹部疼痛。若化物功能失常，可导致消化、吸收障碍，表现为腹胀、腹泻、便溏等。

4.1.2 泌别清浊

泌，即分泌。别，即分别。清，即精微物质。浊，即代谢产物。所谓泌别清浊，是指小肠对承受胃初步消化的饮食物，在进一步消化的同时，并随之进行分别水谷精微和代谢产物的过程。分清，就是将饮食物中的精华部分，包括津液和食物化生的精微，进行吸收，再通过脾之升清散精的作用，上输心肺，输布全身，供给营养。别浊，则体现为两个方面：其一，将饮食物的残渣糟粕，通过阑门传送到大肠，形成粪便，经肛门排出体外；其二，将剩余的水分经肾脏气化作用渗入膀胱，形成尿液，经尿道排出体外。因为小肠在泌别清浊过程中，参与了人体的水液代谢，故有"小肠主液"之说。

小肠分清别浊的功能正常，则水液和糟粕各走其道，二便正常。若小肠功能失调，清浊不分，水液归于糟粕，即可出现水谷混杂，便溏泄泻等。因"小肠主液"，故小肠分清别浊功能失常不仅影响大便，而且也影响小便，表现为小便短少。

5. 三焦

三焦是脏象学说中的一个特有名称。三焦是上焦、中焦、下焦的合称，为六腑之一，属脏腑中最大的腑，又称外腑、孤脏。主升降诸气和通行水液，在五行属火，其阴阳属性为阳。

总观三焦，膈以上为上焦，包括心与肺；横膈以下到脐为中焦，包括脾与胃；脐以下至二阴为下焦，包括肝、肾、大小肠、膀胱、女子胞等。其中肝脏，按其部位来说，应划归中焦，但因它与肾关系密切，故将肝和肾一同划归下焦。三焦的功能实际上是五脏六腑全部功能的总括。

5.1 三焦的生理功能

5.1.1 通行元气

元气，又名原气，是人体最根本的气，根源于肾，由先天之精所化，赖后天之精以养，为人体脏腑阴阳之本，生命活动的原动力。元气通过三焦而输布到五脏六腑，充沛于全身，以激发、推动各个脏腑组织的功能活动。所以说，三焦是元气运行的通道。

5.1.2 疏通水道

三焦能"通调水道"（《医学三字经》），调控人体整个水液代谢过程，在水液代谢过程中起着重要作用。三焦为水液生成敷布、升降出入的道路。三焦在水液代谢过程中的协调平衡作用，称之为"三焦气化"。三焦通行水液的功能，实际上是对肺、脾、肾等脏腑参与水液代谢功能的总括。

5.2 三焦的生理特性

5.2.1 上焦如雾

上焦如雾是指上焦主宣发卫气，敷布精微的作用。上焦接受来自中焦脾胃的水谷精微，通过心肺的宣发敷布，布散于全身，发挥其营养滋润作用，若雾露之溉，故称为"上焦如雾。"（《灵枢·营卫生会篇》）

5.2.2 中焦如沤

中焦如沤是指脾胃运化水谷，化生气血的作用。胃受纳腐熟水谷，由脾之运化而形成水谷精微，以此化生气血，并通过脾的升清转输作用，将水谷精微上输于心肺以濡养周身。因为脾胃有腐熟水谷、运化精微的生理功能，故称"中焦如沤。"（《灵枢·营卫生会篇》）

5.2.3 下焦如渎

下焦如渎是指肾、膀胱、大小肠等脏腑主分别清浊，排泄废物的作用。下焦将饮食物的残渣糟粕传送到大肠，变成粪便，从肛门排出体外，并将体内剩余的水液，通过肾和膀胱的气化作用变成尿液，从尿道排出体外。这种生理过程具有向下疏通，向外排泄之势，故称"下焦如渎。"（《灵枢·营卫生会篇》）

6. 膀胱

膀胱又称净腑，位于下腹部，在脏腑中，居最下处。主贮存尿液及排泄尿液，与肾相表里，在五行属水，其阴阳属性为阳。

膀胱的生理功能

贮存和排出尿液：在人体津液代谢过程中，没有被利用的水液下归于肾，经肾的气化作用，升清降浊，清者回流体内，浊者下输于膀胱，变成尿液。尿液贮存于膀胱，达到一定容量时，通过肾的气化作用，使膀胱开阖适度，则尿液可及时地从尿道排出体外。

◆奇恒之腑

1. 脑

脑，脑由精髓汇集而成，又名髓海。脑深藏于头部，位于人体最上部，其外为头面，内为脑髓，是精髓和神明高度汇集之处，为元神之府。

1.1 脑的生理功能

1.1.1 主宰生命活动

"脑为元神之府"（《本草纲目》），是生命的枢机，主宰五脏六腑的生命活动。脑受伤，则威胁生命。

1.1.2 主精神意识

中医学一方面强调心是思维的主要器官；另一方面也认识到脑是精神、意识、思维活动的枢纽，"为一身之宗，百神之会。"（《修真十书》）脑主精神意识的功能正常，则精神饱满，意识清楚，思维灵敏，记忆力强，语言清晰，情志正常。否则，便出现神志异常。

2. 女子胞

女子胞，又称胞宫、子宫、子脏、胞脏，位于小腹正中部，是女性的内生殖器官，有主持月经和孕育胎儿的作用。

3. 胆

胆为六腑之首，其形中空，呈囊状，与其他的腑相类，故为六腑之一。但胆中贮藏精汁（胆汁），满而不能实，与五脏的功能类似，所以胆又属于奇恒之腑。

4. 髓

髓分为骨髓、脊髓和脑髓等，骨髓可以充养骨骼，脑髓则充养大脑。中医的"髓"概念不应与现代医学定义的"骨髓"混淆。在中医理论中，髓的作用是滋养大脑和脊髓，形成骨髓。肾精与骨髓关系密切，因为肾藏精，精能生髓，肾精不足，骨髓生化乏源。

5. 骨

骨，像所有其他奇恒之腑一样，也与肾脏有关。骨被认为是奇恒之腑之一，因为它们储存着骨髓。肾主骨生髓，骨髓充养骨骼，骨的生长发育与肾精密切相关。肾精不足，骨髓空虚，骨若失养，无力久立和行走。临床实践中利用肾与骨的关系，通过补肾加快骨折的愈合。

6. 脉

脉被认为是一种特殊的奇恒之腑，为气血运行的通路，与肾间接相关。肾藏精，精生髓，精血同源，肾气有助于水谷精微转化为气血。

知识点 5　气血理论

气与血为人体不可脱离的最宝贵的基本物质，它不仅是四肢百骸、脏腑经络的能源和动力，也是营卫津液、精神情志的气化源泉和物质基础。

1. 气

1.1 气的基本含义

中医学从气是宇宙的本原，是构成天地万物的最基本元素这一基本观点出发，认为气是真实存在而至精至微的生命物质，是构成人体的最基本物质，也是维持人体生命活动的最基本物质。生命的基本物质，除气之外，尚有血、津液、精等，但血、津液和精均是由气所化生的。所以说，气是构成人体和维持人体生命活动的最基本物质。人体通过五脏六腑呼吸清气，受纳水谷，将其变为人体生命活动需要的气血津液等各种生命物质，由经脉运送至全身。

另一方面，中医学在论述人体的生命活动时，气这个概念不仅仅具有生命物质这一种含义，同时还具有生理功能的含义。人体生命物质的气是通过人体脏腑组织经络的功能活动而表现出来的。

1.2 气的生成

人体的气，源于先天之精气和后天摄取的水谷精气与呼吸获得的自然界清气，通过肺、脾胃和肾等脏腑生理活动作用而生成。

1.3 气的分类

1.3.1 元气（先天之气）

元气是人体最根本、最原始，源于先天而根于肾的气，是人体生命活动的原动力。因元气来源于先天，故又称先天之气。元气根源于肾，由先天之精所化生，并赖后天脾胃运化之水谷精微充养而成。

1.3.2 营气

营气是血脉中具有营养作用的气。因其富含营养，故称为营气。由于营气行于脉中，又能化生血液，故常常"营血"并称。营气与卫气相对而言，属于阴，故又称为"营阴"。营气是由来自脾胃运化的水谷精微中的精粹部分和肺吸入的自然界清气相结合所化生的。

1.3.3 卫气

卫，有"护卫""保卫"之义。卫气是行于脉外之气。卫气与营气相对而言，属于阳，故又称"卫阳"。卫气，其性剽疾滑利，活动力强，流动迅速。卫气同营气一样，也是由水谷精微和肺吸入的自然的清气所化生。所以说："人受气于谷，谷入于胃，以传与肺，五脏六腑，皆以受气。其清者为营，浊者为卫。营在脉中，卫在脉外。营周不休，五十而复大会。阴阳相贯，如环无端。"（《灵枢·营卫生会》）

1.4 气的功能

气是构成人体和维持人体生命活动的最基本物质，它对于人体具有十分重要的多种生理功能。不同的脏腑组织之气的作用不尽相同，这里将气的生理功能概括为以下几个方面。

1.4.1 推动作用

气的推动作用，指气具有激发和推动作用。气是活力很强的精微物质，能激发和促进人体的生长发育以及各脏腑、经络等组织器官的生理功能，能推动血液的生成、运行，以及津液的生成、输布和排泄等。

1.4.2 温煦作用

气的温煦作用是指气有温暖作用。气是机体热量的来源，是体内产生热量的物质基础。其温煦作用是通过激发和推动各脏腑器官生理功能，促进机体的新陈代谢来实现的。气分阴阳，气具有温煦作用者，谓之阳气。具体言之，气的温煦作用是通过阳气的作用表现出来的。

1.4.3 防御作用

气的防御作用是指气护卫肌肤、抗御邪气的作用。气的防御作用主要体现在两个方面。其一，护卫肌表，抵御外邪。皮肤是人体的藩篱，具有屏障作用。肺合皮毛，肺宣发卫气于皮毛，发挥其防御外邪侵袭的作用。其二，正邪交争，驱邪外出。邪气侵入机体之后，机体的正气奋起与之抗争，正盛邪祛，邪气随即被祛除体外，如是疾病便不能发生。

1.4.4 固摄作用

气的固摄作用，指气对血、津液、精液等液态物质的稳固、统摄，以防止无故流失的作用。气的固摄作用具体表现为：气能摄血，约束血液，使之循行于脉中，而不致逸出脉外；气能摄津，约束汗液、尿液、唾液、胃肠液、粪便等，调控其分泌量或排泄量，防止其异常丢失；固摄精液，使之不因妄动而频繁遗泄；固摄脏腑器官，使其保持相对稳定的位置。

1.4.5 气化作用

气化，泛指人体内气的运行变化。气化是在气的作用下，脏腑的功能活动，精、气、血、津液等不同物质之间的相互化生，以及物质与功能之间的转化，包括了体内物质的新陈代谢，以及物质转化和能量转化等过程。首先，通过进食和呼吸，身体从自然界获得清气和水谷精微，并通过气化的作用，转化为身体必需的精、气、血和津液。之后，代谢废物通过气化作用，转变成汗液、尿液和粪便。此外，在整个生命过程中，精、气、血、津液通过气化作用，相互转化，互相滋养，从而推动了人体生命活动的延续。

2. 血

2.1 血的基本概念

血，即血液，是循行于脉中的富有营养的红色液态物质，是构成人体和维持人体生命活动的基本物质之一。血主于心，藏于肝，统于脾，布于肺，根于肾，有规律地循行脉管之中，在脉内营运不息，充分发挥灌溉全身的生理效应。

2.2 血的生成

脾胃化生的水谷精微是血液生成的最基本物质。水谷精微通过脾的转输升清作用，上输于心肺，在肺吐故纳新之后，复注于心脉，化赤而变成新鲜血液。除此之外，肾藏精，精生髓，精髓也是化生血液的基本物质。在脾胃、心肺、肝肾等脏腑的协同作用下化生为血。

2.3 血的生理功能

2.3.1 营养滋润全身

血的营养作用是由其组成成分所决定的。血循行于脉内，是其发挥营养作用的前提；血沿脉管循行于全身，为全身各脏腑组织的功能活动提供营养。全身各部（内脏、五官、九窍、四肢、百骸）无一不是在血的濡养作用下发挥功能的。

2.3.2 神志活动的物质基础

血主神志的作用是古人通过大量的临床观察而认识到的。无论何种原因形成的血虚或运行失常，均可以出现不同程度的神志方面的症状。心血虚、肝血虚，常有惊悸、失眠、多梦等神志不安的表现，失血甚者还可出现烦躁、恍惚、癫狂、昏迷等神志失常的改变。由此可见，血与神志活动有着密切关系。

2.4 血的循行

2.4.1 血液循行的方向

脉为血之府，脉管是一个相对密闭、如环无端、自我衔接的管道系统。血液在脉管中运行不息，流布于全身，环周不休，以营养人体的周身内外上下。

2.4.2 血液运行的机制

血液正常循行必须具备两个条件：一是脉管系统的完整性；二是全身各脏腑发挥正常生理功能，特别是与心、肺、肝、脾四脏的关系尤为密切。

正常的血液循环来自于心、肺、脾和肝的共同作用。心主血脉，心气是推动血液循行的原动力；肺司呼吸而主一身之气，调节着全身的气机，辅助心脏，推动和调节血液的运行；脾主统血，统摄血液流于脉管之中，防止其外溢；肝主藏血，具有贮藏血液和调节血流量的功能。如果以上所说的任何一脏不能正常行使其功能的话，就会发生异常的血液循行。例如，心气不足可以导致心血凝滞；脾气不足无法收摄血液导致出血等；肝气不调、血液循行紊乱则会出现血瘀、血肿、女性痛经或闭经。

3. 气血的关系

3.1 气为血之帅

气为血帅，一方面因为气是血液形成的原动力；另一方面是由于气可生血。血由营气和津液形成，后两者都源于水谷。而以上这些都离不开气的作用。血液循行依赖气的推动功能；另一方面，气摄血，维持血行于脉中不致外逸。气的此项功能由脾气来执行。气虚不能摄血可导致出血。

3.2 血为气之母

血为气之母，一方面，气无形而血有形，血以载气；另一方面，血为气提供充足的营养。血是气的物质基础，离开了血，气也就不复存在。

知识点 6　病因学说

导致人体发生疾病的原因，称之为病因，又称作"致病因素""病原"（古作"病源"）"病邪"。疾病是人体在一定条件下，由致病因素所引起的有一定表现形式的病理，包括发病形式、病机、发展规律和转归的一系列完整的过程。

本章根据疾病的发病途径及形成过程，将病因分为外感病因：六淫、疠气；内伤病因：七情内伤、饮食失节、劳逸适度；病理产物形成的病因：痰饮、瘀血、结石；以及其他病因：外伤、虫兽伤、寄生虫。

1. 六淫

所谓六淫，是风、寒、暑、湿、燥、火六种外感病邪的统称。阴阳相移，寒暑更作，气候（中医学又称为六气，即风、寒、暑、湿、燥、火六种正常的自然界气候）变化都有一定的规律和限度。如果气候变化异常，六气发生太过或不及，或非其时而有其气（如春天当温而反寒，冬季当寒而反热），以及气候变化过于急骤（如暴寒暴暖）超过了一定的限度，使机体不能与之相适应的时候，就会导致疾病的发生。于是，六气由对人体无害而转化为对人体有害，成为致病的因素。能导致机体发生疾病的六气便称为"六淫"。

六淫致病的一般规律如下：（1）由于六淫本为四时主气发生太过或不及，故容易形成季节性多发病。（2）六淫邪气既可单独致病又可相兼为害。（3）六淫致病以后，在疾病发展过程中，不仅可以互相影响，而且在一定条件下，其病理性质可向不同于病因性质的方向转化。（4）六淫为病，多有由表入里的传变过程。六淫之邪多从肌表或口鼻而入，侵犯人体而发病。故六淫致病，多有由表及里的传变过程。即使直中入里，没有表证，也都称为"外感病"。所以，称六淫为外感病的病因。

1.1 风

风具有轻扬开泄，善动不居的特性，为春季的主气。因风为木气而通于肝，故又称春季为风木当令的季节。风虽为春季的主气，但终岁常在，四时皆有。故风邪引起的疾病虽以春季为多，但不限于春季，其他季节均可发生。

风邪的性质和致病特征：风性轻扬，善行数变，为百病之长。

1.1.1 风为阳邪，轻扬开泄

风邪，其性轻扬升散，具有升发、向上、向外的特性。所以风邪致病，易于伤人上部，易犯肌表、腰背部等阳位。

1.1.2 善行数变

风善动不居，易行而无定处。"善行"是指风邪具有易行而无定处的性质，故其致病有病位游移，行无定处的特性。"数变"是指风邪致病具有变化无常和发病急骤的特性。

1.1.3 风为百病之长

风邪是外感病因的先导，寒、湿、燥、热等邪往往都依附于风而侵袭人体。临床上风邪为患较多，又易与六淫诸邪相合而为病。故称风为百病之长，六淫之首。

1.2 寒

寒具有寒冷、凝结特性，为冬季的主气。寒为水气而通于肾，故称冬季为寒水当令的季节。因冬为寒气当令，故冬季多寒病，但也可见于其他季节。由于气温骤降，防寒保温不够，人体易感受寒邪而为病。

寒邪性质和致病特征：寒冷、凝滞、收引。

1.2.1 寒为阴邪，易伤阳气

寒为阴邪，当阴寒偏盛，阳气不足以祛除寒邪，就会反为被阴寒所侮。寒邪最易损伤人体阳气。阳气受损，失于温煦之功，故全身或局部可出现明显的寒象。

1.2.2 寒性凝滞

凝滞，即凝结阻滞之谓。人身气血津液的运行，赖阳气的温煦推动，才能畅通无阻。寒邪侵入人体，经脉气血失于阳气温煦，易使气血凝结阻滞，涩滞不通，不通则痛，故疼痛是寒邪致病的重要特征。

1.2.3 寒性收引

收引，即收缩牵引之意。寒性收引是指寒邪具有收引拘急之特性，"寒则气收"。寒邪侵袭人体，可使气机收敛，腠理闭塞，经络筋脉收缩而挛急；若寒客经络关节，则筋脉收缩拘急，以致拘挛作痛、屈伸不利或冷厥不仁；若寒邪侵袭肌表，则毛窍收缩，卫阳闭郁，故发热恶寒而无汗。

1.3 暑

暑为火热之邪，为夏季主气。暑邪有明显的季节性，主要发生在夏至以后，立秋以前。

暑邪的性质和致病特征：暑为火所化，主升散，且多挟湿。

1.3.1 暑性炎热

暑为夏月炎暑，盛夏之火气，具有酷热之性，火热属阳，故暑属阳邪。暑邪伤人多表现出一系列阳热症状，如高热、心烦、面赤、烦躁、脉象洪大等，称为伤暑（或暑热）。

1.3.2 暑性升散

升散,即上升发散之意。升,指暑邪易于上犯头目,内扰心神,易上扰心经。散,指暑邪为害,易于伤津耗气。暑为阳邪,阳性升发,故暑邪侵犯人体,多直入气分,可致腠理开泄而大汗出。汗多伤津,津随气泄,故暑邪易耗气伤津,出现气阴两伤的症状。

1.3.3 暑多挟湿

暑季不仅气候炎热,且常多雨而潮湿,热蒸湿动,湿热弥漫空间,人身之所及,呼吸之所受,均不离湿热之气。暑令湿胜必多兼感。其临床特征,除发热、烦渴等暑热症状外,常兼见四肢困倦、胸闷呕恶、大便溏泄不爽等湿阻症状。

1.4 湿

湿具有重浊、黏滞、趋下特性,为长夏主气。夏秋之交,湿热熏蒸,水气上腾,湿气最盛,故一年之中长夏多湿病。湿亦可因涉水淋雨、居处伤湿,或以水为事。湿邪为患,四季均可发病,且其伤人缓慢难察。

湿邪的性质和致病特征:湿为阴邪,阻碍气机,易伤阳气,其性重浊黏滞、趋下。

1.4.1 湿性重浊

湿为重浊有质之邪。所谓"重",即沉重、重着之意。故湿邪致病,其临床症状有沉重的特性,如头重身困、四肢酸楚沉重等。所谓"浊",即秽浊垢腻之意。故湿邪为患,易于出现排泄物和分泌物秽浊不清的现象。如湿气下注,则小便浑浊、妇女黄白带下过多。

1.4.2 湿为阴邪,易阻滞气机

湿性属水,水属于阴,故湿为阴邪。湿邪侵及人体,留滞于脏腑经

络，最易阻滞气机，从而使气机升降失常。

1.4.3 湿性黏滞

"黏"，即黏腻；"滞"，即停滞。所谓黏滞是指湿邪致病具有黏腻停滞的特性。这种特性主要表现在两个方面：一是症状的黏滞性，即湿病症状多黏滞而不爽，如大便黏腻不爽；二是病程的缠绵性，起病缓慢隐袭，病程较长，往往反复发作或缠绵难愈。

1.4.4 湿性趋下

水性就下，湿类于水，其质重浊，故湿邪有下趋之势，易于伤及人体下部。其病多见下部的症状，如水肿多以下肢较为明显。

1.5 燥

燥具有干燥、收敛清肃特性，为秋季主气。
燥邪的性质和致病特征：燥胜则干，易于伤肺。

1.5.1 干涩伤津

燥为秋季肃杀之气所化，其性干涩枯涸，故曰"燥胜则干"。燥邪为害，最易耗伤人体的津液，形成阴津亏损的病变，表现出各种干涩的症状和体征，诸如皮肤干涩皲裂、鼻干咽燥、口唇燥裂等。

1.5.2 燥易伤肺

肺为五脏六腑之华盖，性喜清肃濡润而恶燥，称为娇脏。肺主气而司呼吸，直接与自然界大气相通，且外合皮毛，开窍于鼻，燥邪多从口鼻而入。燥为秋令主气，与肺相应，故燥邪最易伤肺。燥邪犯肺，使肺津受损，宣肃失职，从而出现干咳少痰，或痰黏难咯，或痰中带血，以及喘息胸痛等。

1.6 火 （热）

火具有炎热特性，旺于夏季。但是火并不像暑那样具有明显的季节性，也不受季节气候的限制。

火邪的性质和致病特征：燔灼、炎上、耗气伤津、生风动血。

1.6.1 火性燔灼炎上

燔即燃烧；灼，即烧烫。燔灼，是指火热邪气具有焚烧而熏灼的特性。故火邪致病，机体以阳气过盛为其主要病理机制，临床上表现出高热、恶热、脉洪数等热盛之征。火为阳邪，其性升腾向上，故火邪致病具有明显的炎上特性，其病多表现于上部。

1.6.2 伤津耗气

火热之邪，蒸腾于内，最易迫津外泄，消烁津液，使人体阴津耗伤。故火邪致病，其临床表现除热象显著外，往往伴有口渴喜饮、咽干舌燥、小便短赤、大便秘结等津伤液耗之征。

1.6.3 生风动血

火邪易于引起肝风内动和血液妄行。生风，即肝风内动。火热之邪侵袭人体，往往燔灼肝经，劫耗津血，使筋脉失于濡养，而致肝风内动，称为热极生风。风火相煽，症状急迫，临床上表现为高热、神昏谵语、四肢抽搐、颈项强直、角弓反张、目睛上视等。动血，即出血。火热之邪，灼伤脉络，并使血行加速，迫血妄行，易于引起各种出血，如吐血、衄血、便血、尿血，以及皮肤发斑，妇女崩漏等。

1.6.4 易致肿疡

火热之邪入于血分，聚于局部，腐肉败血，则发为痈肿疮疡。

1.6.5 易扰心神

火与心气相应，心主血脉而藏神。故火之邪伤于人体，最易扰乱神明，出现心烦失眠、狂躁妄动，甚至神昏谵语等证。

2. 七情

2.1 七情的概念

七情是指喜、怒、忧、思、悲、恐、惊七种正常的情志活动，是人的精神意识对外界事物的反应。七情与人体脏腑功能活动有密切的关系。七情分属于五脏，以喜、怒、思、悲、恐为代表，就称为五志。

七情是人对客观事物的不同反应，在正常的活动范围内，一般不会使人致病。只有突然强烈或长期持久的情志刺激，超过人体本身的正常生理活动范围，使人体气机紊乱，脏腑阴阳气血失调，才会导致疾病的发生。因此，作为病因，七情是指过于强烈、持久或突然的情志变化，导致脏腑气血阴阳失调而发生疾病的情志活动。

2.2 七情的致病特点

2.2.1 直接伤及脏腑

七情过激可影响脏腑功能失调而产生病理变化。不同的情志刺激可伤及不同的脏腑，产生不同的病理变化。

2.2.2 影响脏腑气机

气出入有序，升降有常，周流一身，循环无端，而无病。若七情变化，五志过极而发，则气机失调，或为气不周流而郁滞，或为升降失常而逆乱。不同的情志变化，其气机逆乱的表现也不尽相同。怒则气上，喜则气缓，悲则气消，思则气结，恐则气下，惊则气乱。

2.2.3 情志波动，可致病情改变

异常情志波动，可使病情加重或迅速恶化，如眩晕患者，因阴虚阳亢，肝阳偏亢，若遇恼怒，可使肝阳暴张，气血并走于上，出现眩晕欲

仆，甚则突然昏仆不语、半身不遂、口眼歪斜，发为中风。

3. 饮食失宜

饮食是健康的基本条件。饮食所化生的水谷精微是化生气血，维持人体生长、发育，完成各种生理功能，保证生命生存和健康的基本条件。正常饮食是人体维持生命活动之气血阴阳的主要来源之一，但饮食失宜，常是导致许多疾病的原因。饮食物主要依靠脾胃消化吸收，如饮食失宜，首先可以损伤脾胃，导致脾胃的腐熟、运化功能失常，引起消化机能障碍；其次，还能生热、生痰、生湿，产生种种病变，成为疾病发生的一个重要原因。

4. 痰饮

痰饮是机体水液代谢障碍所形成的病理产物。一般说来，痰得阳气煎熬而成，炼液为痰，浓度较大，其质稠黏；饮得阴气凝聚而成，聚水为饮，浓度较小，其质清稀。

痰饮停留在人体的不同部位，产生的临床表现也有所不同。若痰饮流注经络，易使经络阻滞，气血运行不畅，出现肢体麻木、屈伸不利，甚至半身不遂等。痰饮停肺，使肺失宣肃，可出现胸闷、咳嗽、喘促等。胃气宜降则和，痰饮停留于胃，使胃失和降，则出现恶心呕吐等。痰浊上扰，蒙蔽清阳，则会出现头昏目眩、精神不振、痰迷心窍，或痰火扰心、心神被蒙，则可导致胸闷心悸、神昏谵妄，或引起癫狂等疾病。

5. 瘀血

瘀血，又称蓄血、恶血、败血。瘀乃血液停积，不能活动之意。所谓瘀血，是指因血行失度，使机体某一局部的血液凝聚而形成的一种病理产物。

5.1 瘀血的形成

凡是能引起血液运行不畅、或致血离经脉而郁积的内外因素，均可导致瘀血的形成。具体可以分为血出致瘀、气滞血瘀、因虚致瘀、寒凝血瘀和血热致瘀。

5.2 瘀血的致病特点

瘀血形成之后，不仅失去正常血液的濡养作用，而且反过来影响全身或局部血液的运行，其临床表现的共同特点可概括为以下几点：疼痛，一般多刺痛，固定不移；长期血瘀可导致肿块形成，固定不移；瘀血可以导致血行不畅而发生出血，血色紫暗或夹有瘀块。血瘀证患者面部、口唇、爪甲青紫；舌质紫暗；脉细涩沉弦或结代。

知识点 7　中医四诊

中医四诊是中医诊察收集病情资料的基本方法，主要包括望、闻、问、切四诊。通过四诊所收集到的临床资料，尤其是各种症状，作为判断病种、辨别证候的主要依据。四诊各有其特定的诊察内容，不能互相取代，必须四诊合参，才能系统而全面地获得临床资料，为辨证提供可靠依据。

1. 舌诊

望诊，是医生运用视觉对病人的全身和局部，舌象及排出物的变化等进行有目的观察，收集临床资料，以了解健康状况或疾病状况的一种常用诊断手段。主要内容有观察人的神、色、形、态、舌象、脉络、皮肤、五官、九窍等情况，以及排泄物、分泌物、分泌物的形、色、量、质等。这里重点介绍望诊中重要的环节，望舌（舌诊）。望舌是通过观察舌体与舌苔的变化，了解患者生理功能状态和病理变化过程的诊察方法，也是望诊的重要内容，是中医诊法的特色之一。

1.1 舌与五脏的关系

舌质候五脏病变为主，侧重血分；舌苔候六腑病变为主，侧重气分。舌尖多反映上焦心肺的病变；舌中多反映中焦脾胃的病变；舌根多反映下焦肾的病变；舌两侧多反映肝胆的病变。舌的不同部位分候不同脏腑。

1.2 舌诊的方法

医者姿势可略高于患者，患者可以采用坐位或仰卧位，面向自然光线，头略抬起，以便医者俯视口舌部位。病人自然地将舌伸出口外，舌体放松，舌面平展，舌尖略向下，尽量张口使舌体充分暴露。

望舌应当先看舌质，再看舌苔；先看舌尖，再看舌中、舌边，最后看舌根部。必要时还可察看舌下静脉。

1.3 正常舌象

正常舌象的特征概括为淡红舌、薄白苔。即舌色淡红鲜明，舌质滋润，大小适中，柔软灵活；舌苔均匀薄白，干湿适中。提示脏腑机能正常，气血津液充盈，胃气旺盛。

1.4 舌象解读

不同舌象的临床意义，是通过望舌体和望舌苔两个方面综合分析而获得。

1.4.1 望舌质（体）

舌质（舌体）是舌的肌肉和脉络组织。望舌质的内容包括舌色、舌形和舌态。

（1）舌色指舌质的颜色，有淡红、淡白、红（绛）、青紫四种。

（2）舌形是指舌质的形状，包括老嫩、胖瘦、点刺、裂纹、齿痕等方面。

（3）舌态即舌体的动态。正常舌态，舌体伸缩自如，运动灵活，提示脏腑机能旺盛，气血充足，经脉调匀。病理舌态包括痿软、强硬、歪斜、颤动、吐弄、短缩等。

1.4.2 望舌苔

舌苔是舌面上的一层苔状物，由脾胃之气蒸化胃中食浊而产生。正常舌苔，薄白均匀，干湿适中，不滑不燥，紧贴舌面上，与舌质如同一体，舌面的中部和根部稍厚。病理舌苔，多为胃气挟邪气上蒸而成，因患者胃气有强弱，病邪有寒热，故可形成各种不同的病理性舌苔。望舌苔要注意苔质和苔色两方面的变化。

（1）苔质，舌苔的质地、形态。

苔质包括舌苔的厚薄、润燥、腻腐、剥落、真假等。

（2）苔色，舌苔的颜色。

苔色的变化主要有白苔、黄苔、灰黑苔。苔色在临床上可单独出现，亦可相兼出现。各种苔色变化需要同苔质、舌色和舌的形态变化结合起来综合分析。

2. 闻诊

2.1 听声音

听声音是指听辨病人言语气息的高低、强弱、清浊、缓急变化以及咳嗽、呕吐、肠鸣等脏腑病理变化所发出的异常声响，以判断病变寒热虚实等性质的诊病方法。一般来说，如果声音粗大、响亮，则为实证；如果声音低弱，呼吸微弱，则为虚证。

2.2 闻气味

嗅辨与疾病有关的气味，以诊察疾病的方法。嗅气味包括嗅病体气味（口气、汗气、痰涕之气、二便之气、经带恶露之气）和病室气味（病体本身或排出物、分泌物散发之气）。一般来说，腐臭味通常为实热证，鱼腥味则为虚寒证。

3. 问诊

问诊是医生通过对病人或陪诊者进行有目的、有步骤地询问，了解疾病的发生、发展、诊治经过、现在症状和其他与疾病有关的情况，以诊察疾病的方法。问诊的内容包括一般情况、主诉、现病史、既往史、家族史、个人史等。

4. 切诊

切诊是指医生用手对患者体表某些部位进行触、摸、按、压，从而获得病情资料的一种诊察方法。其内容分脉诊和按诊两部分。

4.1 脉诊

脉诊又称切脉，是医生用手指对患者身体某些特定部位的动脉进行切按，体验脉动应指的形象，以了解健康或病情，辨别病证的一种诊察方法。

4.1.1 脉诊的部位

脉诊的常用部位为寸口。寸口是手腕部桡骨茎突内侧的一段动脉（桡动脉），又称气口、脉口。寸口脉分为寸、关、尺三部，以腕后高骨（桡骨茎突）为标记，其内侧的部位为关，关前（腕侧）一指为寸，关后（肘侧）一指为尺。寸关尺共长一寸九分。两手各有寸、关、尺三部，共六部脉。寸口分候脏腑：左寸候心，右寸候肺，左关候肝，右关候脾胃，左右尺候肾。

4.1.2 脉诊的方法

（1）时间

诊法常以平旦，以清晨（平旦）未起床、未进食时为最佳。但这样的要求一般很难做到，一般要求是诊脉时应保持诊室安静，病人在比较安静的环境中休息片刻，以减少各种因素的干扰，这样才能诊察到比较真实的脉象。

（2）平息

医者在诊脉时要保持呼吸自然调匀，清心宁神，以医生自己正常的一呼一吸的时间，去计算病人脉搏的至数。

（3）体位

诊脉时病人的正确体位是正坐、仰卧均可，心脏与寸口同水平，直腕、仰掌。

（4）指法

医生诊脉时选择食指、中指和无名指。手指呈弓形，以指目取脉。三指平齐，中指定关，食指定寸，无名指定尺，布指疏密适度。

4.1.3 平脉（正常脉象）

平脉是指正常人在生理条件下出现的脉象，既具有基本的特点，又有一定的变化规律和范围，而不是指固定不变的某种脉象。脉象不浮不沉，不快不慢，不强不弱，从容和缓，为"有胃"；节律整齐，柔和有力，为"有神"；尺脉沉取有力，为"有根"。脉贵有胃、有神、有根，提示机体气血充盈，气机健旺，阴阳平衡，精神安和的生理状态，是健康的象征。

4.1.4 病脉（病理脉象）

病脉，疾病反映于脉象的变化，叫病理脉象，简称"病脉"。一般说来，除了正常生理变化范围以内及个体生理特异变化之外的脉象，均属病脉。病理脉象一般在脉位、脉次、脉形、脉势四个方面出现不同于平脉的异常表现。近代临床所提及的脉象，有浮、沉、迟、数、洪、细、虚、实、滑、涩、弦、紧、结、代、促、长、短、缓、濡、弱、微、散、芤、伏、牢、革、动、疾等。

4.2 按诊

按诊是医生用手直接触摸或按压病人某些部位，以了解局部冷热、润燥、软硬、压痛、肿块或其他异常变化，从而推断疾病部位、性质和病情轻重等情况的一种诊断方法。按诊是切诊的重要组成部分，是诊法中不容忽视的一环。按诊不仅可以进一步确定望诊之所见，补充望诊之不足，而且亦可为问诊提示重点，特别是对脘腹部疾病的诊断有着更为重要的作用。

知识点 8　辨证原则

1. 辨证的概念

中医辨证即分析、辨识疾病的证候，即以脏腑、经络、病因、病机等基础理论为依据，对四诊所收集的症状、体征，以及其他临床资料进行分析、综合，辨清疾病的原因、性质、部位，以及邪正之间的关系，进而概括、判断为何种证候，为论治提供依据。正确的辨证是确定治疗原则和方法的基础。

中医有许多辨证的方法，如根据八纲辨证、气血津液辨证、卫气营血辨证和脏腑辨证等。每种方法都有自己的特点和侧重点，必须准确灵活应用才能综合地了解疾病，从而为治疗提供基础。

2. 辨证原则

2.1 八纲辨证

八纲辨证是把四诊所收集的资料，经过综合分析，概括病变为阴、阳、表、里、寒、热、虚、实八个部分，从而辨清病变部位、性质和正邪盛衰类别的辨证方法。

病证大体上分为阴证和阳证两类；从病位上分为表证、里证；从性质上分为寒证、热证；从邪正盛衰上分为虚证、实证。阴阳是八纲辨证的总纲，八纲辨证又是其他辨证原则的总纲。

2.2 气血津液辨证

运用气血津液理论，综合病人的病情资料，进行临证辨别、分析、判断，从而确定其气、血、津液的具体病机、证型的思维过程和辨证方法，就是气血津液辨证。

气证，分为气虚、气陷、气滞和气逆四类；血证，分为血虚、血瘀、血热和血寒四类。在生理上，它们相互补充；在病理上，它们相互影响。因此形成了同一疾病的气血辨证。临床上，有气滞血瘀、气不摄血、气血亏虚、气虚血瘀和气随血脱五类。津液的证候可以归为两类：津液亏虚和水液潴留。

2.3 卫气营血辨证

卫气营血辨证是叶天士针对温病创立的辨证方法。将温病在其病程发展过程中表现出的证候，进行分析、归纳，概括为卫分、气分、营分和血分四个不同阶段的证候类型，用以说明其病位深浅、病情轻重以及各个阶段病理变化及传变的规律。

2.4 脏腑辨证

脏腑辨证是根据脏腑生理功能、病理表现，结合八纲、病因、气血等理论，对四诊收集的资料，进行分析归纳，借以探求病因病机，判断疾病的部位、性质、正邪盛衰状况的一种辨证方法。

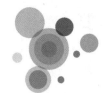

第二部分

针灸学概要

学习目标

学习掌握经络腧穴学、刺法灸法学和针灸治疗学的基本知识点。

知识点目录

❖知识点1　经络总论知识点概要

❖知识点2　腧穴总论知识点概要

❖知识点3　腧穴的定位方法

❖知识点4　人体主要经络及常用腧穴

❖知识点5　刺法灸法学知识点概要

❖知识点6　针灸治疗学知识点概要

知识点 1 经络总论知识点概要

1. 经络的概念

经络是经脉和络脉的统称，是运行气血、联络脏腑和体表及沟通全身各部的通道，是人体各种功能的调控系统。经络是"经"和"络"的统称。经脉，经络系统中的主干。"经"有路径的含义，贯通上下，沟通内外。络脉，经脉别出的分支。"络"有网络之意，较经脉细小，纵横交错，遍布全身。

2. 经络系统的组成

经络分为经脉和络脉两大部分。其中，经脉包括十二经脉、奇经八脉，以及附属于十二经脉的十二经别、经筋、皮部。十二经脉又分为手三阴经、手三阳经、足三阴经和足三阳经；奇经八脉分为任、督、冲、带、阴跷、阳跷、阴维、阳维八脉；经别、皮部、经筋与十二经脉一样，也分别以手、足之三阴、三阳归类；络脉分为十五络、浮络、孙络。

3. 经络系统简介

3.1 十二经脉 （十二正经）

十二脏腑所属经脉，即手三阴经、手三阳经、足三阴经、足三阳经的总称，是经络系统的主体，所以又称为"正经"。

3.1.1 十二经脉的体表分布

四肢部：阴经分布于四肢内侧，上肢内侧者为手三阴，下肢内侧者为足三阴经。手足三阴经为"太阴"在前，"厥阴"在中，"少阴"在后。（足三阴经在内踝上 8 寸以下是"厥阴"在前，"太阴"在中，"少阴"在后。）阳经分布于四肢外侧，上肢外侧者为手三阳经，下肢外侧者为足三阳经。手足三阳经为"阳明"在前，"少阳"在中（侧），"太阳"在后。

躯干部：手三阳经行于肩胛部，手三阴经均从腋下走出。足三阳经为阳明经行于前（胸、腹面），太阳经行于后（背面），少阳经行于侧面。足三阴经均行于腹面。

头面部：头为"诸阳之会"，六条阳经均循行于头部。总的分布规律为：阳明在前，少阳在侧，太阳在后。手足阳明经行于前部、前额；手足少阴经行于侧部、侧头；手足太阳经行于后部、后头；督脉和足厥阴肝经行于巅顶部。

3.1.2 十二经脉的表里络属关系

十二经脉在体内与脏腑相络属，其中阴经属脏主里络腑，阳经属腑主表络脏。一脏配一腑，一阴配一阳，构成脏腑阴阳表里属络关系。如手太阴肺经，属肺络大肠；手阳明大肠经属大肠络肺。十二经脉阴阳相配，与脏腑之阴阳相一致。因此，它们的关系也是根据脏与腑的阴阳搭配来分表里，如肺与大肠相表里，则手太阴肺经与手阳明大肠经相表里。以此类推，其他经亦是如此。互为表里的两经相联系，在生理、病理上相互影响，治疗时相互为用。

3.1.3 十二经脉的走向、循环流注和交接规律

（1）十二经脉的走向

手之三阴从胸走手，手之三阳从手走头，足之三阳从头走足，足之

三阴从足走腹（胸）。

（2）十二经脉流注次序

十二经脉通过阴阳表里、手足同名经的连接，从手太阴至足厥阴，再复从手太阴相接诸经，从而构成了周而复始，如环无端的传注系统。交接顺序：手太阴→手阳明→足阳明→足太阴→手少阴→手太阳→足太阳→足少阴→手厥阴→手少阳→足少阳→足厥阴→手太阴。（图2－1－1）

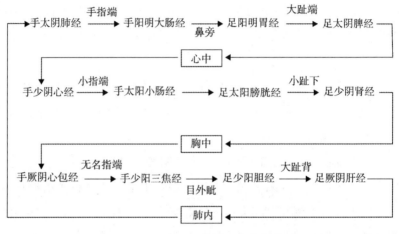

图2－1－1　十二经脉循环流注次序

（3）十二经脉的交接规律

十二经脉的交接规律是"表里、同名相接，阴阳相承"。阴经与阳经在四肢末端交接，阳经与阳经在头面交接，阴经与阴经在胸中交接。手三阴接手三阳，手三阳接足三阳，足三阳接足三阴，足三阴又接手三阴。手之阴阳经交接在手指末端，手之阳经与足之阳经在头面部，足之阳经与阴经交接在足趾末端，足之三阴与手之三阴在胸腹部。阴阳交接是表里经相接，阳经与阳经交接是同名经交接。

3.2 十二经别

十二经别是十二正经离、入、出、合的别行部分，是正经别行深入体腔的支脉。

3.2.1 循行特点

十二经别多从四肢肘膝上下的正经别出（离），经过躯干深入体腔与相关的脏腑联系（入），再浅出于体表上行头项部（出），在头项部，阳经经别合于本经的经脉，阴经经别合于相表里的阳经经脉（合），故有"六合"之称。

3.2.2 主要功能

由于十二经别有离、入、出、合于人体表里之间的特点，加强了十二经脉的内外联系及所属络的脏腑在体腔深部的联系；补充了十二经脉在体内外循环的不足；扩大了经穴的治疗范围；加强了十二经脉与头面的关系，突出了头面部经穴的重要性。

3.3 十二经筋

十二经筋是十二经脉之气濡养筋肉骨节的体系，是附属于十二经脉的筋肉系统。

3.3.1 分布特点

十二经筋循行分布均起始于四肢末端，结聚于关节骨骼部，而走向头面躯干，行于体表，不入内脏。

3.3.2 主要功能

经筋具有约束骨骼、屈伸关节、维持人体正常运动功能的作用。

3.4 十二皮部

十二皮部是十二经脉功能活动反映于体表的部位，也是络脉之气散布之所在。

3.4.1 分布特点

十二皮部的分布区域是以十二经脉体表的分布范围为依据的。

3.4.2 主要功能

皮部是机体的卫外屏障，起着保卫机体、抗御外邪的作用。

3.5 奇经八脉

奇经八脉指别道奇行的经脉。不直接隶属于十二脏腑，也无阴阳表里属络关系。包括督脉、任脉、冲脉、带脉、阴维脉、阳维脉、阴跷脉、阳跷脉。

3.5.1 奇经八脉与十二正经的区别

奇经八脉中除了任督二脉以外，均与十二经脉相伴而行，没有明确的腧穴，它们不像十二经脉是气血循行的通道，而只是起到积蓄和渗灌十二经脉气血的作用。

3.5.2 奇经八脉的功能

（1）进一步加强十二经脉之间的联系。如奇经八脉中的任脉称为阴脉之海，督脉称为阳脉之海，冲脉称为血海或十二经脉之海，带脉约束身体各经，阴阳跷脉则主持人体的阴气和阳气，阴阳维脉维系人体的阴经和阳经。

（2）对十二经脉气血有着蓄积和渗灌的调节作用。十二经脉气有余时，则蓄藏于奇经八脉；十二经脉气血不足时，则由奇经"溢出"及时给予补充。

3.6 十五络脉

十二经脉和任督二脉各自别出一支络脉，加上脾之大络，共计十五条，总称十五络脉。

3.6.1 分布特点

十五络脉的分布特点：十二经脉的别络分别从本经肘膝关节以下的络穴别出后，均走向其相表里经脉（阴经别络于阳经，阳经别络于阴经）。任脉的别络从鸠尾（络穴）分出后散布于腹部，以沟通腹部的经气。督脉的别络从长强（络穴）分出后散布于头部，向左右别走足太阳经，以沟通背部经气。脾之大络从胁下的大包穴分出后散布于胸胁。此外，还有从络脉分出浮行于浅表的孙络和浮现于皮肤表层能看到的浮络，它们遍布全身，难以计数，其作用主要是输布气血于经筋和皮部。

3.6.2 主要功能

四肢部的十二经别络沟通了阴阳表里二经的经气，加强了表里二经的联系和经脉之气的交接传注，补充了十二经循行的不足且扩大了主治范围。躯干部的任脉别络、督脉别络和脾之大络，分别沟通了腹、背和胸胁及全身经气，从而起到输布气血、濡养全身的作用。

4. 经络系统的功能与经络学说的临床应用

4.1 经络系统的功能

4.1.1 联络脏腑、沟通肢窍

由于十二经脉内属五脏六腑，外联四肢百骸，通达五官九窍，再加上奇经八脉、十五络脉、经筋、经别、皮部和浮络、孙络遍布全身，形如网络，纵横交错，入里出表，上通下达，从而把人体各脏腑器官、肢体官窍、筋骨皮肉联系成了一个有机的整体，实现了各组织器官在功能活动之间的联系沟通和协调统一，保证了人体生命活动的正常进行。

4.1.2 运行气血、濡养周身

经络有运行气血、调节阴阳、营养全身的作用。经络是气血运行的通道，气血是人体生命活动的物质基础。人体各个脏腑、组织、器官均需要气血的温养和濡润，才能发挥其正常作用。而气血必须依赖经络系统的循环传注，才能输布周身，以温养濡润全身各脏腑组织器官，维持机体的正常机能。

4.1.3 抗御外邪、保卫机体

由于经络能"行血气而营阴阳"，营气运行于脉中，卫气行于脉外，使营卫之气密布于周身，加强了机体的防御能力，起到了抗御外邪、保卫机体的屏障作用。

4.1.4 传导感应、调整虚实

传导感应是指经络系统对于针刺或其他刺激的感受和应答及各种信息的传递作用。当人体的外部受到某种刺激后，人体就会对这种刺激做出反应，并将相关信息通过经络传递至体内有关脏腑，使该脏腑的功能发生变化。如针刺治疗中的得气现象，就是这个功能的一种表现。反之，脏腑受到某种刺激而功能发生变化时，也可以通过经络将信息传递而反映于体表。调整虚实是指经络在沟通联系、运行气血、感应传递信息的基础上，对各脏腑形体官窍的功能活动具有调节作用，从而使人体复杂的生理活动相互协调，以保持相对平衡的健康状态。此时可以用针刺、艾灸、推拿等治疗方法激发经气，调节机能，使机体重新恢复到平衡协调的状态，以达到治愈疾病的目的。

4.2 经络学说的临床应用

4.2.1 说明病理变化

由于经络里通外达，联络脏腑、四肢百骸，当机体正处于正虚邪实的情况下，经络又是病邪传注的途径。由于脏腑之间有经脉沟通，所以其病变可通过经络相互传变。

4.2.2 揭示针灸的治疗作用

针灸治疗疾病是通过经络的传导感应来调节经气，以恢复脏腑经络的正常功能。这一功能的发挥是以其运行气血、调节阴阳的生理功能为基础的。

4.2.3 指导临床诊断

由于经络的循行分布各有分野，脏腑官窍络属各有差异。所以，可根据体表病变发生部位与经络循行分布的关系，推断疾病所在的经脉。此外，医生还可以根据经络循行线路上的敏感点、压痛点、结节、索状物等经络的特殊反应和变化来诊断疾病。

4.2.4 指导疾病治疗

一方面，经络学说可以指导针灸选穴配穴。根据疾病所涉及的经络，可选用与该疾病有关的经络腧穴来治疗；也可选取相互表里经络的腧穴来治疗；也可根据经络之间的相互联系或选取同名经，或选取相克或相生经络来治疗。另一方面，经络学说可以指导临床用药。按照药物归经选择对证治疗的药物可以提高疗效。

知识点 2　腧穴总论知识点概要

1. 腧穴的定义

腧穴是人体脏腑经络之气输注于体表的部位，是针灸治疗疾病的刺激点。"腧"通"输"，有转输、输注的含义；"穴"即孔隙。所以，腧穴的本义是指人体脏腑经络之气转输或输注于体表的分肉腠理和骨节交会特定的孔隙。

2. 腧穴的分类

人体的腧穴很多，总括起来可分成三类：十四经穴、奇穴、阿是穴。

十四经穴：简称"经穴"，是指归属于十二正经和任脉、督脉循行路线上的腧穴。其特点是均有固定的名称、固定的位置、固定的归经和相对固定的主治功用，而且多具有主治本经病候的共同作用，是腧穴的主要部分。

经外奇穴：指未列入十四经系统的有固定名称和定位的腧穴。其特点：有固定的名称、定位和主治，但无归经。它们的主治范围比较单一，多数对某些病证有特殊疗效。有些穴位命名和取穴方法也奇特，故名经外奇穴。

阿是穴：又称"不定穴""天应穴""压痛点"等。这类腧穴既无固定名称，也无固定的位置和主治，而是以压痛敏感点或其他反应点作为针灸施术部位。这种"以痛为腧"的针灸治疗方法叫"阿是之法"，由孙思邈所著的《千金要方》最早记载并流传后世，用此法所取的穴位统称为阿是穴。

3. 腧穴的治疗作用

腧穴是接受刺激，防治疾病的部位。通过刺激穴位，通经脉调气血，使阴阳平衡，脏腑和调，扶正祛邪。腧穴的治疗作用主要体现在以下三个方面：

3.1 近治作用

腧穴的近治作用是指腧穴均能治疗其所在部位及邻近脏腑、组织、器官的病证。这是所有腧穴主治作用所具有的共同特点，即"腧穴所在，主治所在"。

3.2 远治作用

腧穴的远治作用指某些腧穴不仅能治局部病证，而且还能治疗本经循行所达的远隔部位的脏腑、组织、器官的病证。具有远治作用的腧穴，主要指十二经脉在四肢肘膝关节以下的腧穴，即"经络所及，主治所及"。

3.3 特殊治疗作用

腧穴的特殊治疗作用是指某些腧穴具有良性双向调节或相对的特异性治疗作用。

3.3.1 良性双向调节作用

针刺某些腧穴时，对其相应所治疗的某器官或某机能活动的病理状态具有双向调节作用。如腹泻时针天枢穴可止泻，便秘时针天枢穴则可通便。

3.3.2 相对特异性作用

临床实践证明，有些腧穴对某脏腑器官疾病或某病理状态有相对特异的治疗作用。如大椎穴退热，至阴穴矫正胎位，胆囊穴治疗胆绞痛等，均有较好的效果和较高的特异性。

4. 特定穴

特定穴是十四经穴中具有特殊治疗作用并被给以特定名称的腧穴。它们除具有经穴的共同主治特性外，还有某些特殊的性能和功用，在针灸临床中有重要意义。根据特定穴的分布特点、功能意义和治疗作用，可分为以下十类：五输穴、原穴、络穴、郄穴、八脉交会穴、下合穴及背俞穴、募穴、八会穴和交会穴。

4.1 五输穴

十二经中分布在肘膝关节以下，从四肢末端向肘膝方向排列的井、荥、输、经、合五个穴位。"井"穴，分布于指、趾末端，为经气所出，如水流的源头；"荥"穴，分布于掌指或跖趾关节之前，是经气流过之处，如刚出的泉水微流；"输"穴，分布于掌指或跖趾关节之后，为经气灌注之处，如水流由浅入深；"经"穴，分布于前臂或胫部，为经气所行经的畅行部位，经气盛行，如水入江河畅通无阻；"合"穴，位于肘膝关节附近，为经气充盛入合于脏腑之处，如百川汇入湖海。

4.2 原穴

原穴是脏腑原气经过和留止的部位。十二经各有一个原穴，共十二原穴，均分布于四肢腕、踝关节附近。脏腑的病变，可以反映到其相应的原穴，有助于诊断；而各经原穴对本经所属脏腑的疾病均有特异性治疗作用。手足六阳经的原穴单独存在，均排列在输穴之后，手足六阴经则以输穴为其原穴。

4.3 络穴

十五络脉从经脉分出的部位各有一个腧穴叫络穴，共十五穴，故称十五络穴。其中十二经的络穴均位于四肢肘膝关节以下，而任脉的络穴鸠尾位于上腹部，督脉的络穴长强位于尾骶部，脾之大络大包穴位于胸胁部。十二经络穴具有联络表里二经的作用，兼治表里二经病候；长强、鸠尾、大包除了治疗本经病候外，还治疗其络脉联络部位的病痛（如背、腹、胸胁各部位的病痛等）。

4.4　郄穴

"郄"即孔隙，郄穴是各经经气深集的部位。十二经脉与奇经八脉中的阴跷、阳跷、阴维、阳维四脉各有一个郄穴，共十六个郄穴，多分布于四肢肘膝关节以下。郄穴对各经急性病痛有较好的治疗作用。

4.5　八脉交会穴

八脉交会穴是十二经脉与奇经八脉相通的八个特定穴。它们分别位于腕、踝关节附近，既能治疗其本经病证，又能治其所通的奇经的病证。

4.6　下合穴

手足三阳六腑之气下合于足三阳经的六个特定穴，称为下合穴，也称六腑下合穴。其中胃、胆、膀胱的下合穴就是其本经合穴，而大肠的下合穴（上巨虚）、小肠的下合穴（下巨虚）均在胃经，三焦的下合穴（委阳）在膀胱经。这六个下合穴是治疗六腑病证的重要穴位，均在膝关节附近或以下。

4.7　背俞穴

俞穴又称背俞穴，是脏腑之气输注于背部的腧穴。五脏六腑各有一个背俞穴，均分布于背腰部足太阳膀胱经第 1 侧线上，其位置与相关脏腑所在部位的排列相接近。

4.8 募穴

募穴是脏腑之气汇聚于胸腹部的腧穴，又称腹募穴。五脏六腑各有一个募穴，其位置也与相关脏腑所在部位相接近。

4.9 八会穴

八会穴是人体脏、腑、气、血、筋、脉、骨、髓精气所聚的八个特定穴。它们均分布在躯干和四肢部，分别与上述的八种脏腑器官或组织有着密切联系，主治相关病证。

4.10 交会穴

交会穴是指两经或数经相交会部位的腧穴，多分布于头面、躯干，也见于四肢部。交会穴不仅能治疗其所属经络（本经）的病证，也能治疗其相交会经络（他经）的病证。

知识点 3　腧穴的定位方法

1. 骨度分寸法

骨度分寸法是以体表骨节为主要标志折量全身各部的长度和宽度，定出分寸，用于腧穴定位的方法。（表 2 – 3 – 1）

表 2 – 3 – 1 常用骨度分寸

	起止点	长度	量用法	说明
头面部	前发际正中至后发际正中	12 寸	直寸	用于确定头部经穴的纵向距离
	眉间（印堂）至前发际正中	3 寸	直寸	
	第 7 颈椎棘突下至后发际正中	3 寸	直寸	
	前两额发角（头维）之间	9 寸	横寸	用于确定头部经穴的横向距离
	耳后两乳突（完骨）之间	9 寸	横寸	
胸腹部	胸剑联合至脐的中心	8 寸	直寸	胸部直量，一般以肋骨计算，每一肋骨相邻距离为 1.6 寸
	脐的中心至耻骨联合上缘	5 寸	直寸	
	两乳头之间	8 寸	横寸	通用于胸腹部
腰背部	第 1 胸椎到骶尾联合	21 椎	直寸	背部直量
	两肩胛骨脊柱缘之间	6 寸	横寸	量时两手应下垂
上肢部	腋前皱襞到肘横纹	9 寸	直寸	通用于手三阴、手三阳经脉
	肘横纹到腕横纹	12 寸		

	起止点	长度	量用法	说明
	耻骨联合上缘至股骨内上髁上缘	18寸	直寸	用于确定下肢内侧足三阴经穴的纵向距离
	胫骨内侧髁下方至内踝尖	13寸		
下肢部	股骨大转子至腘横纹	19寸	直寸	1. 用于确定下肢外侧足三阴经穴的纵向距离 2. 外膝眼到外踝尖适用于屈膝时计算；伸膝则以腘横纹到外踝尖计算
	臀横纹至腘横纹	14寸	直寸	
	腘横纹（外膝眼）至外踝尖	16寸		
	外踝尖至足底	3寸	直寸	

2. 体表标志法

体表标志法是以人体自然标志如五官、毛发、关节、肌肉等定位取穴的方法。

2.1 固定标志

不受人体活动影响而固定不移的标志为固定标志，如五官、毛发、爪甲、乳头、脐部、骨节的凹凸、肌肉的隆起等。如肩胛冈内端平第3胸椎棘突、肩胛骨下角平第7胸椎棘突、髂嵴平第4腰椎棘突。

2.2 活动标志

需要采取相应的动作才能出现的标志为活动标志，如关节、肌肉、皮肤随活动而出现的凹陷、褶皱等。

3. 指寸定位法

指寸定位法是以患者手指的某部位折作一定分寸来定取穴位的

方法。

3.1 中指同身寸法

中指屈曲时，中节掌侧两端纹头之间为 1 寸。用于四肢取穴的直寸、背部的横寸取穴。

3.2 拇指同身寸法

拇指指关节的横度作为 1 寸。用于四肢部取穴。

3.3 横指同身寸法

将食、中、无名、小指并拢，以中指第 2 节横纹处为准，四指的横度为 3 寸，又称"一夫法"。用于下肢直寸和背部的横寸取穴。

知识点 4　人体主要经络及常用腧穴

1. 手太阴肺经

1.1 经脉循行（图 2 - 4 - 1）

手太阴肺经起于中焦，向下联络大肠，回绕过来沿着胃的上口，通过横膈，属于肺脏。从肺系，横出腋下，向下经上臂内侧，行手少阴经和手厥阴经的前面，下行到肘窝中，沿前臂内侧前缘，进入寸口，经过鱼际，沿着鱼际的边缘，出拇指内侧端。

手腕后方的分支，从列缺穴（LU 7）处分出，走向食指内侧端，与手阳明大肠经相接。

联系的脏腑：肺、大肠、胃、中焦。

联系的器官：喉咙、气管。

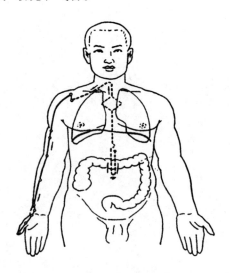

图 2 - 4 - 1　手太阴肺经经脉循行示意图

1.2 主治概要

本经腧穴主要治疗肺、胸、喉、头面和经脉循行部位的其他病证。

1.3 常用腧穴

本经腧穴起于中府穴（LU 1），止于少商穴（LU 11），两侧各 11 个腧穴。

1.3.1 中府（LU 1 募穴）

定位：在胸前壁，第 1 肋间隙的外上方，云门穴下 1 寸，平第 1 肋间隙，距前正中线 6 寸。病人坐直或卧床以定位此点。（图 2 - 4 - 2）

主治：①咳嗽，气喘，胸痛；②肩背痛。

刺法：向外斜刺 0.5 ~ 0.8 寸。不可直刺或向内侧深刺，以免伤及肺脏，引起气胸。

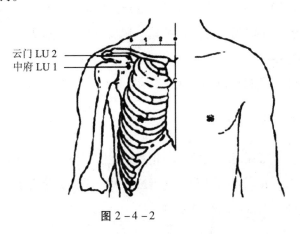

云门 LU 2
中府 LU 1

图 2 - 4 - 2

1.3.2 尺泽（LU 5 合穴）

定位：仰掌，微屈肘。在肘横纹中，肱二头肌腱桡侧凹陷处。（图 2 - 4 - 3）

主治：①咳嗽，气喘，咯血，咽喉肿痛；②中暑；③急性腹痛伴吐泻；④肘臂挛痛。

刺法：直刺 0.8 ~ 1.2 寸。治疗急性腹痛伴腹泻时点刺头静脉出血。

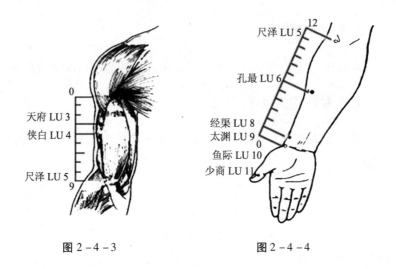

图 2 - 4 - 3   图 2 - 4 - 4

1.3.3 孔最（LU 6 郄穴）

定位：微屈肘，掌心相对，或伸前臂仰掌，在前臂掌面桡侧，当太渊穴（LU 9）与尺泽穴（LU 5）连线上，腕横纹上7寸。（图 2 - 4 - 4）

主治：①咳嗽，咯血，鼻衄，咽喉痛；②热病无汗；③肘关节和前臂痉挛性疼痛。

刺法：直刺 0.5 ~ 1 寸。

1.3.4 列缺（LU 7 络穴 八脉交会穴通于任脉）

定位：微屈肘，侧腕掌心相对。在前臂桡侧缘，桡骨茎突上方，腕横纹上 1.5 寸。当一只手的食指按在另一手桡骨茎突上，食指尖端下边的凹陷即是穴。（图 2 - 4 - 5）

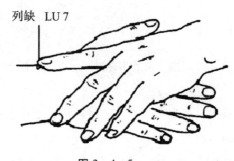

图 2 - 4 - 5

主治：①咳嗽，气喘，咽喉痛；②头痛，颈项强痛，面瘫；③阴茎疼痛和血尿；④腕痛无力。

刺法：向上斜刺 0.3～0.5 寸。

1.3.5 太渊（LU 9 腧穴 原穴 八会穴之脉会）

定位：伸臂仰掌。在腕掌侧横纹桡侧，桡动脉搏动处。（图 2 - 4 - 6）

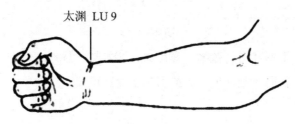

图 2 - 4 - 6

主治：①感冒，咳嗽，痰多，气喘；②手腕痛。

刺法：避开桡动脉，直刺 0.3～0.5 寸。

1.3.6 鱼际（LU 10 荥穴）

定位：第 1 掌骨桡侧的中点，赤白肉际处，第 1 掌指关节近端。（图 2 - 4 - 7）

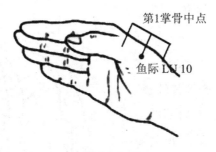

图 2 - 4 - 7

主治：①发热，咽喉痛，失语，咳嗽，哮喘；②手心热。

刺法：直刺 0.5～0.8 寸，可灸。

1.3.7 少商（LU 11 井穴）

定位：伸拇指。在拇指末节桡侧，距指甲角侧方约 0.1 寸。（图 2 - 4 - 8）

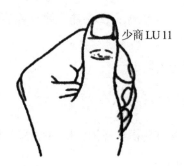

图 2 - 4 - 8

主治：①咽喉痛，咳嗽，鼻出血；②发热，昏迷，癫狂。

刺法：斜向上刺 0.1 寸，或点刺出血；可灸。

2. 手阳明大肠经

2.1 经脉循行 (图 2 - 4 - 9)

手阳明大肠经，起于食指尖端（商阳穴 LI 1），沿食指桡侧向上延伸，出第 1 和第 2 掌骨（合谷穴 LI 4）间，进入两筋（拇长伸肌腱和拇短伸肌腱）之间。沿前臂桡侧进入肘外侧，经上臂外侧前边，上肩部的最高点（肩髃穴 LI 15），出肩峰的前缘，向上交会第 7 颈椎下（手足三阳经的汇合）并向下进入锁骨上窝，与相应的脏腑肺相连，然后穿过膈膜进入大肠。锁骨上窝的分支向上延伸到颈部，穿过脸颊进入下牙龈。然后

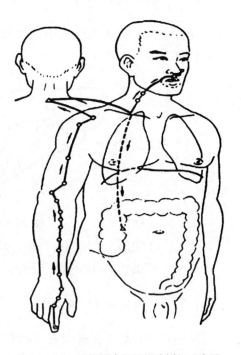

图 2 - 4 - 9　手阳明大肠经经脉循行示意图

回绕至上唇并穿过人中，左边的向右，右边的向左，上夹鼻孔旁的迎香穴（LI 20），与足阳明胃经相接。

联系的脏腑：大肠和胃。

联系的器官：口、下齿和鼻。

2.2 主治概要

口、齿、鼻和咽喉的疾病以及涉及上肢外侧前缘，肩部和颈部前侧的疾病。

2.3 常用腧穴

手阳明大肠经穴起于商阳穴（LI 1），止于迎香穴（LI 20），两侧各 20 个穴位。

2.3.1 合谷（LI 4 原穴）

定位：该穴位于手背部，在第 1 和第 2 掌骨之间，大约在第 2 掌骨桡侧的中点处。（图 2 – 4 – 10）

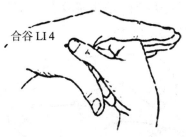

图 2 – 4 – 10

当拇指的指间关节的横向折痕与拇指和另一只手的拇食指之间的指蹼缘重合在一起时，拇指尖端下即是穴。

主治：①头痛、头晕，目赤肿痛，齿痛，鼻衄，面瘫；②恶寒，发烧，无汗证，多汗证；③腹痛，腹泻，便秘，痢疾；④痛经，闭经，难产；⑤小儿惊风，牙关紧闭；⑥荨麻疹，痤疮；⑦上肢痿痹，手指挛痛。

刺法：直刺 0.5～1 寸。妊娠者禁针。

2.3.2 手三里（LI 10）

定位：当阳溪（LI 5）与曲池（LI 11）连线上，肘横纹下 2 寸。（图 2 - 4 - 11）

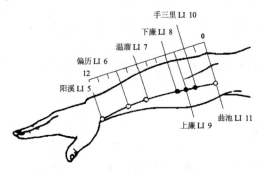

图 2 - 4 - 11

主治：①腹痛，腹泻；②手臂麻木，疼痛，肘挛不伸，上肢不遂。

刺法：直刺 0.8 ~ 1.2 寸；可灸。

2.3.3 曲池（LI 11 合穴）

定位：肘关节屈曲 90°时，在肘横纹上，当尺泽（LU 5）与肱骨外上髁连线的中点。（图 2 - 4 - 12）

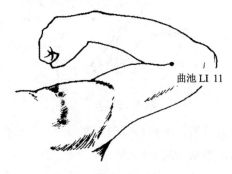

图 2 - 4 - 12

主治：①头痛，咽喉疼痛，目赤肿痛，齿痛；②上肢瘫痪，肘臂疼痛无力；③腹痛，呕吐，腹泻；④湿疹，荨麻疹，痤疮；⑤热病，高血压。

刺法：直刺 1 ~ 1.5 寸；可灸。

2.3.4 肩髃（LI 15 手阳明、阳跷交会穴）

定位：在肩峰前下方，三角肌上，肩峰与肱骨大结节之间。当臂外展时，或向前平伸时，当肩锁关节前下方凹陷处。（图 2 - 4 - 13）

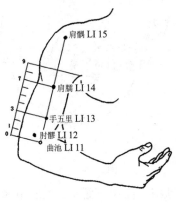

图 2 - 4 - 13

主治：上肢瘫痪，肩臂痛。

刺法：直刺或向下斜刺 0.8 ~ 1.5 寸。

2.3.5 扶突（LI 18）

定位：在颈外侧部，喉结旁，当胸锁乳突肌的胸骨头和锁骨头之间。（图 2 - 4 - 14）

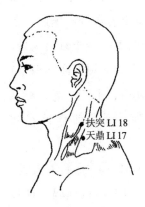

图 2 - 4 - 14

主治：①咽喉疼痛，暴喑，瘰疬，瘿瘤；②上肢痿痹，肩臂疼痛。

刺法：直刺 0.5～0.8 寸。

2.3.6 迎香（LI 20）

定位：该穴位于鼻唇沟，鼻翼外缘中点旁。（图 2 - 4 - 15）

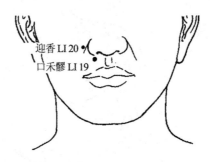

迎香 LI 20
口禾髎 LI 19

图 2 - 4 - 15

主治：①鼻塞，衄血，面痒，面瘫；②胆道蛔虫病。
刺法：直刺 0.1～0.2 寸，或平刺或斜刺 0.3～0.5 寸。

3. 足阳明胃经

3.1 经脉循行 (图 2 - 4 - 16)

足阳明胃经，起于鼻翼两侧迎香穴（LI 20），上行到鼻根部，向下沿着鼻的外侧进入上齿龈内，回出环绕口唇，向下交会于颏唇沟处，再向后沿着口腮后下方，出于下颌大迎（ST 5）处，沿着下颌角颊车（ST 6），上行耳前，经过上关（GB 3），沿着发际，到达前额神庭穴（GV 24）。

面部支脉，从大迎（ST 5）前下走人迎，沿着喉咙进入锁骨上窝，向下经过横膈。锁骨上窝部直行的经脉，经乳头，向下进入少腹两侧气冲（ST 30）。

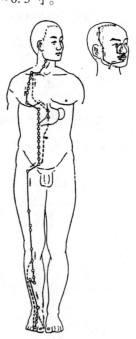

图 2 - 4 - 16　足阳明胃经经脉循行示意图

口部支脉，沿着腹里向下到气冲（ST 30）会合，再由此下行至髀关（ST 31），再穿过伏兔，下至膝盖，沿着胫骨外侧前缘，下经足背，到达第 2 趾尖的侧面。

胫部支脉，从膝盖以下三寸处分出（足三里 ST 36），进入足中趾外侧端。

足背部支脉，从背部冲阳穴（ST 42）分出，终止于大趾内侧端隐白穴（SP 1），在此与足太阴脾经相接。

联系的脏腑：胃和脾。

联系的器官：眼、鼻、齿、耳、口、咽喉、乳房。

3.2 主治概要

本经腧穴主治胃肠病和头面、目、鼻、口齿病和神志病，以及经脉循行部位的其他病证。

3.3 常用腧穴

足阳明胃经起于承泣穴（ST 1），止于厉兑穴（ST 45），左右各 45 穴。

3.3.1 四白（ST 2）

定位：在面部，瞳孔正下方，当眼睛直视前方，眼眶下孔凹陷处。（图 2 – 4 – 17）

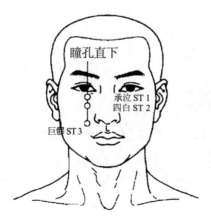

图 2 – 4 – 17

主治：①目赤肿痛，眼睑瞤动，迎风流泪，夜盲；②口眼歪斜，面痛。

刺法：直刺0.3～0.5寸；通常不灸。

3.3.2 地仓（ST 4）

定位：在面部，口角外侧，上直对瞳孔。（图2－4－18）

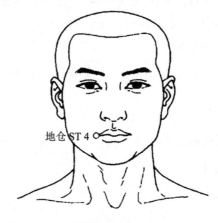

图2－4－18

主治：口眼歪斜，流涎，唇缓不收。

刺法：斜刺或沿皮下刺入0.5～0.8寸或向颊车穴（ST 6）方向透刺。

3.3.3 颊车（ST 6）

定位：在下颌角前上方约一横指（中指）处，当咀嚼时咬肌隆起处。（图2－4－19）

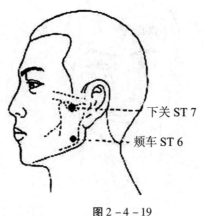

图2－4－19

主治：口眼歪斜，颊肿，齿痛，牙关紧闭。

刺法：直刺0.3～0.5寸，或沿皮下向地仓（ST 4）方向透刺。

3.3.4　下关（ST 7）

定位：在耳前，当颧弓与下颌切迹所形成的凹陷中，口微张时取穴。（图2－4－19）

主治：①齿痛，牙关开阖不利，面痛，口眼歪斜；②耳鸣，耳聋，聤耳，眩晕。

刺法：直刺0.5～1寸。

3.3.5　头维（ST 8）

定位：在头侧面，额角发际上0.5寸，距头正中线4.5寸。（图2－4－20）

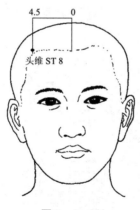

图2－4－20

主治：头痛，眩晕，视物不明，眼睑瞤动。

刺法：沿皮刺入0.5～1寸。

3.3.6　乳根（ST 18）

定位：当乳头直下，乳房根部，第5肋间隙，距前正中线4寸。（图2－4－21）

主治：①乳痛，乳汁少；②咳嗽，气喘，胸痛。

刺法：斜刺或平刺 0.5 ~ 0.8 寸。

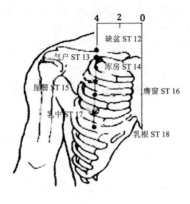

图 2 - 4 - 21

3.3.7 梁门（ST 21）

定位：当脐中上 4 寸，距前正中线 2 寸。（图 2 - 4 - 22）

主治：胃痛，呕吐，食欲不振，腹胀，腹泻。

刺法：直刺 0.8 ~ 1.2 寸。

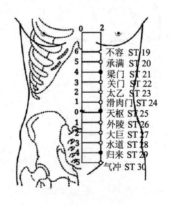

图 2 - 4 - 22

3.3.8 天枢（ST 25 大肠募穴）

定位：在腹中部，距前正中线 2 寸。（图 2 - 4 - 22）

主治：①腹胀，腹痛，绕脐腹痛，便秘，腹泻，痢疾；②月经不调，癥瘕积聚，痛经，闭经。

刺法：直刺 1~1.5 寸。

3.3.9 水道（ST 28）

定位：位于脐下 3 寸，距前正中线 2 寸。（图 2-4-22）
主治：①水肿，小便不利，小腹胀，痛经，疝气；②便秘。
刺法：直刺 1~1.5 寸。

3.3.10 归来（ST 29）

定位：位于脐下 4 寸，距前正中线 2 寸。（图 2-4-22）
主治：①月经不调，痛经，闭经，带下，疝气，小腹痛；②便秘。
刺法：直刺 1~1.5 寸。

3.3.11 伏兔（ST 32）

定位：位于大腿前部，在连接髂前上棘和髌底外侧端的连线上，髌底上 6 寸。（图 2-4-23）

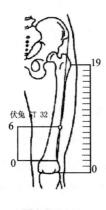
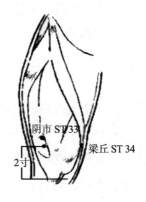

图 2-4-23　　　　　图 2-4-24

主治：腰膝冷痛，下肢麻痹或无力。
刺法：直刺 1~2 寸。

3.3.12 梁丘（ST 34 郄穴）

定位：屈膝，在大腿前面，当髂前上棘与髌底外侧的连线上，髌底

上 2 寸。(图 2 - 4 - 24)

主治:①急性胃痛,呕吐,乳痛;②膝关节疼痛和下肢痿痹。

刺法:直刺 0.5 ~ 1 寸;可灸。

3.3.13 犊鼻 (ST 35)

定位:屈膝,在髌骨与髌韧带外侧凹陷中。(图 2 - 4 - 25)

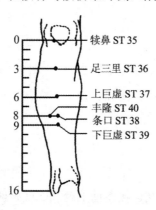

图 2 - 4 - 25

主治:膝关节肿痛,下肢痿痹,脚气。

刺法:向内侧斜刺 0.5 ~ 1 寸。

3.3.14 足三里 (ST 36 合穴 下合穴 强壮要穴)

定位:位于小腿外侧,犊鼻 (ST 35) 下 3 寸,距胫骨前嵴 1 指宽 (中指)。(图 2 - 4 - 25)

主治:①胃痛,呕吐,腹痛,腹胀,肠鸣,泄泻,痢疾,便秘;② 头痛,头晕,失眠,癫狂;③咳嗽,气喘;④心悸,气短;⑤下肢痿 痹,脚气,水肿;⑥全身强壮要穴,常用艾灸能强身健体治疗虚劳 羸瘦。

刺法:直刺 1 ~ 2 寸。

3.3.15 上巨虚 (ST 37 大肠下合穴)

定位:在小腿前外侧,当犊鼻 (ST 35) 下 6 寸,距胫骨前缘一横

指（中指）。(图 2 - 4 - 25)

主治：①腹痛，腹胀，肠鸣，腹泻，痢疾，便秘，肠痈；②下肢痿痹，脚气。

刺法：直刺 1 ~ 1.5 寸。

3.3.16 条口（ST 38）

定位：位于小腿外侧，犊鼻（ST 35）下 8 寸，距胫骨前嵴 1 指宽（中指）。(图 2 - 4 - 25)

主治：①肩臂疼痛；②下肢痿痹，脚气。

刺法：直刺 1 ~ 1.5 寸。

3.3.17 下巨虚（ST 39 小肠下合穴）

定位：位于小腿外侧，犊鼻（ST 35）下 9 寸，距胫骨前嵴 1 指宽（中指）。(图 2 - 4 - 25)

主治：①小腹痛，泄泻，痢疾；②乳痈；③下肢痿痹，脚气。

刺法：直刺 1 ~ 1.5 寸。

3.3.18 丰隆（ST 40 络穴）

定位：位于小腿外侧，外踝尖上 8 寸，条口（ST 38）外侧，距胫骨前嵴外侧 2 指宽（中指）。(图 2 - 4 - 25)

主治：①咳嗽，痰多，哮喘；②头痛，头晕，癫狂；③下肢痿痹。

刺法：直刺 1 ~ 1.5 寸。

3.3.19 解溪（ST 41 经穴）

定位：位于足背和小腿交界处的横纹中央凹陷处，拇长伸肌腱与趾长伸肌腱之间。(图 2 - 4 - 26)

主治：①头痛，眩晕，癫狂；②腹胀，便秘；③下肢痿痹，踝关节疼痛。

刺法：直刺 0.5 ~ 1 寸。

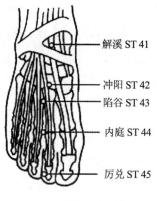

图 2 − 4 − 26

3.3.20 内庭（ST 44 荥穴）

定位：位于足背第 2、3 趾间，趾蹼缘后方赤白肉际处。（图 2 −
4 −26）

主治：①热病，头痛，齿痛，咽喉疼痛，面瘫，鼻衄；②腹胀，便
秘，胃痛；③足背肿痛。

刺法：直刺或斜刺 0.5 ~ 0.8 寸。

4. 足太阴脾经

4.1 经脉循行 (图 2 − 4 − 27)

足太阴脾经，起于足大趾末端，沿着大趾内侧赤白肉际，过大趾本
节后的第 1 跖趾关节后面，上行至内踝前，再上小腿，沿胫骨后交出足
厥阴肝经的前面，上循膝、股部内侧前缘，入腹，属于脾，联络胃，过
横膈上行，挟食管两旁，连系舌根，分散于舌下。

胃部的支脉：向上再通过横膈，流注于心中，与手少阴心经相接。
（图 2 −4 − 27）

联系的脏腑：脾、胃、心。

联系的器官：咽喉、舌。

4.2 主治概要

脾胃疾病、妇科病、前阴病和经脉循行部位的其他病证。

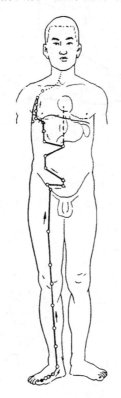

图 2 - 4 - 27 足太阴脾经经脉循行示意图

4.3 常用腧穴

本经腧穴起于隐白穴（SP 1），止于大包穴（SP 21），两侧各 21 个腧穴。

4.3.1 隐白（SP 1 井穴）

定位：位于足大趾末节内侧，距趾甲角 0.1 寸。（图 2 - 4 - 28）

主治：① 月经过多，崩漏，尿血，便血；② 癫狂，多梦，小儿惊风，昏厥。

刺法：斜刺0.1寸或点刺出血。

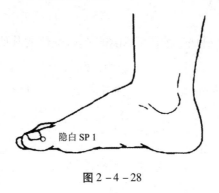

图 2 - 4 - 28

4.3.2 太白（SP 3 输穴 原穴）

定位：在足内侧缘，当足大趾本节（第1跖趾关节）后下方赤白肉际凹陷处。（图 2 - 4 - 29）

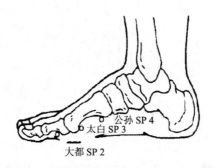

图 2 - 4 - 29

主治：①腹痛，腹胀，呕吐，腹泻，便秘，水肿；②体重节痛，足痛，足肿，痿证。

刺法：直刺0.5～1寸。

4.3.3 公孙（SP 4 络穴 八脉交会穴）

定位：位于足内侧缘，第1跖骨基底的前下方凹陷中，赤白肉际处。（图 2 - 4 - 29）

主治：①胃痛，呕吐，腹胀，腹泻；②心烦，失眠，心痛，心悸。

刺法：直刺0.5～1寸。

4.3.4 三阴交（SP 6 足太阴、足少阴、足厥阴交会穴）

定位：位于小腿内侧，内踝尖正上方 3 寸，胫骨内侧缘后方。（图 2 - 4 - 30）

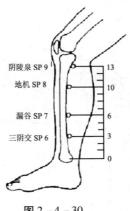

图 2 - 4 - 30

主治：①月经不调，痛经，崩漏，赤白带下，经闭，难产，遗尿，水肿，小便不利；②肠鸣腹胀，泄泻，饮食不化；③心悸，失眠，高血压；④湿疹，荨麻疹；⑤下肢痿痹。

刺法：直刺 1～1.5 寸。孕妇禁针。

4.3.5 地机（SP 8 郄穴）

定位：位于小腿内侧，在连接内踝尖与阴陵泉（SP 9）的连线上。（图 2 - 4 - 30）

主治：①月经不调，痛经，崩漏；②腹痛，泄泻；③小便不利，水肿；④下肢痿痹。

刺法：直刺 1～2 寸。

4.3.6 阴陵泉（SP 9 合穴）

定位：位于小腿内侧，在胫骨内侧髁下缘，胫骨内侧缘的凹陷处。（图 2 - 4 - 30）

主治：①腹胀，泄泻，黄疸；②小便不利，水肿，遗尿；③痛经，前阴痛；④膝关节内侧痛，下肢痿痹。

刺法：直刺1~2寸。

4.3.7 血海（SP 10）

定位：膝关节屈曲，在髌骨内侧端上2寸，位于股四头肌的内侧隆起处。（图2-4-31）

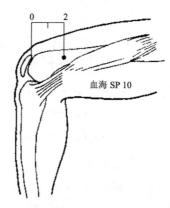

图2-4-31

主治：①月经不调，停经，崩漏，闭经；②荨麻疹，湿疹，丹毒；③膝关节肿痛。

刺法：直刺1~1.5寸。

4.3.8 大包（SP 21 脾之大络）

定位：位于侧胸部，腋中线上，第6肋间隙处。（图2-4-32）

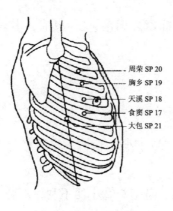

图2-4-32

主治：①胸胁痛，咳嗽，气喘；②全身疼痛，四肢无力。

刺法：斜刺或平刺 0.5~0.8 寸。

5. 手少阴心经

5.1 经脉循行 (图 2 - 4 - 33)

手少阴心经，起于心中，出属于"心系"（心与其他脏器相联系的部位），过横膈，下络小肠。

经脉的分支：从出来，挟着食道上行，系于目（指眼球与脑相联系的脉络）。

经脉直行部分：从"心系"，上行于肺部，横出于腋窝（极泉），沿上臂内侧后缘，至肘窝内侧，沿前臂内侧后缘，到掌后豌豆骨部，入掌，经小指内侧到达指尖，与手太阳小肠经相接。（图 2 - 4 - 33）

联系的脏腑：心、小肠、肺。

联系的器官：眼、舌、咽喉。

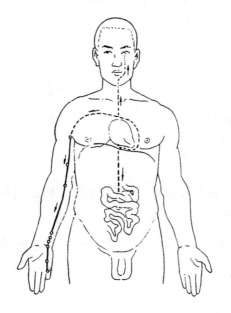

图 2 - 4 - 33　手少阴心经经脉循行示意图

5.2 主治概要

主要治疗心、胸、神志病和经脉循行部位的其他病证。

5.3 常用腧穴

本经腧穴起于极泉穴（HT 1），止于少冲穴（HT 9），两侧各 9 个腧穴。

5.3.1 少海（HT 3 合穴）

定位：屈肘，在肘横纹内侧端与肱骨内上髁连线的中点处。

主治：①心悸，心痛，癫痫；②胸胁痛，肘臂挛痛，臂麻手颤。

刺法：直刺 0.3～0.5 寸。

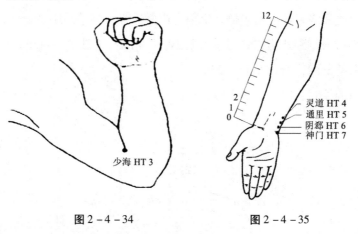

图 2 - 4 - 34   图 2 - 4 - 35

5.3.2 通里（HT 5 络穴）

定位：仰掌，在前臂掌侧，当尺侧腕屈肌腱的桡侧缘，腕横纹上 1 寸。（图 2 - 4 - 35）

主治：①暴喑，舌强不语；②心悸，怔忡；③腕臂痛。

刺法：直刺 0.3～0.5 寸。

5.3.3 阴郄（HT 6 郄穴）

定位：仰掌，尺侧腕屈肌腱的桡侧缘，腕横纹上 0.5 寸。（图 2 - 4 - 35）

主治：①心痛，心悸，惊恐；②吐血，衄血；③骨蒸潮热，盗汗。

刺法：直刺 0.3 ~ 0.5 寸。

5.3.4 神门（HT 7 输穴 原穴）

定位：仰掌，腕掌侧横纹尺侧端，尺侧腕屈肌腱的桡侧凹陷处。（图 2 - 4 - 35）

主治：①心痛，心悸，怔忡，失眠，健忘，多梦，癫狂痫；②手腕痛，手指麻木。

刺法：直刺 0.3 ~ 0.5 寸。

5.3.5 少府（HT 8 荥穴）

定位：在手掌面，第 4、5 掌骨之间，握拳时，当小指尖处。（图 2 - 4 - 36）

主治：①阴痒，小便不利，遗尿；②心痛，胸痛；③小指拘急疼痛。

刺法：直刺 0.3 ~ 0.5 寸。

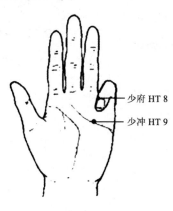

图 2 - 4 - 36

5.3.6 少冲（HT 9 井穴）

定位：在手小指末节桡侧，距指甲角0.1寸。（图2-4-36）

主治：①心痛，心悸；②热病，癫狂痫。

刺法：浅刺0.1寸，或点刺出血。

6. 手太阳小肠经

6.1 经脉循行（图2-4-37）

手太阳小肠经起于手小指尺侧端，沿手背尺侧至腕部，出于尺骨茎突，直上前臂外侧尺骨后缘，经尺骨鹰嘴与肱骨内上髁之间，沿上臂外侧后缘到肩关节，绕行肩胛部，交会于肩上，向下入锁骨上窝，络于心脏，沿食管过横膈，过胃，属于小肠。

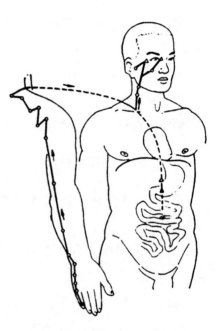

图2-4-37　手太阳小肠经
经脉循行示意图

锁骨上窝支脉：沿颈部上面颊，至目外眦，转入耳中。

颊部支脉：上行目眶下，抵于鼻旁，至眼内角，与足太阳膀胱经相接。

联系的脏腑：小肠，心，胃。

联系的器官：喉咙，耳，鼻，眼。

6.2 主治概要

主要治疗头面病，咽喉病，热病及上肢外侧、肩胛背部等疾病。

6.3 常用腧穴

本经腧穴起于少泽穴（SI 1），止于听宫穴（SI 19），两侧各 19 个腧穴。

6.3.1 少泽（SI 1 井穴）

定位：在手小指末节尺侧，距指甲根角约 0.1 寸。（图 2 - 4 - 38）
主治：①乳少，乳痈；②热病，中风，昏迷。
刺法：浅刺 0.1 寸或点刺出血。

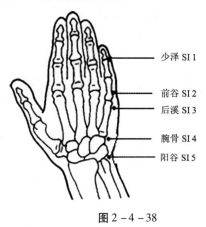

少泽 SI 1

前谷 SI 2
后溪 SI 3

腕骨 SI 4
阳谷 SI 5

图 2 - 4 - 38

6.3.2 后溪（SI 3 输穴 八脉交会穴）

定位：微握拳，在手掌尺侧，第 5 掌指关节近端，掌横纹头赤白肉际。（图 2 - 4 - 38）
主治：①热病，疟疾，癫狂痫；②头项强痛、腰背痛、手指及肘臂挛痛；③耳聋，目赤。
刺法：直刺 0.5 ~ 1 寸。

6.3.3 养老（SI 6 郄穴）

定位：在前臂背面尺侧，当尺骨小头近端桡侧凹陷中。（图 2 - 4 - 39）
主治：①目视不明；②肩、背、肘、臂酸痛。

刺法：向肘方向斜刺 0.5～0.8 寸。

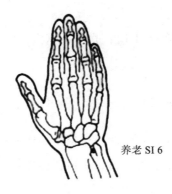

养老 SI 6

图 2 - 4 - 39

6.3.4 小海（SI 8 合穴）

定位：微屈肘。在肘外侧，当尺骨鹰嘴与肱骨内上髁之间凹陷处。（图 2 - 4 - 40）

主治：①肘臂疼痛，麻木；②头痛，耳鸣，癫痫。

刺法：直刺 0.3～0.5 寸；可灸。

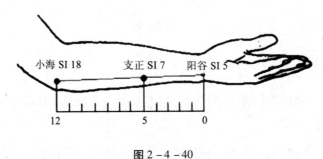

小海 SI 18　　　支正 SI 7　　　阳谷 SI 5

12　　　　　　5　　　　　　0

图 2 - 4 - 40

6.3.5 天宗（SI 11）

定位：在肩胛下窝部，肩胛冈中点与肩胛骨下角连线的上 1/3 与下 2/3 的交点凹陷中。（图 2 - 4 - 41）

主治：①咳嗽，气喘，乳痈；②肩胛背痛。

刺法：直刺或斜刺 0.5～1 寸。

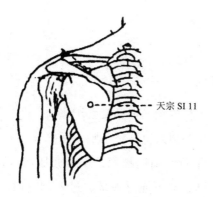

图 2 - 4 - 41

6.3.6 颧髎 (SI 18)

定位：位于目外眦正下方，颧骨下缘凹陷处。（图 2 - 4 - 42）

主治：口眼歪斜，眼睑瞤动，齿痛，颊肿。

刺法：直刺 0.3 ~ 0.5 寸，斜刺或皮下刺入 0.5 ~ 0.8 寸。

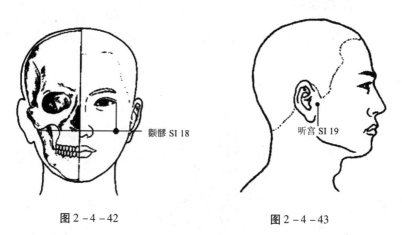

图 2 - 4 - 42   图 2 - 4 - 43

6.3.7 听宫 (SI 19)

定位：位于耳屏前，下颌骨髁状突后方，张口时呈凹陷处。（图 2 - 4 - 43）

主治：耳鸣，耳聋，聤耳，齿痛。

刺法：张口直刺 1 ~ 1.5 寸。

7. 足太阳膀胱经

7.1 经脉循行 (图2-4-44)

足太阳膀胱经，起于目内眦，上额交会于巅顶。

巅顶部直行支脉：从头顶入里联络于脑，回出分开下行项后，沿肩胛部内侧向下，与脊柱平行，到达腰部，从脊旁肌肉进入体腔联络肾脏，属于膀胱；腰部支脉：向下通过臀部，进入腘窝内；后项部支脉：通过肩胛骨内缘直下，经过臀部，沿大腿后外侧下行，与腰部下来的支脉会合于腘窝中。从此向下，通过腓肠肌，出于外踝后，至小趾外侧端，与足少阴肾经相接。

联系的脏腑：膀胱、肾、脑。

联系的器官：目、鼻、耳。

7.2 主治概要

主要治疗头、目、项、背、腰、下肢部病证，神志病及相关脏腑疾病。

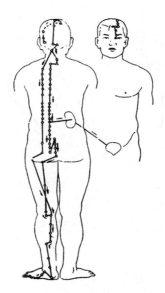

图2-4-44 足太阳膀胱经经脉循行示意图

7.3 常用腧穴

本经腧穴起于睛明穴（BL 1），止于至阴穴（BL 67），两侧各 67 个腧穴。

7.3.1 睛明（BL1）

定位：目内眦角稍上方凹陷处。（图 2 – 4 – 45）

主治：目赤肿痛，近视，迎风流泪，夜盲。

刺法：嘱患者闭目，左手轻轻将眼球推向外侧，右手缓慢沿眼眶边缘直刺 0.5 ~ 1 寸；不宜捻转、提插（或仅轻微捻转、提插）；以避免出血，起针后立刻按压针孔。

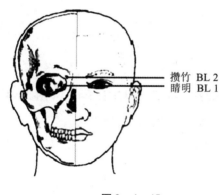

图 2 – 4 – 45

7.3.2 攒竹（BL 2）

定位：位于眉头的凹陷处或眶上切迹处。（图 2 – 4 – 45）

主治：①视物不明，目赤肿痛，迎风流泪，眼睑𥆧动；②头痛，眉棱骨痛，面瘫；③呃逆。

刺法：皮下刺入 0.5 ~ 0.8 寸或点刺出血。

7.3.3 天柱（BL 10）

定位：位于斜方肌外缘之后发际凹陷中，距后发际正中线 1.3 寸。

（图 2 - 4 - 46）

主治：①热病，头痛，眩晕，鼻塞；②项强，肩背痛。

刺法：直刺或斜刺 0.5～0.8 寸。请勿将针向内上方深刺，以免伤及延髓。

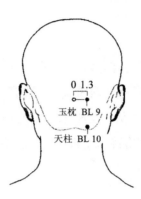

图 2 - 4 - 46

7.3.4 大杼（BL 11 八会穴之骨会）

定位：位于第 1 胸椎棘突下，旁开 1.5 寸。（图 2 - 4 - 47）

主治：①热病，咳嗽；②项强，肩背痛。

刺法：斜刺 0.5～0.8 寸。

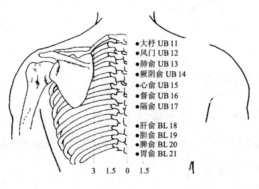

图 2 - 4 - 47

7.3.5 风门（BL 12）

定位：当第 2 胸椎棘突下，旁开 1.5 寸。（图 2 - 4 - 47）

主治：①感冒，发热，头痛，咳嗽；②颈项强痛，肩背痛。

刺法：斜刺0.5~0.8寸。

7.3.6　肺俞（BL 13 背俞穴）

定位：在背部，第3胸椎棘突下，旁开1.5寸。（图2－4－47）

主治：①咳嗽，气喘，咯血；②骨蒸潮热，盗汗；③荨麻疹，痤疮。

刺法：斜刺0.5~0.8寸。

7.3.7　厥阴俞（BL 14 背俞穴）

定位：在背部，当第4胸椎棘突下，旁开1.5寸。（图2－4－47）

主治：①心痛，心悸；②咳嗽，气喘。

刺法：斜刺0.5~0.8寸。

7.3.8　心俞（BL 15 背俞穴）

定位：在背部，当第5胸椎棘突下，旁开1.5寸。（图2－4－47）

主治：①心痛，心悸；②咳嗽，气喘，盗汗；③失眠，健忘，多梦，癫痫。

刺法：斜刺0.5~0.8寸。

7.3.8　膈俞（BL 17 八会穴之血会）

定位：在背部，当第7胸椎棘突下，旁开1.5寸。（图2－4－47）

主治：①胃痛，呃逆，饮食不下；②咳嗽，气喘；③潮热，盗汗；④荨麻疹，痤疮。

刺法：斜刺0.5~0.8寸。

7.3.9　肝俞（BL 18 背俞穴）

定位：当第9胸椎棘突下，旁开1.5寸。（图2－4－47）

主治：①胁痛，黄疸，呕吐；②目赤肿痛，视物模糊；③癫狂痫。

刺法：斜刺 0.5～0.8 寸。

7.3.10 胆俞（BL 19 背俞穴）

定位：在背部，当第 10 胸椎棘突下，旁开 1.5 寸。（图 2 - 4 - 47）
主治：①胁痛，黄疸，口苦；②肺痨，潮热盗汗。
刺法：斜刺 0.5～0.8 寸。

7.3.11 脾俞（BL 20 背俞穴）

定位：在背部，当第 11 胸椎棘突下，旁开 1.5 寸。（图 2 - 4 - 47）
主治：腹胀，腹泻，呕吐，黄疸，痢疾。
刺法：斜刺 0.5～0.8 寸。

7.3.12 胃俞（BL 21 背俞穴）

定位：当第 12 胸椎棘突下，旁开 1.5 寸。（图 2 - 4 - 47）
主治：胃痛，呕吐，腹胀，肠鸣。
刺法：斜刺 0.5～0.8 寸。

7.3.13 肾俞（BL 23 背俞穴）

定位：在腰部，当第 2 腰椎棘突下，旁开 1.5 寸。（图 2 - 4 - 48）
主治：① 遗精，阳痿，遗尿，小便不利，水肿，月经不调，带下；
②头痛，头晕，耳聋，耳鸣，齿痛，腰膝酸痛；③咳嗽，气喘；④洞泄
不化，五更泄泻。
刺法：直刺 0.5～1 寸。

7.3.14 气海俞（BL 24 背俞穴）

定位：在腰部，当第 3 腰椎棘突下，旁开 1.5 寸。（图 2 - 4 - 48）
主治：①腹胀，肠鸣；②遗尿，小便不利，水肿；③腰痛。
刺法：直刺 0.5～1 寸。

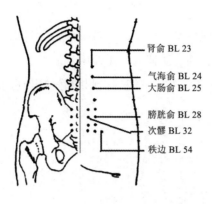

肾俞 BL 23

气海俞 BL 24
大肠俞 BL 25

膀胱俞 BL 28
次髎 BL 32
秩边 BL 54

图 2 - 4 - 48

7.3.15 大肠俞（BL 25 背俞穴）

定位：俯卧，在腰部，当第 4 腰椎棘突下，旁开 1.5 寸。（图 2 - 4 - 48）

主治：①腹胀，腹泻，便秘，痔疮；②腰痛。

刺法：直刺 0.8 ~ 1.2 寸。

7.3.16 膀胱俞（BL 28 背俞穴）

定位：在骶部，当骶正中嵴旁 1.5 寸，平第 2 骶后孔。（图 2 - 4 - 48）

主治：①遗尿，小便不利，水肿；②腰骶疼痛，下肢痿痹。

刺法：直刺 0.8 ~ 1.2 寸。

7.3.17 次髎（BL 32 背俞穴）

定位：在骶部，当髂后上棘内下方，正对第 2 骶后孔中。大约在第 2 骶后孔和背部正中线的中点。（图 2 - 4 - 48）

主治：①阳痿，遗精，月经不调，痛经，带下；②腰骶痛，下肢痿痹。

刺法：直刺 1 ~ 1.5 寸。

7.3.18 委中（BL 40 下合穴）

定位：在腘横纹中点，当股二头肌腱与半腱肌肌腱的中间。（图 2 -

4 - 49)

主治：①腰痛，腘肌痉挛，偏瘫，下肢痿痹；②丹毒，隐疹，周身瘙痒；③腹痛，呕吐，腹泻；④遗尿，小便困难。

刺法：直刺 1 ~ 1.5 寸，或用三棱针点刺腘静脉出血。

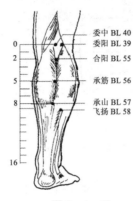

图 2 - 4 - 49

7.3.19 膏肓（BL 43）

定位：在背部，当第 4 胸椎棘突下，旁开 3 寸。（图 2 - 4 - 50）

主治：①肺痨，咳嗽，气喘；②健忘，遗精，羸瘦虚劳；③肩背痛。

刺法：斜刺 0.5 ~ 0.8 寸。

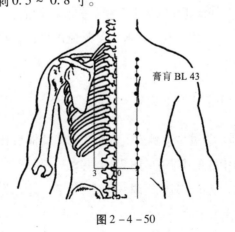

图 2 - 4 - 50

7.3.20 秩边（BL 54）

定位：在臀部，平第 4 骶后孔，骶正中嵴旁开 3 寸。（图 2 - 4 - 48）

主治：①腰骶痛，下肢痿痹；②痔疾，便秘，脱肛；③小便不利，前阴痛。

刺法：直刺1～2寸。

7.3.21 承山（BL 57）

定位：在小腿腓肠肌肌腹下出现尖角凹陷处，委中（BL 40）与昆仑（BL 60）之间，当伸直小腿或足跟抬高时，大约在委中与跟腱的中点。（图2－4－49）

主治：①痔疮，便秘；②腰腿痛；③脚气。

刺法：直刺1～2寸。

7.3.22 飞扬（BL 58 络穴）

定位：在小腿后侧，当外踝后，昆仑穴（BL 60）直上7寸，承山（BL 57）外下方1寸处。（图2－4－49）

主治：①头痛，目眩，鼻衄；②腰背痛，下肢痿痹。

刺法：直刺1～2寸。

7.3.23 昆仑（BL 60 经穴）

定位：在足外踝后方，当外踝尖与跟腱之间的凹陷处。（图2－4－51）

主治：①头痛，项强，鼻衄；②腰痛，足跟肿痛；③难产。

刺法：直刺0.5～1寸。

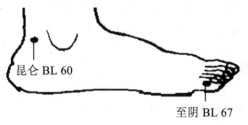

昆仑 BL 60

至阴 BL 67

图2－4－51

7.3.24 至阴（UB 67 井穴）

定位：在足小趾末节外侧，距趾甲角0.1寸。（图2－4－51）

主治：①头痛，目痛，鼻塞，鼻衄；②胎位不正，难产。

刺法：浅刺0.1寸或点刺出血；艾灸治疗胎位不正。

8. 足少阴肾经

8.1 经脉循行 (图2-4-52)

足少阴肾经，起于足小趾下，斜走足心（涌泉穴 KI 1），出于舟骨粗隆下，沿内踝后，进入足跟，再向上行于腿肚内侧，出于腘窝内侧半腱肌腱与半膜肌之间，上经大腿内侧后缘，通过脊柱，属于肾，络于膀胱。

肾脏直行支脉：从肾脏向上通过肝和横膈，进入肺中，沿喉咙，挟于舌根两旁。

肺部支脉：从肺出，联络心脏，流注胸中，与手厥阴心包经相接。

联系的脏腑：肾、膀胱、心、肺、肝、髓。

联系的器官：喉咙、舌根。

8.2 主治概要

妇科病，前阴病，肾、心、肝、脑病，肺和咽喉病以及经脉循行部位的其他病证。

8.3 常用腧穴

本经腧穴起于涌泉穴（KI 1），止于俞府穴（KI 27），左右各27个腧穴。

8.3.1 涌泉（KI 1）

定位：正坐或仰卧，跷足。在足底部，卷足时足前部凹陷处，约当

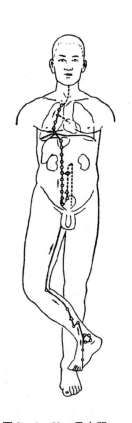

图2-4-52 足少阴肾经经脉循行示意图

足底第2、3趾趾缝纹头端与足跟连线的前1/3与后2/3交点上。（图
2-4-53）

主治：①头痛，眩晕，失眠，昏厥，小儿惊风，癫狂痫；②便秘，
小便不利；③咽喉肿痛，舌干，失音；④咽喉肿痛，舌干；⑤足心热，
下肢瘫痪。

刺法：直刺0.5~1寸。

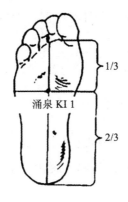

图2-4-53

8.3.2 太溪（KI 输穴 原穴）

定位：位于足内侧，内踝后方，位于内踝与跟腱之间凹陷处。（图
2-4-54）

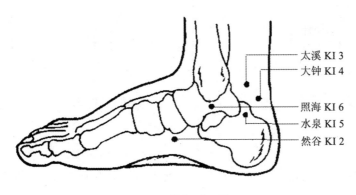

图2-4-54

主治：①阳痿，遗精，消渴，小便频数；②头痛，头晕，视物模

糊，耳聋，耳鸣，齿痛，咽干；③咳嗽，哮喘；④失眠，健忘；⑤下肢厥冷，内踝痛，足跟痛。

刺法：直刺0.5～1寸。

8.3.3 照海（KI 6 八脉交会穴）

定位：在足内侧，内踝尖下方凹陷处。（图2-4-54）

主治：①咽干，咽痛；②月经不调，赤白带下，便秘，小便不利；③失眠，癫痫。

刺法：直刺0.3～0.5寸。

8.3.4 复溜（KI 7 经穴）

定位：在小腿内侧，跟腱的前方，太溪直上2寸。（图2-4-55）

主治：①腹痛，腹胀，肠鸣，腹泻，水肿；②盗汗，身热无汗；③腰脊强痛，下肢痿痹。

刺法：直刺0.5～1寸。

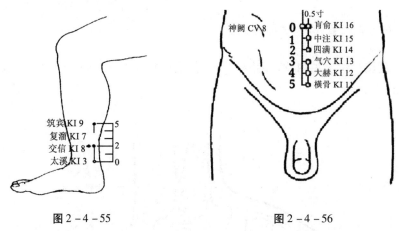

图2-4-55　　　　　　　　图2-4-56

8.3.5 大赫（KI 12）

定位：在下腹部，当脐中下4寸，前正中线旁开0.5寸。（图2-4-56）

主治：月经不调，带下，阳痿，遗精，疝气。

刺法：直刺 1~1.5 寸。

8.3.6 肓俞（KI 16）

定位：位于腹部正中，前中线旁开 0.5 寸。（图 2 - 4 - 56）
主治：①脐周痛，腹胀，腹泻，痢疾，便秘；②月经不调；③疝气。
刺法：直刺 1~1.5 寸。

8.3.7 俞府（KI 27）

定位：在胸部，当锁骨下缘，前正中线旁开 2 寸。（图 2 - 4 - 57）
主治：咳嗽，气喘，胸痛。
刺法：斜刺或平刺 0.5~0.8 寸。

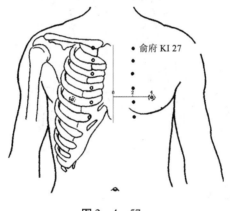

俞府 KI 27

图 2 - 4 - 57

9. 手厥阴心包经

9.1 经脉循行（图 2 - 4 - 58）

手厥阴心包经起于胸中，出属心包络，向下通过横膈，从胸至腹依次联络上、中、下三焦。胸部的支脉：沿着胸中，出于胁部，至腋下三寸处（天池），上行抵腋窝中，沿上臂内侧，行于手太阴和手少阴之间，进入肘窝中，向下行于前臂两筋之间，进入掌中，沿着中指到指端。另一分支起源于手掌，沿着无名指一直延伸到指尖，与手少阳三焦经相连。

联系的脏腑：心包和三焦。

联系的器官：心、心包、胃。

9.2 主治概要

主要治疗心、胸、胃、神志病以及经脉循行部位的其他病证。

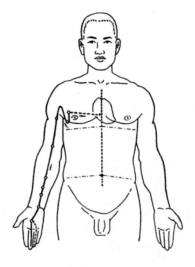

图 2 – 4 – 58

9.3 常用腧穴

手厥阴心包经起点为天池穴（PC 1），终点为中冲穴（PC 9），两侧各有 9 个穴位。

9.3.1 曲泽（PC 3 合穴）

定位：位于前臂内侧，在肘横纹中，当肱二头肌腱的尺侧缘。（图 2 – 4 – 59）

主治：①心痛，心悸，癫狂痫；②胃痛，呕吐，腹泻；③热病，中暑；④肘臂挛痛。

刺法：直刺 1~1.5 寸，或三棱针放血。

9.3.2 郄门（PC 4 郄穴）

定位：仰掌。在前臂掌侧，腕横纹上 5 寸，掌长肌腱与桡侧腕屈肌腱之间。（图 2 - 4 - 59）

主治：①心痛，心悸，癫狂痫；②咳血，咯血，吐血。

刺法：直刺 0.5 ~ 1 寸。

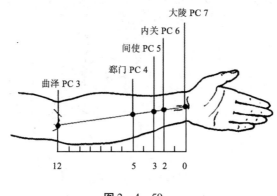

图 2 - 4 - 59

9.3.3 间使（PC 5 经穴）

定位：仰掌。在前臂掌侧，腕横纹上 3 寸，掌长肌腱与桡侧腕屈腱之间。（图 2 - 4 - 59）

主治：①心痛，心悸，癫狂痫；②胃痛，呕吐，呃逆；③热病，疟疾。

刺法：直刺 0.5 ~ 1 寸。

9.3.4 内关（PC 6 络穴 八脉交会穴）

定位：仰掌。在前臂掌侧，腕横纹上 2 寸，掌长肌腱与桡侧腕屈肌腱之间。（图 2 - 4 - 59）

主治：①心痛，心悸，心烦，失眠，郁证，癫狂痫；②胃痛，呕吐，呃逆；③中风，偏瘫，眩晕，偏头痛。

刺法：直刺 0.5 ~ 1 寸。

9.3.5 劳宫（PC 8 荥穴）

定位：仰掌。在手掌心，当第 2、3 掌骨之间偏于第 3 掌骨，握拳屈指时中指尖处。（图 2 - 4 - 60）

主治：①心痛，心悸，中风昏迷，癫狂痫；②口臭，口疮；③鹅掌风。

刺法：直刺 0.3 ~ 0.5 寸。

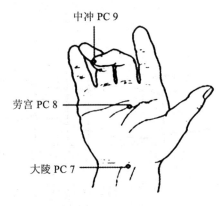

图 2 - 4 - 60

9.3.6 中冲（PC 9 井穴）

定位：在手中指末节尖端中央。（图 2 - 4 - 60）

主治：①心痛，中风昏迷，中暑，晕厥，小儿惊风；②热病，舌强肿痛。

刺法：浅刺 0.1 寸；或用三棱针点刺出血。

10. 手少阳三焦经

10.1 经脉循行 （图 2 - 4 - 61）

手少阳三焦经起于环指末端，向上行于小指与环指之间，沿着手背，出于前臂外侧桡骨和尺骨之间，向上通过肘尖，沿上臂外侧，上达肩部，交出足少阳经的后面，向上进入缺盆部，分布于胸中，散络于心包，向下通过横膈，从胸至腹，属上、中、下三焦。

胸部的支脉：从胸向上，出于缺盆部，上走颈旁，联系耳后，沿耳后直上，出于耳部，上行额角，再屈而下行至面颊部，到达眶下部。

耳部的支脉：从耳后进入耳中，出走耳前，过足少阳经上关穴的前方，与前一支脉交会于面颊部，到达目外眦，与足少阳胆经相接。

联系的脏腑：三焦和心包。

联系的器官：眼和耳。

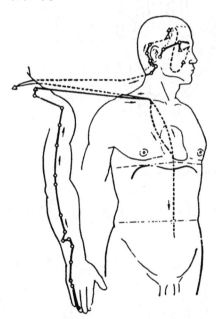

图2-4-61 手少阳三焦经经脉循行示意图

10.2 主治概要

主要治疗侧头、耳、眼和喉疾病，以及经脉循行部位的其他病证。

10.3 常用腧穴

手少阳三焦经起于关冲穴（TE 1），止于丝竹空穴（TE 23），两侧各由23个穴位组成。

10.3.1 关冲（TE 1 井穴）

定位：在手环指末节尺侧，距指甲根角 0.1 寸。（图 2 - 4 - 62）

主治：①热病，中风昏迷；②咽喉肿痛，目赤，耳鸣，耳聋。

刺法：浅刺 0.1 寸，或用三棱针点刺出血。

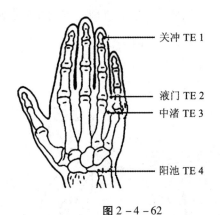

关冲 TE 1

液门 TE 2
中渚 TE 3

阳池 TE 4

图 2 - 4 - 62

10.3.2 中渚（TE 3 输穴）

定位：握拳时，第 4、5 掌骨间凹陷处，液门后方 1 寸处。（图 2 - 4 - 62）

主治：①耳鸣，耳聋，头痛，目赤肿痛，咽喉疼痛；②肩、背、肘臂疼痛以及手指挛痛。

刺法：直刺 0.3 ~ 0.5 寸。

10.3.3 阳池（TE 4 原穴）

定位：在腕背横纹中，当指伸肌腱的尺侧缘凹陷处。（图 2 - 4 - 63）

主治：①耳鸣，耳聋，咽喉肿痛；②消渴，疟疾；③腕痛，上肢痿痹。

刺法：直刺 0.3 ~ 0.5 寸。

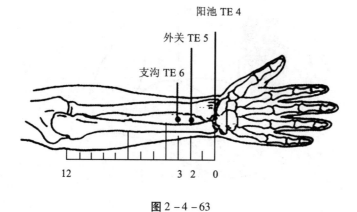

图 2 - 4 - 63

10.3.4 外关（TE 5 络穴 八脉交会穴）

定位：腕背横纹上 2 寸，尺骨与桡骨之间。（图 2 - 4 - 63）

主治：①热病，头痛，目赤肿痛，耳鸣，耳聋；②胸胁痛；③上肢痿痹。

刺法：直刺 0.5 ~ 1 寸。

10.3.5 支沟（TE 6 经穴）

定位：腕背横纹上 3 寸，尺骨与桡骨之间。（图 2 - 4 - 63）

主治：①热病，便秘；②耳聋，耳鸣；③胁肋痛，肩背痛。

刺法：直刺 0.5 ~ 1 寸。

10.3.6 肩髎（TE 14）

定位：当臂外展时，于肩峰后下方呈现凹陷，在肩髃后方 1 寸处。（图 2 - 4 - 64）

主治：肩臂挛痛。

刺法：直刺 1 ~ 1.5 寸。

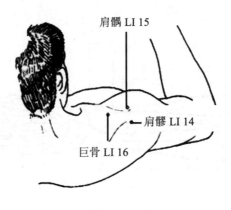

肩髃 LI 15

肩髎 LI 14

巨骨 LI 16

图 2 - 4 - 64

10.3.7 翳风（TE 17）

定位：正坐，侧伏或侧卧。在耳垂后方，当乳突与下颌角之间的凹陷处。（图 2 - 4 - 65）

主治：①耳鸣，耳聋，聤耳，口眼歪斜，齿痛，牙关紧闭，颊肿；②呃逆。

刺法：直刺 0.8 ~ 1.2 寸。

10.3.8 角孙（TE 20）

定位：正坐，侧伏或侧卧。在头部，折耳郭向前，当耳尖直上入发际处。（图 2 - 4 - 65）

主治：①目翳，齿痛，疟腮；②偏头痛，项强。

刺法：平刺 0.3 ~ 0.5 寸；小儿腮腺炎宜用灯火灸。

10.3.9 耳门（TE 21）

定位：正坐，侧伏或侧卧。在面部，当耳屏上切迹的前方，下颌骨髁突后缘凹陷处。（图 2 - 4 - 65）

主治：耳鸣，耳聋，聤耳，齿痛。

刺法：微张口，直刺 0.5 ~ 1 寸。

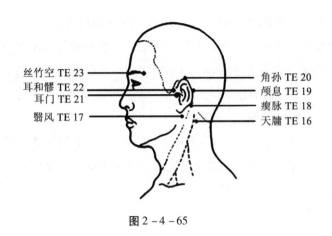

丝竹空 TE 23
耳和髎 TE 22
耳门 TE 21
翳风 TE 17

角孙 TE 20
颅息 TE 19
瘈脉 TE 18
天牖 TE 16

图 2 - 4 - 65

10.3.10 丝竹空（TE 23）

定位：位于眉毛外侧部凹陷处。（图 2 - 4 - 65）

主治：目赤肿痛，眼睑瞤动。

刺法：避开动脉，斜刺或平刺 0.3 ~ 0.5 寸。

11. 足少阳胆经

11.1 足少阳胆经循行（图 2 - 4 - 66）

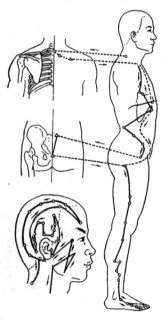

足少阳胆经起于目外眦（瞳子髎 GB 1），上行到额角部（颔厌 GB 4），然后向下折返至耳后区（风池 GB 20），沿颈旁，行手少阳三焦经之前，至肩上再向后交出手少阳三焦经之后，向下进入锁骨上窝。

耳部支脉：从耳后，进入耳中，出走耳前，到目外眦后。

目外眦支脉：起于目外眦，下至大迎穴（ST 5），在眶下与手少阳三焦经交汇。下行经过颊车（ST 6），下颈，与前脉在锁骨上窝

图 2 - 4 - 66　足少阳胆经经脉循行示意图

处会和，再进一步下降到胸部，穿过膈肌与肝脏连接，进入胆囊，再沿

胁肋内下行至腹股沟动脉部，经过外阴部毛际横行入臀部（环跳 GB 30）。

缺盆部直行脉：从锁骨上窝向下延伸，沿着胸部的外侧通过腋窝前方，并通过胁肋部到达髋部，与前脉会和。再沿着大腿外侧下行到膝盖的外侧，下行经腓骨前侧，直下到达腓骨下端，下出外踝前，沿着足背部，到第 4 趾的外侧。

足背支脉：从足临泣（GB 41）分出，沿第 1 和第 2 跖骨之间，出于大趾端，穿过趾甲，回过来到趾甲后的毫毛部，与足厥阴肝经相连。

联系的脏腑：胆、肝。

联系的器官：目、耳。

11.2 主治概要

主要治疗侧头、耳、目、咽喉、神志病、热病以及经脉循行部位的其他病证。

11.3 常用腧穴

本经腧穴起于瞳子髎穴（GB 1），止于足窍阴穴（GB 44），两侧各 44 个腧穴。

11.3.1 瞳子髎（GB 1）

定位：目外眦外侧 0.5 寸，位于眼眶外侧凹陷处。（图 2 - 4 - 67）
主治：①目赤肿痛，目翳，青盲；②偏头痛，眩晕。
刺法：平刺 0.3 ~ 0.5 寸。

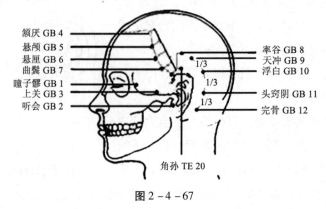

图 2 - 4 - 67

11.3.2 听会 (GB 2)

定位：当耳屏间切迹的前方，下颌骨髁突的后缘，张口凹陷处。（图 2－4－67）

主治：①耳鸣，耳聋；②口眼㖞斜。

刺法：张口，直刺 0.5～1 寸。

11.3.3 率谷 (GB 3)

定位：耳尖直上入发际 1.5 寸。（图 2－4－67）

主治：①偏头痛，眩晕；②急慢性小儿惊风。

刺法：平刺 0.5～0.8 寸。

11.3.4 阳白 (GB 14)

定位：当患者直视前方时，该点位于瞳孔直上，眉上 1 寸。（图2－4－68）

主治：①口眼㖞斜，眼睑下垂，视物模糊，目赤肿痛，眼睑瞤动；②前额痛，眩晕。

刺法：平刺 0.3～0.5 寸。

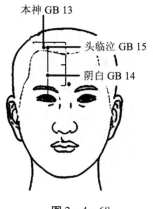

图 2－4－68

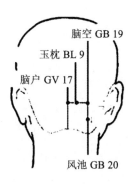

图 2－4－69

11.3.5 风池 (GB 20)

定位：在项部，当枕骨之下，与风府 (GV 16) 相平，胸锁乳突肌与斜方肌上端之间的凹陷处。(图 2 – 4 – 69)

主治：①感冒，鼻塞，头痛，口眼歪斜，目赤肿痛；②中风，高血压，癫痫，头痛，眩晕，耳鸣，耳聋；③颈项强痛，肩背痛。

刺法：针尖略微向下，向鼻尖方向刺入 0.8 ~ 1.2 寸，或平刺透风府穴 (GV 16)。穴位深层是延髓，必须严格控制进针的角度和深度。

11.3.6 肩井 (GB 21)

定位：这一穴位于肩部，在大椎 (GV 14) 与肩峰连线的中点处。(图 2 – 4 – 70)

主治：①头项强痛，肩背疼痛，上肢不遂；②乳痛，乳汁不下；③滞产。

刺法：直刺 0.5 ~ 0.8 寸，内有肺尖，不可深刺，孕妇禁刺。

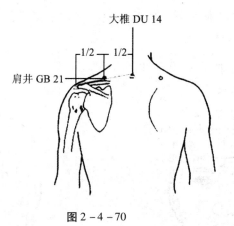

图 2 – 4 – 70

11.3.7 日月 (GB 24)

定位：乳头直下，第 7 肋间隙。(图 2 – 4 – 71)

主治：胁痛，黄疸，呕吐，吞酸。

刺法：斜刺或平刺 0.5 ~ 0.8 寸。

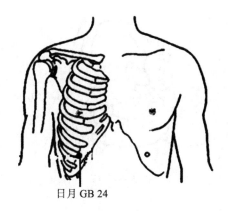

日月 GB 24

图 2 - 4 - 71

11.3.8 带脉 (GB 26)

定位：位于第 11 肋骨的游离端下方，与脐部齐平。（图 2 - 4 - 72）

主治：①月经不调，闭经，带下，疝气；②腰胁痛。

刺法：直刺 0.5 ~ 1 寸。

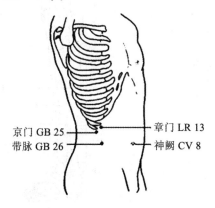

京门 GB 25 ——　　—— 章门 LR 13
带脉 GB 26 ——　　—— 神阙 CV 8

图 2 - 4 - 72

11.3.9 环跳 (GB 30)

定位：当股骨大转子顶点与骶管裂孔连线的外 1/3 与内 2/3 交点处。（图 2 - 4 - 73）

主治：腰胯疼痛，半身不遂，下肢痿痹。

刺法：直刺 2 ~ 3 寸。

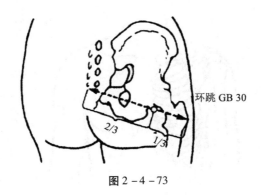

图 2 - 4 - 73

11.3.10 风市（GB 31）

定位：在大腿外侧部的中线上，当腘横纹上 7 寸。（图 2 - 4 - 74）

主治：①半身不遂，下肢痿痹，脚气；②周身瘙痒；③突发性耳聋。

刺法：直刺 1～2 寸。

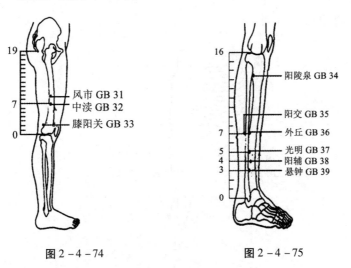

图 2 - 4 - 74   图 2 - 4 - 75

11.3.11 阳陵泉（GB 34 合穴 胆之下合穴　八会穴之筋会）

定位：当腓骨小头前下方凹陷处。（图 2 - 4 - 75）

主治：①胁痛，黄疸，口苦，呕吐，吞酸；②膝关节肿痛，下肢痿痹，半身不遂，脚气；③小儿惊风。

刺法：直刺 1～1.5 寸。

11.3.12 光明（GB 37 络穴）

定位：当外踝尖上5寸，腓骨前缘。（图2－4－75）
主治：①目痛，夜盲，近视；②乳房胀痛；③下肢痿痹。
刺法：直刺1～1.5寸。

11.3.13 悬钟（GB 39 八会穴之髓会）

定位：外踝尖上3寸，腓骨后缘。（图2－4－75）
主治：①项强，胸胁胀痛，下肢痿痹，半身不遂，脚气；②头晕，耳鸣，耳聋。
刺法：直刺1～1.5寸。

11.3.14 丘墟（GB 40 原穴）

定位：在足外踝的前下方，当趾长伸肌腱的外侧凹陷处。（图2－4－76）
主治：①胸胁胀痛，下肢痿痹，足跗肿痛；②热病，疟疾；③目赤肿痛，目翳。
刺法：直刺0.3～0.5寸。

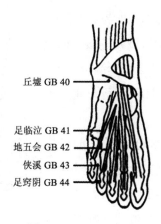

图2－4－76

11.3.15 足临泣（GB 41 输穴 八脉交会穴通于带脉）

定位：在第4和第5跖骨的交界处之前，在小趾伸肌腱外侧的凹陷处。（图2-4-76）

主治：①偏头痛，目赤肿痛；②足背疼痛，脚趾麻木；③月经不调，乳痈。

刺法：直刺0.3~0.5寸。

12. 足厥阴肝经

12.1 经脉循行（图2-4-77）

足厥阴肝经，起于大脚趾背面毫毛部，沿着足背上行，穿过内踝前1寸，向上行小腿内侧，至内踝上8寸处，交出足太阴脾经的后面，上行腘内侧，沿着大腿内侧进入阴毛中，环绕阴部，上达小腹，挟胃旁，属于肝，联络胆，向上通过横膈，分布于胁肋，沿喉的后部上升到鼻咽部，并与"眼部"（眼球与大脑连接的区域）连接。向上出于前额头，与督脉会合于巅顶。

目系支脉：从目系下行颊里，环绕唇内。

肝部支脉：从肝分出，通过横膈，向上流注于肺部并与手太阴肺经相接。

联系的脏腑：肝、胆、肺、胃。

联系的器官：生殖器、喉咙、鼻咽部、目和唇。

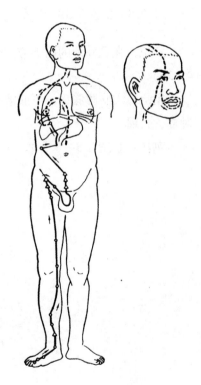

图2-4-77 足厥阴肝经经脉循行示意图

12.2 主治概要

主要治疗肝病、妇科病，以及经脉循行部位的其他病证。

12.3 常用腧穴

本经腧穴起于大敦穴（LR 1），止于期门穴（LR 14），两侧各 14 个腧穴。

12.3.1 大敦（LR 1 井穴）

定位：在大脚趾背侧，距趾甲角侧后方 0.1 寸。（图 2 - 4 - 78）

主治：①中风昏迷，癫痫；②疝气，遗尿，月经不调，经闭，崩漏，阴挺。

刺法：斜刺 0.1~0.2 寸，或点刺出血。

12.3.2 行间（LR 2 荥穴）

定位：在足背侧，当第 1、2 趾骨间，趾蹼缘后方赤白肉际处。（图 2 - 4 - 78）

主治：①头痛，眩晕，目赤肿痛，青盲；②胁痛，口苦，黄疸；③失眠，癫痫；④疝气，小便不利，月经不调，痛经，崩漏，月经不调。

刺法：直刺 0.5~0.8 寸。

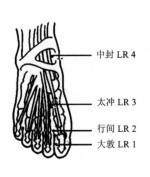

图 2 - 4 - 78

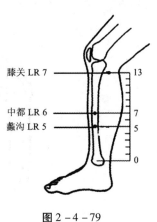

图 2 - 4 - 79

12.3.3 太冲 （LR 3 输穴 原穴）

定位：在足背侧，当第 1 跖骨和第 2 趾骨结合前方凹陷处。（图 2 - 4 - 78）

主治：①头痛，眩晕，目赤肿痛，口眼歪斜；②胁痛，黄疸，腹胀，呕逆；③月经不调，疝气，小便不利；④中风，癫痫，小儿惊风；⑤下肢痿痹，足跗肿痛。

刺法：直刺 0.5 ~ 0.8 寸。

12.3.4 蠡沟 （LR 5 络穴）

定位：在小腿内侧，当足内踝尖上 5 寸，胫骨内侧中央。（图 2 - 4 - 79）

主治：①外阴瘙痒，疝气，月经不调，带下，小便不利；②腰痛，下肢痿痹。

刺法：平刺 0.5 ~ 0.8 寸。

12.3.5 曲泉 （LR 8 合穴）

定位：在膝内侧，屈膝，腘横纹内侧端，股骨内侧髁的后缘，半腱肌肌腱内缘凹陷中。（图 2 - 4 - 80）

主治：①月经不调，痛经，带下，遗精，小便不利；②膝肿痛。

刺法：直刺 1 ~ 1.5 寸。

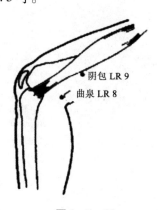

图 2 - 4 - 80

12.3.6 章门（LR 13 脾募穴 八会穴之脏会）

定位：在侧腹部，当第 11 肋游离端的下方。（图 2 - 4 - 81）

主治：①腹痛，腹胀，泄泻，呕吐；②胁肋痛。

刺法：斜刺 0.5 ~ 0.8 寸。

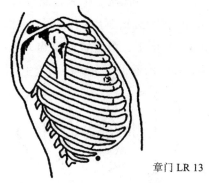

章门 LR 13

图 2 - 4 - 81

12.3.7 期门（LR 14 募穴）

定位：在胸部，乳头正下方，第 6 肋间隙。（图 2 - 4 - 82）

主治：胸胁胀痛，口苦，呕吐，呃逆。

刺法：斜刺 0.5 ~ 0.8 寸；可灸。

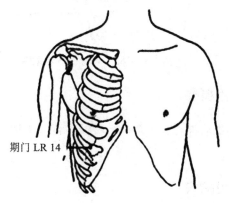

期门 LR 14

图 2 - 4 - 82

13. 督脉

13.1 经脉循行（图 2 - 4 - 83）

督脉起于小腹部（胞中）当骨盆的中央，女性进入尿道口的外端，男性进入阴茎周围，由此分出络脉，分布于阴部，会合于会阴，绕向肛门之后，从长强穴（GV 1）向上，沿着脊柱里边，上行至风府穴（GV 16），进入脑部。上至巅顶，沿额下行至鼻柱，止于齿龈。

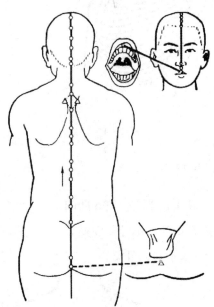

图 2 - 4 - 83　督脉循行示意图

13.2 主治概要

本经腧穴主治神志病，热病，腰骶、背、头项局部病证，以及相应的内脏疾病。

13.3 常用腧穴

本经腧穴始于长强穴（GV 1），止于龈交穴（GV 28），共 28 个穴位组成。

13.3.1 长强穴（GV 1 络穴）

定位：跪伏或胸膝位。在尾骨端下，当尾骨端与肛门连线的中点处。（图 2 - 4 - 84）

主治：①泄泻，便秘，痔疾，脱肛；②癫狂痫；③腰痛，尾骶骨痛。

刺法：斜刺，针尖向上与骶骨平行刺入 0.8 ~ 1 寸。不得直刺，以防刺穿直肠。

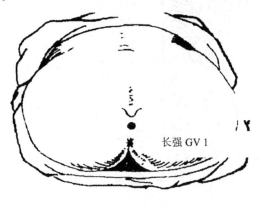

图 2 - 4 - 84

13.3.2 腰阳关（GV 3）

定位：在腰部，当后正中线上，第 4 腰椎棘突下凹陷中。（图 2 - 4 - 85）

主治：①月经不调，遗精，阳痿；②腰骶痛，下肢痿痹。

刺法：斜刺 0.5 ~ 1 寸。

13.3.3 命门（GV 4）

定位：在腰部，当后正中线上，第 2 腰椎棘突下凹陷中。（图 2 - 4 - 85）

主治：①月经不调，白带，不孕，遗精，阳痿；②泄泻；③腰脊强痛，下肢痿痹。

刺法：斜刺 0.5 ~ 1 寸。

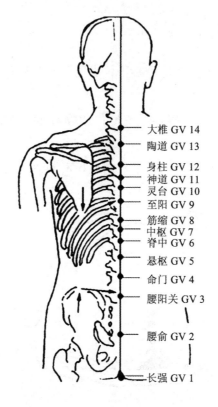

大椎 GV 14
陶道 GV 13
身柱 GV 12
神道 GV 11
灵台 GV 10
至阳 GV 9
筋缩 GV 8
中枢 GV 7
脊中 GV 6
悬枢 GV 5
命门 GV 4
腰阳关 GV 3
腰俞 GV 2
长强 GV 1

图 2 - 4 - 85

13.3.4 至阳 （GV 9）

定位：在背部，当后正中线上，第 7 胸椎棘突下凹陷中。（图 2 - 4 - 85）

主治：①胸胁胀痛，黄疸，胃痛；②咳嗽，气喘；③背痛，脊强。

刺法：斜刺 0.5 ~ 1 寸；可灸。

13.3.5 身柱 （GV 12）

定位：在背部，当后正中线上，第 3 胸椎棘突下凹陷中。（图 2 - 4 - 85）

主治：①咳嗽，气喘；②癫痫，小儿惊风；③脊背强痛。

刺法：斜刺 0.5 ~ 1 寸；可灸。

13.3.6 大椎 (GV 14)

定位：在后正中线上，第7颈椎棘突下凹陷中。（图2-4-85）

主治：①热病，疟疾，感冒，发热，盗汗，咳嗽，气喘；②癫狂痫；③头痛项强，肩背痛，腰脊强痛。

刺法：斜刺0.5~1寸。

13.3.7 哑门 (GV 15)

定位：正坐位，在项部，当后发际正中直上0.5寸，第1颈椎下。（图2-4-86）

主治：①暴喑，舌强不语；②头痛，项强；③癫狂痫。

刺法：垂直刺入或向下颌方向缓慢刺入0.5~1寸，不要向上斜刺或深刺，以防刺伤延髓。

13.3.8 风府 (GV 16)

定位：在项部，当后发际正中直上1寸，枕外隆凸直上，两侧斜方肌之间凹陷中。（图2-4-86）

主治：①癫狂痫，中风不语；②头痛，项强。

刺法：直刺或斜向下颌方向缓慢刺入0.5~1寸。针尖不可向上，以免刺入枕骨大孔，误伤延髓。

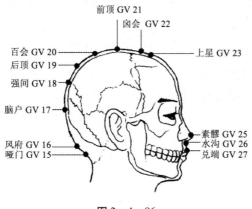

图2-4-86

13.3.9 百会（GV 20）

定位：在头部，当后发际正中直上 7 寸处。（图 2 - 4 - 86）

主治：①头痛，头晕，耳鸣，耳聋，鼻塞，视物模糊；②失眠，健忘，癫狂痫，中风，半身不遂，失语；③脱肛，子宫脱垂。

刺法：平刺 0.5 ~ 0.8 寸。

13.3.10 上星（GV 23）

定位：仰靠坐位。在头部，当前发际正中直上 1 寸。（图 2 - 4 - 86）

主治：①头痛，眩晕，鼻塞，鼻衄，目痛，迎风流泪；②热病，疟疾；③癫狂痫。

刺法：平刺 0.5 ~ 1 寸；可灸。

13.3.11 神庭（GV 24）

定位：仰靠坐位。在头部，当前发际正中直上 0.5 寸。（图 2 - 4 - 86）

主治：①头痛，眩晕，鼻塞，鼻衄，目痛，迎风流泪；②失眠，癫狂痫。

刺法：平刺 0.5 ~ 1 寸；可灸。

13.3.12 水沟（GV 26）

定位：仰靠坐位，在面部，当人中沟的上 1/3 与中 1/3 交点处。（图 2 - 4 - 86）

主治：①昏迷，晕厥，中暑，中风，癫狂痫，小儿惊风；②面肿，口角歪斜；③腰脊强痛。

刺法：向上斜刺 0.3 ~ 0.5 寸。

14. 任脉

14.1 任脉循行 (图2-4-87)

任脉起于小腹内,下出会阴,向上行于耻骨,沿着腹内,向上经过关元(CV 4)等穴,到达咽喉部,进一步上升,环绕嘴唇,穿过面颊,进入目眶下。

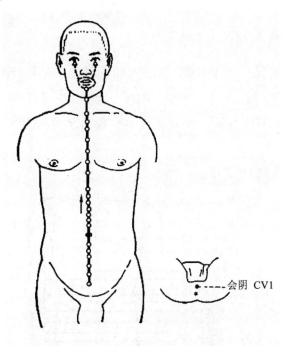

图2-4-87 任脉循行示意图

14.2 主治概要

主治腹、胸、颈、头面的局部病证及相应的内脏器官疾病。部分腧穴具有保健作用。

14.3 常用腧穴

14.3.1 中极（CV 3 膀胱募穴）

定位：仰卧位，在下腹部，脐中上4寸，前正中线上。（图2-4-88）

主治：①遗尿，小便不利，疝气；②月经不调，崩漏，带下，遗精，阳痿。

刺法：直刺1~1.5寸。

14.3.2 关元（CV 4 小肠募穴）

定位：仰卧位，在下腹部，前正中线上，脐中下3寸。（图2-4-88）

主治：①崩漏，带下，痛经，阳痿、遗精，遗尿，小便不利；②腹泻、脱肛；③中风脱证，虚劳羸瘦。本穴为全身强壮穴之一，为保健要穴。

刺法：直刺1~2寸。

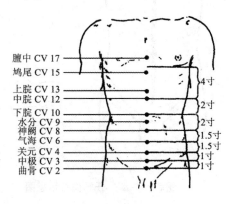

膻中 CV 17
鸠尾 CV 15
上脘 CV 13
中脘 CV 12
下脘 CV 10
水分 CV 9
神阙 CV 8
气海 CV 6
关元 CV 4
中极 CV 3
曲骨 CV 2
4寸
2寸
2寸
1.5寸
1.5寸
1寸
1寸

图2-4-88

14.3.3 气海（CV 6 肓之原穴）

定位：位于下腹部，前正中线上，脐下1.5寸。（图2-4-88）

主治：①腹痛，腹泻，便秘；②月经不调，闭经，遗尿，疝气，遗精，阳痿；③中风脱证，虚劳羸瘦。为全身强壮穴之一，为保健要穴。

刺法：直刺 1 ~ 2 寸。

14.3.4 神阙（CV 8）

定位：仰卧位，在脐中央。（图 2 - 4 - 88）

主治：①腹痛，腹泻，便秘，痢疾，脱肛；②中风脱证、四肢厥冷；③水肿，小便不利。

刺法：禁刺。直接灸或间接灸（隔姜、隔盐）。

14.3.5 水分（CV 9）

定位：在上腹部，脐中上 1 寸，前正中线上。（图 2 - 4 - 88）

主治：①腹痛，腹泻；②水肿，小便不利。

刺法：直刺 1 ~ 2 寸，可灸。

14.3.6 中脘（CV 10 胃之募穴 八会穴之腑会）

定位：位于上腹部，前正中线上，脐上 4 寸。（图 2 - 4 - 88）

主治：①胃痛，腹痛，腹胀，肠鸣泄泻，黄疸，反胃，呕逆，食不化，纳呆，疳积；②咳喘痰多，失眠，脏躁，癫狂痫。

刺法：直刺 1 ~ 1.5 寸。

14.3.7 膻中（CV 17 心包募穴 八会穴之气会）

定位：前正中线上，平第 4 肋间隙。（图 2 - 4 - 88）

主治：①咳嗽，气喘，胸痛，胸闷；②心痛，心悸，心烦；③乳少，乳痈；④呕吐，呃逆，噎膈。

刺法：平刺 0.3 ~ 0.5 寸。

14.3.8 天突（CV 22）

定位：前正中线上，胸骨上窝的中点。（图 2 - 4 - 89）

主治：①咳嗽，气喘、咽喉疼痛，梅核气，失音，声音嘶哑；②瘰疬，瘿气。

刺法：先直刺 0.2 寸，当针尖超过胸骨柄内缘，即向下沿胸骨柄后缘刺入 1~1.5 寸。必须严格注意进针的角度和深度，以免刺伤肺脏。

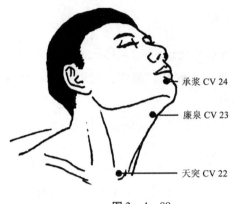

承浆 CV 24

廉泉 CV 23

天突 CV 22

图 2 - 4 - 89

14.3.9 廉泉（CV 23）

定位：位于前正中线上，微仰头，喉结上方，舌骨上缘凹陷处。
（图 2 - 4 - 89）

主治：舌下肿痛，中风失语，暴暗，吞咽困难。

刺法：斜刺 0.5~1 寸，可灸。

14.3.10 承浆（CV 24）

定位：位于精神颏唇沟的中心。（图 2 - 4 - 89）

主治：①口歪，面部肿胀，牙龈肿胀，流涎；②癫狂痫。

刺法：浅刺 0.3~0.5 寸，可灸。

15. 经外奇穴

15.1 头颈部腧穴

15.1.1 四神聪（EX-HN 1）

定位：正坐位。在头顶部，当百会前后左右各 1 寸，共 4 个腧穴。
（图 2 - 4 - 90）

主治：头痛，眩晕，失眠，健忘，癫狂痫。

刺法：平刺 0.5 ~ 0.8 寸。

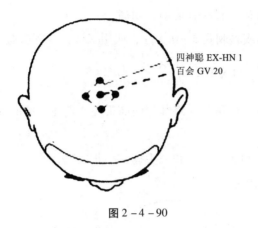

四神聪 EX-HN 1
百会 GV 20

图 2 - 4 - 90

15.1.2 印堂（EX-HN 3）

定位：正坐仰靠位或仰卧位。在额部，两眉头的中点。（图 2 - 4 - 91）

主治：①头痛，眩晕，失眠，小儿惊风；②鼻渊，鼻衄，鼻塞，目痛，眉棱骨痛。

刺法：提捏局部皮肤，向下平刺，或向左右透刺攒竹、睛明等，0.5 ~ 1 寸。

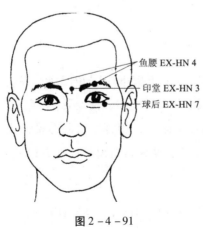

鱼腰 EX-HN 4
印堂 EX-HN 3
球后 EX-HN 7

图 2 - 4 - 91

15.1.3 太阳（EX-HN 5）

定位：正坐或侧伏坐位。在颞部，当眉梢与目外眦之间，向后约一

横指的凹陷处。（图2－4－92）

主治：偏头痛，目疾，齿痛，面痛。

刺法：直刺或斜刺0.3～0.5寸；或用三棱针点刺出血。

15.1.4 耳尖（EX-HN 6）

定位：在耳郭的顶部，将耳郭向前折叠，点在耳郭的顶端。（图2－4－92）

主治：目赤肿痛，麦粒肿，头痛，小儿惊风。

刺法：点刺出血。

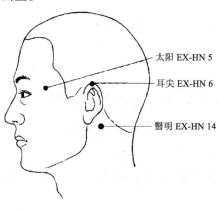

太阳 EX-HN 5

耳尖 EX-HN 6

翳明 EX-HN 14

图 2－4－92

15.1.5 球后（EX-HN 7）

定位：仰靠坐位。当眶下缘外1/4与内3/4交界处。（图2－4－91）

主治：视神经炎、视神经萎缩、青光眼、早期白内障、近视等目疾。

刺法：选30号以上毫针，用押手将眼球推向上方，沿眶下缘从外下向内上，针身成弧形沿眼球刺向视神经孔方向刺0.5～1寸，不宜捻转，可轻度提插。

15.1.6 金津、玉液（EX-HN 12、EX-HN 13）

定位：正坐张口，卷舌，在舌面下，舌系带两旁静脉上取穴。左称金津，右称玉液。（图2－4－93）

主治：①舌强不语，口疮，舌肿；②消渴，呕吐。

刺法：点刺出血。

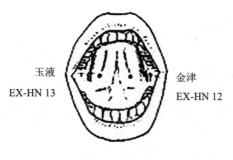

玉液
EX-HN 13

金津
EX-HN 12

图 2 - 4 - 93

15.1.7 翳明（EX-HN 14）

定位：正坐位，头略前倾。在项部，当翳风后 1 寸。（图 2 - 4 - 92）

主治：目疾，耳鸣，失眠，头痛。

刺法：直刺 0.5 ~ 1 寸。

15.2 胸腹部腧穴

子宫（EX-CA 1）

定位：位于下腹部，脐中下 4 寸，前正中线旁开 3 寸。（图 2 - 4 - 94）

主治：月经不调，痛经，闭经，崩漏，疝气，阴挺。

刺法：直刺 0.8 ~ 1.2 寸，可灸。

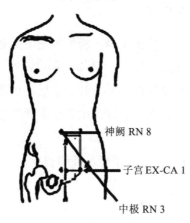

神阙 RN 8

子宫 EX-CA 1

中极 RN 3

图 2 – 4 –94

15.3 背部腧穴

15.3.1 定喘（EX-B 1）

定位：在脊柱区，横平第 7 颈椎棘突下，后正中线旁开 0.5 寸。（图 2 – 4 –95）

主治：哮喘，咳嗽。

刺法：直刺 0.3 ~ 0.5 寸。

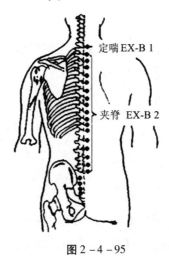

定喘 EX-B 1

夹脊 EX-B 2

图 2 – 4 –95

15.3.2 夹脊穴（EX-B 2）

定位：在脊柱区，第 1 胸椎至第 5 腰椎棘突下两侧，后正中线旁开 0.5 寸，一侧 17 穴，左右共 34 穴。（图 2 – 4 –95）

主治：上背部的穴位主要治疗心、肺、上肢的疾病；下背部的穴位主要治疗肝、胆、脾、胃的疾病；腰部的穴位主要治疗泌尿生殖系统和肠道的疾病。

刺法：直刺 0.3 ~ 0.5 寸，或用梅花针叩刺。

15.3.3 胃脘下俞

定位：位于脊柱旁开 1.5 寸，横平第 8 胸椎棘突下。（图 2 – 4 –96）

主治：腹痛，胃痛，消渴。

刺法：斜刺 0.3~0.5 寸。

15.3.4 腰眼（EX-B 6）

定位：在腰部，横平第 4 腰椎棘突下，后正中线旁开约 3.5 寸凹陷中。（图 2 - 4 - 97）

主治：①月经不调，白带过多；②腰痛。

刺法：直刺 0.5~1 寸。

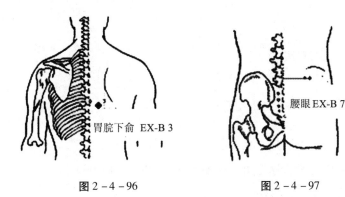

胃脘下俞 EX-B 3

腰眼 EX-B 7

图 2 - 4 - 96   图 2 - 4 - 97

15.3.5 十七椎（EX-B 7）

定位：在脊柱区，位于后正中线上，第 5 腰椎棘突下。（图 2 - 4 - 98）

主治：①腰部疼痛；②月经不调，崩漏，痛经。

刺法：直刺 0.5~1 寸。

15.3.6 腰奇（EX-B 8）

定位：位于骶部，当尾骨端直上 2 寸。（图 2 - 4 - 98）

主治：①癫痫；②头痛，失眠。

刺法：斜向上刺 1~1.5 寸。

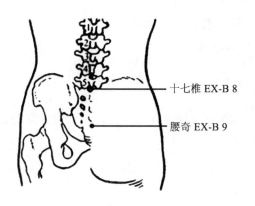

十七椎 EX-B 8

腰奇 EX-B 9

图 2 – 4 – 98

15.4 上肢穴

15.4.1 腰痛点（EX-UE 7）

定位：位于手背，腕关节和掌指关节的中点，在第 2 和第 3 掌骨之间，第 4 和第 5 掌骨之间，双手 4 穴。（图 2 – 4 – 99）

主治：急性腰扭伤。

刺法：直刺 0.3 ~ 0.5 寸。

15.4.2 外劳宫（EX-UE 8）

定位：在手背上，在第 2 掌骨和第 3 掌骨之间，掌指关节后方的 0.5 寸。（图 2 – 4 – 99）

主治：颈项强痛，落枕。

刺法：直刺 0.3 ~ 0.5 寸。

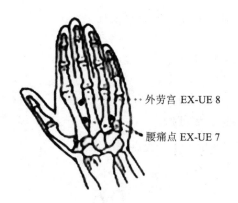

图 2 - 4 - 99

15.4.3 八邪（EX-UE 9）

定位：位于手背，第 1 ~ 5 指间，指蹼缘后方赤白肉际处，左右共有 8 穴，用微握拳可定位。（图 2 - 4 - 100）

主治：手指肿胀，手指麻木，毒蛇咬伤引起的肿胀和手臂疼痛。

刺法：直刺 0.3 ~ 0.5 寸。

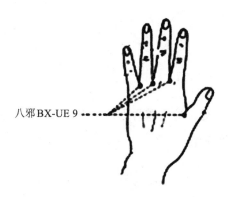

图 2 - 4 - 100

15.4.4 四缝（EX-UE 10）

定位：位于掌面，指间近端关节横向折痕的中点，每只手有 4 个穴位。（图 2 - 4 - 101）

主治：小儿疳积，百日咳。

刺法：点刺出血或挤出一些黄色液体。

15.4.5 十宣（EX-UE 11）

定位：位于十个指尖上，距指甲大约 0.1 寸。（图 2 – 4 – 101）
主治：中风昏迷，癫狂痫。
刺法：直刺 0.1～0.2 寸，或点刺出血。

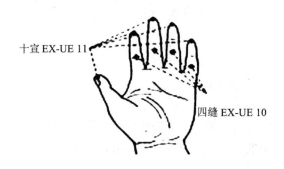

十宣 EX-UE 11

四缝 EX-UE 10

图 2 – 4 – 101

15.5 下肢穴

15.5.1 鹤顶（EX-LE 2）

定位：位于膝盖处，位于髌骨上缘中点的凹陷处。（图 2 – 4 – 102）
主治：膝关节疼痛。
刺法：直刺 0.8～1 寸。

15.5.2 膝眼（EX-LE 5）

定位：当膝盖弯曲时，该穴位于髌韧带内侧和外侧的两个凹陷内，
这两个穴位也分别称为内侧膝眼和外侧膝眼。（图 2 – 4 – 102）
主治：膝关节疼痛。
刺法：斜刺 0.5～1 寸。

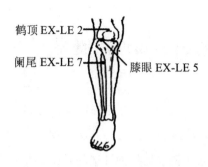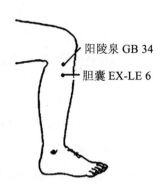

图 2 - 4 - 102　　　　　　　图 2 - 4 - 103

15.5.3 胆囊（EX-LE 6）

定位：该穴位于腓骨小头正下方的凹陷下 2 寸。（图 2 - 4 - 103）

主治：急慢性胆囊炎，胆结石，胆道蛔虫病，下肢痿痹。

刺法：直刺 1.5 ~ 2 寸。

15.5.4 阑尾（EX-LE 7）

定位：在胫骨的前上方，在犊鼻下 5 寸，胫骨前缘外 1 横指。（图 2 - 4 - 102）

主治：急慢性阑尾炎，消化不良，下肢瘫痪。

刺法：直刺 1.5 ~ 2 寸。

15.5.5 八风（EX-LE 10）

定位：在足背，第 1 ~ 5 趾间，趾蹼缘后方赤白肉际处，一足 4 穴，左右 8 穴。（图 2 - 4 - 104）。

主治：足趾疼痛，肿胀，毒蛇咬伤。

刺法：斜刺 0.5 ~ 0.8 寸，或用三棱针点刺出血。

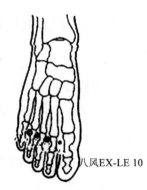

图 2 - 4 - 104

知识点 5　刺法灸法学知识点概要

刺法，古称"砭刺"，又称"针法"，指采用各种针具，通过一定的手法刺激人体的腧穴或部位，以防治疾病的方法。刺法依据针具的不同分为毫针刺法和特种针具刺法。毫针刺法是各种针法的基础，是针灸医师必须掌握的基本方法和操作技能。临床上常用的特种针具包括三棱针、皮肤针、皮内针等，一般针对特定病证进行治疗，具有针对性强、疗效确切的特点。刺法依据部位的不同又可以分为传统经穴刺法和特定部位刺法，例如头针和耳针。

灸法，古称"灸焫"，又称"艾灸"，指采用以艾绒或其他易燃材料烧灼、熏熨人体的一定部位或腧穴，以防治疾病的方法。依据施灸材料的不同，灸法又分为艾灸法和非艾灸法。艾灸法包括艾炷灸、艾卷灸、温针灸和温灸器灸等。非艾灸法包括天灸、灯火灸、黄蜡灸、药锭灸、药捻灸、药笔灸和药线灸等。

1. 毫针刺法操作

1.1 毫针结构和规格

毫针的结构，分为针尖、针身、针根、针柄、针尾五个部分。毫针的不同规格，主要以针身的直径和长度区分。临床一般以粗细为 0.30 ～ 0.45mm（26 ～ 30 号）和长短为 25 ～ 75mm（1 ～ 3 寸）者常用。短毫针主要用于肌肉浅薄部位的腧穴或在浅刺时应用，长毫针多用于肌肉丰厚部位的腧穴或在深刺时应用；毫针的粗细与针刺的刺激强度有关，供辨证施治时选用。

1.2 毫针操作的基本训练

毫针的操作练习，基本是对指力和手法的锻炼。

1.2.1 纸垫练针法

用松软的细草纸或毛边纸，折叠成厚约 2cm，长和宽分别为 8cm、5cm 的纸垫，外用棉线呈"井"字形扎紧。在此纸垫上可练习进针指力和捻转动作。

1.2.2 棉球练针法

取棉絮一团，用棉线缠绕，外紧内松，做成直径为 6~7cm 的圆球，外包白布一层缝制，即可练针。因棉球松软，可以练习提插、捻转、进针、出针等各种毫针操作手法的模拟动作。

1.2.3 自身练针法

通过纸垫、棉球等物体练针，具有了一定的指力基础后，可以在自己身上进行试针练习，以亲身体会进针、行针、得气的感觉。

1.3 针刺前的准备

1.3.1 器械准备

按照治疗需要选择恰当规格的毫针、托盘、镊子、艾绒、火罐、消毒棉球、75% 的酒精、1.5% 的碘酒、2% 的龙胆紫溶液等。在刺灸操作前应仔细检查以上器具是否完备。

1.3.2 患者体位

接受针刺治疗的过程中，患者体位选择是否合适，对腧穴是否准确定位，针刺的施术操作，持久的留针，以及防止晕针、滞针、弯针，甚至折针等针刺意外的发生具有重要意义。对部分重症和体质虚弱，或精神紧张、畏惧针刺的患者，其体位选择尤为重要。

临床常用体位有以下几种：仰卧体位、俯卧体位、侧卧体位、仰靠坐位、俯伏坐位和侧伏坐位。

1.3.3 消毒

（1）针具、器械消毒

针灸临床提倡"一针一穴一棉球"，以减少反复使用可能造成的感染。临床最好使用一次性无菌针。器械的消毒方法有很多，首选高压蒸汽灭菌法。此外还有药液浸泡消毒法和煮沸消毒法。

（2）医师手指消毒

在针刺操作之前，医师应按照标准洗手法将手洗刷干净，待干后再用75%乙醇棉球擦拭，方可持针操作。持针施术时，医师应尽量避免手指直接接触针身，如某些刺法需要触及针身时，必须用消毒干棉球作为间隔物，以确保针身无菌。

（3）针刺部位消毒

患者针刺部位，可用75%乙醇棉球或棉签擦拭消毒；或先用2%碘酊涂擦，再用75%乙醇棉球或棉签擦拭脱碘。擦拭时应从针刺部位的中心点向外绕圈消毒；当针刺部位消毒后，切忌接触污物，保持洁净，防止再次污染。

1.4 进针

1.4.1 进针方法

针刺治疗时，持针进行操作的手称为"刺手"，一般为右手；配合刺手按压穴位局部、协同刺手进针、行针的手称为"押手"，一般为左手。进针法是医师采用各种方法将毫针刺入腧穴皮下的操作方法。常用的进针法有以下几种：

（1）指切进针法

又称爪切进针法，用押手拇指或示指的指甲切按腧穴处皮肤，刺手持针，针尖紧靠押手指甲缘，将针迅速刺入。此法适宜于短针的进针，亦可用于腧穴局部紧邻重要的组织器官者。

（2）夹持进针法

押手拇、示两指持消毒干棉球，裹于针体下端，露出针尖，使针尖接触腧穴，刺手持针柄，刺手、押手同时用力将针刺入腧穴。此法适用于长针的进针。

（3）舒张进针法

押手示、中两指或拇、示两指将所刺腧穴部位的皮肤撑开绷紧，刺手持针，使针从刺手示、中两指或拇、示两指的中间刺入。此法主要用于皮肤松弛部位的腧穴。

（4）提捏进针法

用押手拇示两指将腧穴部位的皮肤捏起，刺手持针从捏起部的上端刺入。此法主要用于皮肉浅薄的穴位，特别是面部腧穴的进针。

1.4.2 针刺的角度和深度

（1）针刺角度

针刺角度是指针刺时针身与皮肤表面所形成的夹角。可根据腧穴部位的解剖特点和针刺治疗要求而确定。一般分为直刺、斜刺和平刺三种。

（2）针刺深度

针刺深度指针身刺入穴位内的深度。主要根据腧穴部位的解剖特点和治疗需要确定。同时还要结合患者年龄、体质、时令等因素综合考虑。

1.4.3 行针手法

毫针进针后，为了使患者产生针感，或进一步调整针感的强弱，或使针感向某一方向扩散、传导而采取的操作方法，称为"行针"，亦称"运针"。行针手法包括基本手法和辅助手法两类。

（1）基本行针手法

提插法　指将针刺入腧穴一定深度后，施以上提下插的操作手法。

将针向上引退为提，将针向下刺入为插，如此反复地做上下纵向运动就构成了提插法。

捻转法 指将针刺入腧穴一定深度后，施以向前、后捻转动作，使针在腧穴内反复前后来回旋转的行针手法。

（2）辅助行针手法

循法 医师用手指顺着经脉的循行径路，在腧穴的上下部轻柔循按的方法。此法能推动气血，激发经气，促使针后易于得气，此外循法还具有一定的行气作用。

飞法 医师用刺手拇、示两指持针，细细捻搓数次，然后张开两指，一搓一放，反复数次，状如飞鸟展翅，故称飞法。本法的作用在于催气、行气，并使针感增强，适用于肌肉丰厚部位的腧穴。

刮法 毫针刺入一定深度后，以拇指或示指的指腹抵住针尾，用拇指、示指或中指指甲，由下而上或由上而下频频刮动针柄，或者用拇指、中指固定针柄，以示指指尖由上至下刮动针柄的方法称为刮法。本法在针刺不得气时用之可激发经气，如已得气者可以加强针感的传导和扩散。

弹法 针刺后在留针过程中，以手指轻弹针尾或针柄，使针体微微振动的方法称为弹法。本法有催气、行气的作用。

摇法 毫针刺入一定深度后，刺手手持针柄，将针轻轻摇动的方法称摇法（图2-2-29）其法有二：一是直立针身而摇一是直立针身而摇，以泻实清热；二是卧倒针身而摇，使经气向一定方向传导。

震颤法 针刺入一定深度后，刺手拇、示两指夹持针柄，用小幅度、快频率的提插、捻转手法，使针身轻微震颤的方法称震颤法。本法可促使针下得气，增强针感。

1.4.4 针刺得气

得气是指医师将毫针刺入腧穴一定深度后，施以一定的行针手法，使针刺部位产生经气感应，这种针下的经气感应又称"气至"或"针感"。针刺得气后，患者方面的感觉主要有酸、麻、胀、重、凉、热、触电、跳跃、蚁行，以及特定条件下的疼痛等。医师方面的感觉主要指针下沉、涩、紧等感觉的变化。

得气是针刺产生治疗作用的关键，是判定医师针刺操作正确与否、患者经气盛衰、疾病预后转归、临床治疗效果有无的重要依据，也是针刺过程中进一步实施手法的基础。如果针刺未能得气，则应从以下几方面寻找原因：医师因素包括取穴失准，行针手法不熟练，针刺角度、方向、深浅把握不当，医师注意力不集中等；患者因素包括个体禀赋、体格强弱，以及机体状态等原因；还有环境因素等。

1.4.5 补泻手法

针刺补泻，是指在针刺得气的基础上，采用适当的针刺手法补益正气或疏泄病邪，从而调节人体脏腑经络功能，促使阴阳平衡，恢复人体健康的针刺方法。

（1）常用的补泻手法

捻转补泻 捻转补泻是主要依据向不同方向捻转时用力轻重的不同以区分补泻的针刺手法。针刺得气后，在针下得气处反复施行捻转手法，拇指向前捻转时用力重（左转），指力下沉，拇指向后还原时用力轻，为补法。针刺得气后，在针下得气处反复施行捻转手法，拇指向后捻转时用力重（右转），指力上浮，拇指向前还原时用力轻，为泻法。

提插补泻 提插补泻是主要依据实施提、插手法时用力轻重的变化来区分补泻的针刺手法。针刺得气后，在针下得气处反复施行小幅度的重插轻提手法，以下插用力为主，为补法；在针下得气处反复施行小幅度的轻插重提手法，以上提用力为主，为泻法。

徐疾补泻 徐疾补泻是主要依据针刺速度快慢，以及出针、按闭穴位的快慢来区分补泻的针刺手法。针刺得气后，徐进缓退，是为补法；缓进徐退，是为泻法。

开阖补泻 开阖补泻是主要依据出针时是否按闭针孔以区分补泻的针刺手法。缓慢退针，出针后迅速按压针孔片刻，为补法；疾速出针，出针时摇大针孔且不加按压，为泻法。

迎随补泻 迎随补泻是主要依据针刺方向与经脉气血运行方向的顺逆以区分补泻的针刺手法。进针时针尖随着经脉循行方向刺入为补法，针尖迎着经脉循行方向刺入为泻法。

呼吸补泻 呼吸补泻是主要依据针刺进退与患者呼吸状态配合以区分补泻的针刺手法。

（2）影响针刺补泻的因素

影响针刺补泻的因素包括：机体的功能状态、腧穴主治功用的相对特异性和针刺手法三方面的因素。

1.4.6 留针和出针

（1）留针

将针刺入腧穴并施行手法后，使针留置穴内称为留针。留针的目的是为了加强针刺的作用和便于继续行针施术。一般病证只要针下得气而施以适当的补泻手法后，即可出针或留针 10～30 分钟。但对一些特殊病证，如急性腹痛、破伤风、角弓反张，以及寒性、顽固性疼痛或痉挛性病证，可适当延长留针时间，有时留针可达数小时，以便在留针过程中做间歇性行针，以增强、巩固疗效。留针方法可分为静留针法和动留针法两种，临床中留针与否及选用何种留针方法要根据患者的疾病性质和身体状况灵活选用。

（2）出针

出针，又称起针、退针。在施行针刺手法或留针达到预定针刺目的和治疗要求后，即可出针。出针时，医师先以押手持消毒干棉球轻轻按压于针刺部位，刺手持针做轻微提捻动作，感觉针下松动后，将针缓慢退至皮下，再将针迅速退出；然后用消毒干棉球按压针孔片刻。如刺针深度较浅，针下无紧涩感，也可迅速将针退出。

1.4.7 针刺异常情况的预防与处理

针刺是一种既简便又安全的治疗方法，但若操作不慎、疏忽大意，或犯刺禁，或针刺手法不当，或对人体解剖部位缺乏全面的了解，也会出现晕针、滞针、弯针、折针、皮下血肿、创伤性气胸等异常情况。一旦出现异常情况，应立即进行有效的处理。

（1）晕针

晕针是指在针刺过程中患者发生晕厥的现象。

【表现】

在针刺过程中，患者出现神情异常、头晕目眩、恶心欲吐等；甚见心慌气短、面色苍白、冷汗出、四肢厥冷、脉沉细等；重者出现神志昏迷、唇甲青紫、大汗淋漓、二便失禁、脉微欲绝等。

【原因】

晕针多见于首次接受针刺、恐针、畏痛、情绪紧张者；或素体虚弱，或劳累过度，或空腹者，或大汗、大泻、大出血者；或体位不当，或刺激手法过强，或诊室闷热，或过于寒冷等。

【处理】

立即停止针刺，迅速全部出针。患者平卧，头部放低，松解衣带，保温；服用糖类饮料或制品（可能影响患者自身原有疾病者慎用）或温开水；通畅空气。重者在行上述处理后，可选水沟、素髎、内关、合谷、太冲、涌泉、足三里等穴指压或针刺之，亦可灸百会、气海、关元等穴；一般患者可逐渐恢复正常。若见不省人事、呼吸微弱、脉微欲绝者，可配合急救措施。如出针后患者有晕针现象，应休息观察并做相应处理。

【预防】

对于初次接受针刺治疗，特别是精神紧张者，要先做好解释工作，消除其恐惧心理；对体质虚弱、大汗、大泻、大出血等患者，取穴宜精，手法宜轻。对于饥饿或过度疲劳者，应推迟针刺时间，待其体力恢复、进食后再行针刺。注意患者体位的舒适自然，尽可能选取卧位。注意室内空气流通，消除过热、过冷因素。医师在治疗施术过程中，应守神入微，密切观察患者的神态，随时询问其感觉，如有不适立即处理。

（2）滞针

滞针是指在行针或出针时，医师捻转、提插、出针均感困难，且患者感觉疼痛或疼痛加剧的现象。

【表现】

在行针或出针时，医师捻转、提插和出针均感困难。若强行捻转、提插时，患者痛不可忍。

【原因】

针刺入腧穴后，引起局部肌肉痉挛；进针后患者移动体位；医师向单一方向捻针太过，肌纤维缠绕于针身所致。若留针时间过长，也可出现滞针。

【处理】

如患者精神紧张而致肌肉痉挛引起者，需做好耐心解释，消除其紧张情绪；患者体位移动者，需帮助其恢复原来体位；单向捻转过度者，需向反方向捻转；或用手指在滞针邻近部位做循按手法，或弹动针柄，或在针刺邻近部位再刺一针，以宣散邪气、解除滞针。

【预防】

对于初诊患者和精神紧张者，要做好针刺前解释工作，消除紧张情绪。针刺时选择较舒适体位，避免留针时移动体位。痉挛性疾病行针时手法宜轻巧，不可捻转角度过大。若用搓法时，应注意防止滞针。

（3）弯针

弯针是指进针、行针或留针时，针身在患者体内出现弯曲的现象。

【表现】

针柄改变了进针时或留针时的方向和角度，医师提插、捻转和出针均感困难，患者感觉针刺部位疼痛。

【原因】

医师手法不熟练，进针用力过猛、过速，或针下碰到坚硬组织；进针后患者改变了体位；或外力碰击或压迫针柄；或针刺部位处于痉挛状态；或滞针处理不当等。

【处理】

出现弯针后，不得再行手法，切忌强拔针、猛退针，以防引起折针、出血等。若体位移动所致者，须先恢复原来体位，局部放松后始可退针。若针身弯曲度较小者，可按一般的起针方法，随弯针的角度将针慢慢退出。若针身弯曲度大者，可顺着弯曲的方向轻微地摇动退针。如针身弯曲不止一处，须结合针柄扭转倾斜的方向逐次分段退出，切勿急拔猛抽，以防断针。

【预防】

首先医师手法要熟练、轻巧，避免进针过猛、过速。患者的体位选择应适当，留针期间不可移动体位。防止针刺部位和针柄受外力碰压。另外，针刺痉挛状态的部位时应尤宜慎重。

（4）断针

断针又称折针，是指针刺过程中，毫针针身折断在患者体内的现象。

【表现】

在行针、出针时，发现针身折断，或部分针身浮露于皮肤之外，或全部没于皮肤之下。

【原因】

针具检查疏忽或使用劣质针具。针刺或留针时患者改变了体位。针刺时将针身全部刺入；行针时强力提插、捻转，引起肌肉痉挛。遇弯针、滞针等异常情况处理不当，并强力出针。外物碰撞、压迫针柄等。

【处理】

医师应冷静、沉着，并告诫患者不要恐惧，保持原有体位，以防残端向深层陷入。若残端尚有部分露于皮肤之外，可用镊子钳出。若残端与皮肤相平或稍低，而折面仍可看见，可用左手拇、示两指垂直向下挤压针孔两旁皮肤，使残端露出皮肤之外，右手持镊子将针拔出。若残端深入皮下，须采用外科手术方法取出。

【预防】

针刺前必须仔细检查针具，尤其是针根部，对于不符合质量的针具应剔除不用。避免过猛、过强地行针。选择的毫针长度必须大于行针深度，针刺时切勿将针身全部刺入腧穴，更不能进至针根，应留部分针身在体外。行针和退针时，如果发现有弯针、滞针等异常情况，应及时处理，不可强力硬拔。

针刺导致血管损伤包括出血和皮下血肿。出血是指出针后针刺部位出血；皮下血肿是指针刺部位因皮下出血而引起肿痛等现象。

【表现】

出针后针刺部位出血或肿胀疼痛，甚见皮肤呈青紫等现象。

【原因】

针刺过程中刺伤血管，或者患者凝血机制障碍所致。

【处理】

出血者，可用干棉球行长时间按压。若微量的皮下出血而出现局部小块青紫时，一般不必处理，可自行消退。若局部肿胀疼痛较剧，青紫面积大而且影响到活动功能时，在 24 小时内先冷敷止血，24 小时之后再做热敷或在局部轻轻按揉，使局部瘀血吸收消散。

【预防】

术前仔细检查针具，熟悉腧穴解剖结构，避开血管针刺。针刺时避免针刺手法过重，并嘱患者不可随意移动体位。分层延时出针，出针时立即用消毒干棉球按压针孔。有出血倾向者，针刺时要慎重。

（5）气胸

针刺引起创伤性气胸是指针刺入胸腔，使胸膜破损，空气进入胸膜腔所造成的气胸。

【表现】

患者突感胸闷、胸痛、心悸、气短、呼吸不畅、刺激性干咳，严重者呼吸困难、发绀、冷汗、烦躁、精神紧张，甚至出现血压下降、休克等危急症状。

体格检查：视诊可见患侧肋间隙变宽、胸廓饱满，叩诊患侧呈鼓音，听诊患侧呼吸音减弱或消失，触诊或可见气管向健侧移位。

影像学检查可见患侧肺组织被压缩。部分患者出针时并不立即出现症状，而是过一小段时间才逐渐感到胸闷、疼痛、呼吸困难等。

【原因】

针刺胸部、背部及邻近腧穴不当，刺伤胸膜，空气聚于胸腔而造成气胸。

【处理】

一旦发生气胸，应立即出针；患者采取半卧位休息，避免屏气、用力、高声呼喊，应平静心情，尽量减少体位翻转。轻者可自然吸收，如有症状，可对证处理，如给予镇咳、消炎等药物，以防止因咳嗽扩大创孔，避免加重和感染；重者，如出现呼吸困难、发绀、休克等现象，应立即组织抢救。

【预防】

为患者选择合适体位。对于胸部、背部及邻近腧穴，根据患者体形，严格掌握针刺的角度、方向和深度，施行提插手法的幅度不宜过大。

1.4.8 针刺治疗的注意事项

（1）患者过于饥饿、疲劳，精神过度紧张时，不宜立即针刺。体弱年迈、气虚血亏的患者，针刺时手法不宜过强，并应尽量选用卧位。

（2）妇女怀孕腹部、腰骶部的腧穴不宜针刺。三阴交、合谷、昆仑、至阴等一些能引起子宫收缩的腧穴，在孕期禁针。妇女经期，若非为了调经，亦不应针刺。

（3）小儿囟门未合时，头顶部的腧穴不宜针刺。

（4）自发性出血或损伤后出血不止的患者，不宜针刺。

（5）皮肤有感染、溃疡、瘢痕的部位，不宜针刺。

（6）对于尿潴留的患者，在针刺小腹部腧穴时，应掌握适当的方向、角度、深度等，以免误伤膀胱。

2. 灸法

灸法是指利用艾叶等易燃材料或药物，点燃后在穴位上或患处进行烧灼或熏熨，借其温热性刺激及药物的药理作用，以达到防病治病目的的一种外治方法。

2.1 灸法的作用

2.1.1 温通经络，祛散寒邪

灸法以温热性刺激为主，灸火的热力能透达组织深部，温热之力能助阳通经，又能散寒逐痹。

2.1.2 补虚培本，回阳固脱

灸能增强脏腑的功能，补益气血，填精益髓。因此，凡先天不足、后天失养及大病、久病导致的脏腑功能低下、气血虚弱、中气下陷皆为灸法的适应病证。另外，灸法对阳气虚脱而出现的大汗淋漓、四肢厥冷、脉微欲绝的脱证有显著的回阳固脱的作用。

2.1.3 行气活血，消肿散结

灸之温热刺激，可使气血调和，营卫通畅，起到行气活血、消肿散结的作用。因此，凡气血凝滞及形成肿块者均是灸法的适宜病证，如乳痈初起、瘰疬、瘿瘤等。特别是疮疡阴证之日久不溃、久溃不敛者，使用灸法治疗，更显示出独特的治疗效果。

2.1.4 预防保健，益寿延年

灸法不仅能治病，而且还可以激发人体正气，增强抗病能力，起到预防保健作用。对于中老年人，于无病时或处于亚健康的状态下，长期坚持灸关元、气海、足三里等穴可以延缓衰老，达到益寿延年的目的。因此，灸法又有"保健灸法""长寿灸法"之称。

2.2 艾灸的分类

灸法的种类十分丰富，一般依据施灸材料可分为艾灸法和非艾灸法两大类。

2.2.1 艾灸法

（1）艾炷灸

将艾炷放在穴位上施灸，称为艾炷灸。艾炷灸可分为直接灸和间接灸两种。

①直接灸：将艾炷直接放在皮肤上点燃施灸的方法。根据施灸的程度不同，即灸后有无烧伤化脓，又分为化脓灸（瘢痕灸）和非化脓灸（非瘢痕灸）。

化脓灸：化脓灸法灼伤较重，可使局部皮肤溃破、化脓，并留永久瘢痕，故又称烧灼灸、瘢痕灸。

非化脓灸：本法以达到温烫为主，使穴位局部皮肤发生红晕或轻微烫伤，灸后不化脓，不留瘢痕，近现代应用较多。

②间接灸：间接灸也称隔物灸、间隔灸，是将艾炷与皮肤之间衬隔某种物品而施灸的一种方法。本法根据所隔物品的不同，可分为数十种。所隔物品大多为药物，既可用单味药物，也可用复方药物，药物性能不同，临床应用的范围也有所异。临床常用的有隔姜灸、隔蒜灸、隔盐灸、隔附子饼灸等。

隔姜灸：切取厚约 0.2~0.3cm 厚的生姜 1 片。在中心处用针穿刺数孔，上置艾炷，放在穴位上，用火点燃艾炷施灸。本法可根据病情反复施灸，适用于风寒咳嗽、腹痛、泄泻、风寒湿痹、痛经、面神经麻痹等，尤宜于寒证。

隔蒜灸：用独头蒜，或较大蒜瓣横切成 0.2~0.3cm 厚的蒜片，中心处用针穿刺数孔，置于穴位或患处皮肤上，再将艾炷置于蒜瓣上，用火点燃艾炷施灸。本法多用于未溃之化脓性肿块，如乳痈、疖肿，以及瘰疬、牛皮癣、神经性皮炎、关节炎、手术后瘢痕等。

隔盐灸：又称神阙灸，用于脐窝部施灸，用干燥纯净的食盐末适量，将脐窝填平，上置艾炷，用火点燃施灸。本法可治疗急性腹痛、泄泻、痢疾、风湿痹证及阳气虚脱证。

隔附子饼灸：将生附子研为细末，用黄酒调和制饼，直径 1~2cm，厚0.3~0.5cm，中心处用针穿刺数孔，上置艾炷，放于穴位或患处皮肤上，点燃艾炷施灸。附子辛温大热，有温肾益火作用，故此灸法多用来治疗各种阳虚病证。

（2）艾条灸

艾条灸，又称艾卷灸，是用特制的艾条在穴位皮肤上熏烤或温熨的施灸方法。将点燃的艾条悬于施灸部位之上，称为悬起灸。一般艾火距皮肤2~3cm，灸10~15分钟，以灸至皮肤温热红晕，而又不致烧伤皮肤为度。悬起灸又分为温和灸、回旋灸和雀啄灸。

①温和灸：将艾卷的一端点燃，对准应灸的腧穴部位或患处，距离皮肤2~3cm，进行熏烤，使患者局部有温热感而无灼痛为宜，一般每穴灸10~15分钟，至皮肤红晕为度。

②雀啄灸：将点燃的艾卷置于穴位或患处上方约3cm处，施灸时，艾卷点燃的一端与施灸部位的皮肤并不固定在一定的距离，而是像鸟雀啄食一样，将艾卷一上一下地移动。

③回旋灸：施灸时，艾卷点燃的一端与施灸皮肤保持在一定的距离，但位置不固定，而是均匀地向左右方向移动或反复旋转地进行灸治。

（3）温针灸

温针灸是针刺与艾灸相结合的一种方法。适用于既需要针刺留针，又需施灸的疾病。操作方法为，在针刺得气后，将针留在适当的深度，在针柄上穿置一段长约1.5cm的艾卷施灸，或在针尾搓捏少许艾绒点燃施灸。此法是一种简便易行的针灸并用方法。其艾绒燃烧的热力，可通过针身传入体内，使其发挥针与灸的作用，达到治疗的目的。

（4）温灸器灸

温灸器是便于施灸的器械，常用的有3种类型，即温灸盒、温灸筒、温灸架。

温灸盒是一种特制的盒形灸具，内装艾卷或无烟艾条。用温灸盒每次灸15~30分钟。温灸筒为筒状的金属灸具，常用的有平面式和圆锥式两种。平面式底部面积较大，布有许多小孔，内套有小筒，用于放置艾绒施灸，适用于治疗较大面积的皮肤病。圆锥式底面瘦小，只有一个小孔，适用于点灸某一个穴位。温灸架为架状灸具，将艾卷的一端点燃，插入灸疗架的上孔内灸 15～30 分钟。

2.2.2 其他灸法（非艾灸类）

灯火灸

灯火灸，是用灯心草蘸油点燃后快速按在穴位上进行焠烫的方法，又称灯草灸、油捻灸。灯心草，为灯心草科植物，秋季采收，入药者为干燥茎髓，呈细长圆柱形，一般长 50～60cm，表面呈乳白色至淡黄白色，粗糙，有细纵沟纹。

2.3 灸法注意事项

2.3.1 施灸的顺序

一般是先灸上部，后灸下部；先灸背、腰部，后灸腹部；先灸头部，后灸四肢。

2.3.2 灸法的补泻

补法是点燃艾炷后，不吹其火，待其慢慢燃烧、自灭；泻法是点燃艾炷后，以口速吹旺其火，快燃速灭。由此看来，补法火力温和，时间稍长，能使真气聚而不散；泻法火力较猛而时间较短，能促使邪气消散。

2.3.3 施灸的禁忌

凡实热证或阴虚发热、邪热内炽等证，如高热等，均不宜使用艾灸疗法。颜面部、心区、体表大血管部和关节肌腱部位不可用瘢痕灸。妇女妊娠期腰骶部和小腹部禁用瘢痕灸，其他灸法也不宜灸量过重。对昏迷、肢体麻木不仁及感觉迟钝的患者，勿灸过量，以避免烧伤。瘢痕灸之后，需要安静修养，忌高强度劳动，必须保持局部皮肤清洁，以免引起化脓部位的感染。如果发生感染，应立即处理。

3. 拔罐法

拔罐法是一种以罐为工具，利用燃烧、抽吸、蒸汽等方法造成罐内负压，使罐吸附于体表腧穴或患处的一定部位，使局部皮肤充血，产生良性刺激，达到调节脏腑、平衡阴阳、疏通经络、防治疾病目的的方法。

3.1 罐的常见种类

临床上常用的罐有竹罐、陶罐、玻璃罐和抽气罐四类。

3.2 罐的吸拔方法

3.2.1 火罐法

火罐法是利用燃烧时消耗罐中部分氧气，并借火焰的热力使罐内的气体膨胀而排除罐内部分空气，使罐内气压低于罐外气压（统称负压），借以将罐吸附于施术部位的皮肤上。常用的方法有以下几种：

（1）闪火法

用止血钳或镊子等夹住95%乙醇棉球（或用7~8号粗铁丝，一头缠绕石棉绳或线带，做成乙醇棒），一手握罐体，罐口朝下，将棉球点燃后立即伸入罐内摇晃数圈随即退出，迅速将罐扣于应拔部位，此时罐内已成负压即可吸住。此法适用于人体各部位，可留罐、闪罐、走罐等，临床最为常用。

（2）投火法

将易燃软质纸片（卷），或蘸乙醇的棉球点燃后投入罐内，趁火旺时迅速将罐扣于应拔部位。投火时，不论使用纸卷或纸条，都必须高出罐口1寸多，等到燃烧至1寸，纸卷和纸条都能斜立罐内侧面，火焰不会烧着皮肤。此法罐内燃烧物易坠落烫伤皮肤，故多用于身体侧面或横向拔罐、拔单罐、留罐、排罐等。

（3）滴酒法

在罐内壁上中段滴 2～3 滴 95% 的乙醇，再将罐横侧翻滚一下，使乙醇均匀附于罐内壁上（不可流到罐口处），点燃乙醇后，迅速将罐扣在选定的部位，即可吸住。

（4）贴棉法

将直径 1～2cm 的 95% 乙醇棉片，薄蘸乙醇，紧贴于罐内壁，点燃后迅速将罐扣于应拔部位。此法多用于侧面拔，亦用于身体侧面横向拔罐。

3.2.2 水罐法

此法一般使用竹罐。先将竹罐放在锅内加水煮沸（也可在水里加煮中药制成药液使用），使用时将罐子倾倒用镊子夹出，甩去水液，用折叠的湿冷毛巾紧扪罐口，降低罐口温度，乘热按在皮肤上，即能吸住。此法适用于任何部位，吸拔力较小，操作需快捷。

3.2.3 抽气罐法

先将抽气罐紧扣在应拔部位，用抽气筒将罐内的部分空气抽出，使其产生负压，吸拔于皮肤上。或用抽气筒套在塑料杯罐活塞上，将空气抽出，即能吸住。此法适用于任何部位处拔罐。

3.3 拔罐法的应用

3.3.1 走罐

走罐又名推罐法、拉罐法。先于施罐部位涂上润滑剂（常用医用凡士林、医用甘油、液状石蜡或润肤霜等），也可用温水或药液，同时还可将罐口涂上油脂；使用闪火法将罐吸住后，立即用手握住罐体，略用力将罐沿着一定路线反复推拉，至走罐部位皮肤紫红为度，推罐时着力在罐口，用力均匀，防止罐漏气脱落。该法适用于病变范围较广、肌肉丰厚而平整的部位，如背部脊柱两旁、下肢股四头肌处、腰骶部、腹部及肩关节等。

3.3.2 闪罐

用闪火法将罐吸拔于应拔部位，随即取下，再吸拔，再取下，反复吸拔直至局部皮肤潮红，或罐体底部发热为度；动作要迅速而准确。必要时也可在闪罐后留罐；适用于肌肉较松弛，吸拔不紧或留罐有困难之处，以及局部皮肤麻木或功能减退的虚证患者。适用于治疗风湿痹证、中风后遗症，以及肌肤麻木、肌肉萎缩等。

3.3.3 刺络拔罐

用皮肤针、三棱针或粗毫针等，在腧穴或患处点刺出血，或三棱针挑刺后，再行拔罐留罐；起罐后用消毒棉球擦净血迹；挑刺部位用消毒敷料或创可贴贴敷。

3.3.4 留针拔罐

留针时，以针为中心拔罐，留置规定时间后，起罐再起针。此法不宜用于胸背部，因罐内负压易加深针刺深度，从而容易引起气胸。

3.4 启罐法

启罐又名起罐，即将吸拔牢的罐具取下的方法。一般罐具启罐，一手握住罐体底部稍倾斜，将拇指或示指按压罐口边缘的皮肤，使罐口与皮肤之间产生空隙，空气进入罐内即可将罐取下。不可生硬拉拔，以免拉伤皮肤，产生疼痛。

3.5 罐法的适应范围

拔罐法的适应范围非常广泛，尤其对于各种疼痛类疾病、软组织损伤、急慢性炎症、风寒湿痹证，以及脏腑功能失调、经脉闭阻不通所引起的各种病证均有较好的疗效。

3.6 罐法的注意事项

拔罐部位，一般选择肌肉丰满、皮下组织充实及毛发较少的部位为宜。吸拔力过大，吸拔时间过久，可能使拔罐部位的皮肤起水泡。如果水泡较少（小），可以不做处理，自行吸收；如果水泡较多或溃破，则应第一时间处理避免感染。拔罐前应充分暴露应拔部位，有毛发者宜剃去，操作部位应注意防止烫伤。手法要熟练，动作要轻、快、稳、准。若不慎出现烧烫伤，应按外科烧烫伤处理。

高热、抽搐和痉挛发作者不宜拔罐；急性严重疾病、慢性全身虚弱性疾病及接触性传染病患者不宜拔罐；过饥、醉酒、过饱、过度疲劳者不宜拔罐；婴幼儿、孕妇的腰骶及腹部、前后阴、乳房部不宜拔罐；心尖区、体表大动脉搏动处、静脉曲张处不宜拔罐。

4. 三棱针法

三棱针法也称刺络泻血法，是用三棱针刺破血络或腧穴，放出适量血液或挤出少量液体，或挑断皮下纤维组织，以治疗疾病的方法。其中放出适量血液以治疗疾病的方法属刺络法或刺血法，又称放血疗法。

4.1 三棱针操作

三棱针的操作方法一般分为点刺法、刺络法、散刺法、挑治法4种。

4.1.1 点刺法

点刺法即点刺腧穴出血或挤出少量液体的方法。此法是用三棱针点刺腧穴或血络以治疗疾病的方法。针刺前，在预定针刺部位上下用左手拇指、示指向针刺处推按，使血液积聚于点刺部位。常规消毒后，左手拇、示、中三指夹紧被刺部位，右手持针，直刺 2～3mm，快进快出，轻轻挤压针孔周围，使出血数滴，或挤出少量液体。然后用消毒干棉球按压针孔。为了刺出一定量的血液或液体，点刺穴位的深度不宜太浅。此法多用于指（趾）末端、面部、耳部的穴位，如十宣、十二井穴等。

4.1.2 散刺法

用一手固定被刺部位，另一手持针在施术部位点刺多点。根据病变部位大小不同，可刺数针，甚至十余针以上，由病变外缘环形向中心点刺，以促使瘀血或水肿的排泄，达到"宛陈则除之"，通经活络的目的。针刺深浅根据局部肌肉厚薄、血管深浅而定。此法多用于局部瘀血、水肿、顽癣等。

4.1.3 刺络法

即点刺静脉出血的方法。常规消毒后，右手持针垂直点刺，快进快出，动作要求稳、准、快。浅刺用于小静脉显现的部位，如下肢后面、额部、颞部、足背等部位；深刺多用于肘窝、腘窝的静脉及小静脉瘀滞处。

4.1.4 挑治法

此法是以三棱针挑断穴位皮下纤维组织以治疗疾病的方法。局部消毒后，左手捏起施术部位皮肤，右手持针先以 15°～30°角进入皮肤，然后上挑针尖，挑破皮肤或皮下组织，并可挤出一定量的血液或少量液体，然后用无菌敷料保护创口，以胶布固定。对于一些畏惧疼痛者，可先用2%利多卡因局麻后再挑刺。挑刺的部位可以选用经穴，也可选用奇穴，更多选用阿是穴和阳性反应点。在选用阳性反应点时，应注意与痣、毛囊炎、色素斑及背俞穴相鉴别。

4.2 三棱针法适应范围

三棱针刺络放血具有通经活络、开窍泻热、消肿止痛等作用，适用范围较为广泛，凡各种实证、热证、瘀血、疼痛等均可应用。目前较常用于急症，如昏厥、高热、中风闭证、急性咽喉肿痛、中暑等。也可用于某些慢性病，如顽癣、扭挫伤、头痛、肩周炎、丹毒、指（趾）麻木等。

4.3 三棱针法注意事项

对患者要做必要的解释工作，以消除思想顾虑，尤其是对放血量较大者。操作前应严格消毒，防止感染。操作时手法宜轻、稳、准、快，不可用力过猛，防止刺入过深、创伤过大，损害其他组织，更不可伤及动脉。对体弱、贫血、低血压、孕妇和产后等，均要慎重使用。凡有出血倾向和血管瘤的患者，不宜使用本法。使用三棱针法，每日1次或每隔一天1次，3~5次为一个疗程；急症可以增强为每日两次。如放血量大，建议每周1~2次。挑刺法3~7天1次，3~5次为1个疗程，两疗程间休息10~14天。

5. 皮肤针法

皮肤针法是以多支短针浅刺人体一定部位（穴位）的一种针刺方法。皮肤针法通过叩刺皮部，以疏通经络、调和气血，促使机体恢复正常，从而达到防治疾病的目的。皮肤针是针头呈小锤状的一种针具，一般针柄长15~19cm，一端附有莲蓬状的针盘，下边散嵌着不锈钢短针。针柄有软柄和硬柄两种类型，软柄一般用有机玻璃或硬塑料制作。根据所嵌针数的不同，又分别称为梅花针（五支针）、七星针（七支针）、罗汉针（十八支针）等。针尖不宜过锐，应呈松针形。

5.1 皮肤针操作

针刺前针具灭菌。施针前在局部皮肤用2%碘酊进行消毒，再用75%酒精棉脱碘。将针柄末端置于掌心，拇指居上，示指在下，余指呈握拳状固定针柄末端。针尖对准叩刺部位，运用灵活的腕力垂直叩刺，即将针尖垂直叩击在皮肤上，并立刻弹起。如此反复进行。叩刺时要运用灵活的腕力直刺、弹刺、速刺。叩刺速度要均匀，防止快慢不一、用力不匀地乱刺。针尖起落要呈垂直方向，即将针垂直地刺下、垂直地提起，如此反复操作。防止针尖斜着刺入和向后拖拉着起针，这样会增加病人的疼痛。针刺部位须准确，按预定应刺部位下针，每一针之间的距离，一般为1～1.5cm。

5.1.1 叩刺部位

可分为循经叩刺、穴位叩刺和局部叩刺3种。

（1）循经叩刺

指沿着与疾病有关的经脉循行路线叩刺。主要用于项、背、腰、骶部的督脉和膀胱经，其次是四肢肘、膝以下的三阴经、三阳经。可治疗相应脏腑经络病变。

（2）穴位叩刺

指选取与疾病相关的穴位叩刺。主要用于背俞穴、夹脊穴和阳性反应点。

（3）局部叩刺

指在病变局部叩刺。如治疗头面五官、关节及局部扭伤、顽癣等疾病可叩刺病变局部。

5.1.2 叩刺强度

根据患者病情、体质、年龄和叩刺部位的不同，可分别采用弱刺激、中等刺激和强刺激。

（1）弱刺激

用较轻的腕力叩刺，冲力小，针尖接触皮肤的时间愈短愈好，局部皮肤略见潮红，患者无疼痛感觉。适用于年老体弱、小儿、初诊患者，以及头面五官肌肉浅薄处。

（2）强刺激

用较重的腕力叩刺，冲力大，针尖接触皮肤的时间可稍长，局部皮肤可见出血，患者有明显疼痛感觉。适用于年壮体强，以及肩、背、腰、臀、四肢等肌肉丰厚处。

（3）中等刺激

叩刺的腕力介于强、弱刺激之间，冲力中等，局部皮肤潮红，但无出血，患者稍觉疼痛。适用于多数患者，除头面五官等肌肉浅薄处，其他部位均可选用。

5.1.3 皮肤针适应范围

皮肤针可以用于治疗疼痛类疾病，如头痛、肩背痛等；消化系统疾病，如呃逆、胃脘痛、腹痛等；呼吸系统疾病，如鼻塞、哮喘等；其他，如失眠、面瘫、斑秃、荨麻疹、痿证、肌肤麻木等。

5.1.4 皮肤针注意事项

注意检查针具，当发现针尖有钩毛或缺损、针锋参差不齐者，须及时修理。针具及针刺局部皮肤均应消毒。重刺后，局部皮肤需用酒精棉球消毒并应注意保持针刺局部清洁，以防感染。局部皮肤有创伤、溃疡及瘢痕者，不宜使用本法。

6. 耳针

耳针法是指采用毫针或其他方式刺激耳部特定部位，以预防、诊断和治疗全身疾病的一种方法。耳针治疗范围较广，操作方法简单易行，对于疾病的预防和诊治具有一定的意义。

6.1 耳郭表面解剖

耳郭表面解剖部位的名称。（图 2 – 6 – 1）

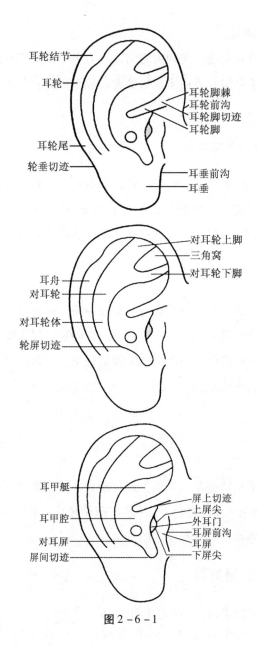

图 2 - 6 - 1

6.2 耳穴分布规律

耳穴在耳郭表面的分布状态形似倒置在子宫内的胎儿（头部朝下，臀部朝上）。其分布规律：与头面相应的穴位分布在耳垂；与上肢相应的穴位分布在耳舟；与躯干相应的穴位分布在对耳轮体部；与下肢相应的穴位分布在对耳轮上、下脚；与腹腔脏器相应的穴位分布在耳甲艇；与胸腔脏器相应的穴位分布在耳甲腔；与盆腔脏器相应的穴位分布在三角窝；与消化道相应的穴位分布在耳轮脚周围。

6.3 耳郭区划定位标准与耳穴

6.3.1 耳轮部位

耳轮部总计分为 12 区，共有 13 穴。（图 2 – 6 – 2，表 2 – 6 – 1）

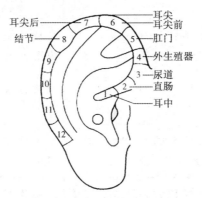

图 2 – 6 – 2 耳轮耳穴分区

表 2 – 6 – 1 耳轮部位的耳穴定位及主治

穴名	定位	主治
耳（HX_1）	在耳轮脚处，即耳轮 1 区	呃逆、荨麻疹、皮肤瘙痒、咯血
直肠（HX_2）	在耳轮脚棘前上方的耳轮处，即耳轮 2 区	便秘、腹泻、脱肛、痔疮
尿道（HX_3）	在直肠上方的耳轮处，即耳轮 3 区	尿频、尿急、尿痛、尿潴留
外生殖器（HX_4）	在对耳轮下脚前方的耳轮处，即耳轮 4 区	睾丸炎、附睾炎、阴道炎、外阴瘙痒
肛门（HX_5）	三角窝前方的耳轮处，即耳轮 5 区	痔疮、肛裂
耳尖前（HX_6）	在耳尖的前部，即耳轮 6 区	发热、结膜炎

（续表）

穴名	定位	主治
耳尖（HX$_{6,7i}$）	在耳郭向前对折的上部尖端处，即耳轮6、7区交界处	发热、高血压、急性结膜炎、睑腺炎、痛证、风疹、失眠
耳尖后（HX$_7$）	在耳尖的后部，即耳轮7区	发热、结膜炎
结节（HX$_8$）	在耳轮结节处，即耳轮8区	头晕、头痛、高血压
轮1（HX$_9$）	在耳轮结节下方的耳轮处，即耳轮9区	扁桃体炎、上呼吸道感染、发热
轮2（HX$_{10}$）	在轮1区下方的耳轮处，即耳轮10区	扁桃体炎、上呼吸道感染、发热
轮3（HX$_{11}$）	在轮2区下方的耳轮处，即耳轮11区	扁桃体炎、上呼吸道感染、发热
轮4（HX$_{12}$）	在轮3区下方的耳轮处，即耳轮12区	扁桃体炎、上呼吸道感染、发热

6.3.2 耳舟部位

耳舟部总计分为6区，共有6穴。（图2-6-3，表2-6-2）

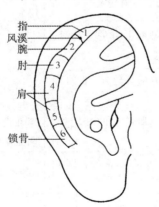

图2-6-3 耳舟耳穴分区

表 2 - 6 - 2 耳舟部位耳穴定位及主治

穴名	定位	主治
指（SF_1）	在耳轮脚处，即耳轮 1 区	呃逆、荨麻疹、皮肤瘙痒、咯血
腕（SF_2）	在指区的下方处，即耳舟 2 区	腕部疼痛
风溪（$SF_{1,2i}$）	在耳轮结节前方，指区与腕区之间，即耳舟 1、2 区交界处	荨麻疹、皮肤瘙痒、过敏性鼻炎、哮喘
肘（SF_3）	在腕区的下方处，即耳舟 3 区	肱骨外上髁炎、肘部疼痛
肩（$SF_{4,5}$）	在肘区的下方处，即耳舟 4、5 区	肩关节周围炎、肩部疼痛
锁骨（SF_6）	在肩区的下方处，即耳舟 6 区	肩关节周围炎

6.3.3 对耳轮部位

对耳轮部总计分为 13 区，共有 14 穴。（图 2 - 6 - 4，表 2 - 6 - 3）

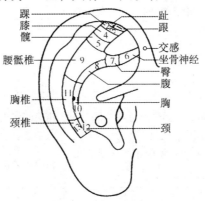

图 2 - 6 - 4 对耳轮耳穴分区

表 2-6-3 对耳轮部位耳穴定位及主治

穴名	定位	主治
跟（AH₁）	在对耳轮上脚前上部，即对耳轮 1 区	足跟痛
趾（AH₂）	在耳尖下方的对耳轮上脚后上部，即对耳轮 2 区	甲沟炎、足趾部麻木疼痛
踝（AH₃）	在趾、跟区下方处，即对耳轮3 区	踝关节扭伤、踝关节炎
膝（AH₄）	在对耳轮上脚中 1/3 处，即对耳轮 4 区	膝关节肿痛
髋（AH₅）	在对耳轮上脚的下 1/3 处，即对耳轮 5 区	髋关节疼痛、坐骨神经痛、腰骶部疼痛
坐骨神经（AH₆）	在对耳轮下脚的前 2/3 处，即对耳轮 6 区	坐骨神经痛、下肢瘫痪
交感（AH₆ₐ）	在对耳轮下脚前端与耳轮内缘交界处，即对耳轮 6 区前端	自主神经功能疾病及胃肠、心、胆、输尿管等疾病
臀（AH₇）	在对耳轮下脚的后 1/3 处，即对耳轮 7 区	坐骨神经痛、臀部疼痛
腹（AH₈）	在对耳轮前部上 2/5 处，即对耳轮 8 区	消化系统、盆腔疾病
腰骶椎（AH₉）	在腹区后方，即对耳轮 9 区	相应部位疾病
胸（AH₁₀）	在对耳轮体前部中 2/5 处，即对耳轮 10 区	相应胸胁部位疾病
胸椎（AH₁₁）	在胸区后方，即对耳轮 11 区	相应部位疾病
颈（AH₁₂）	在对耳轮体前部下 1/5 处，即对耳轮 12 区	落枕等颈项部疾病
颈椎（AH₁₃）	在颈区后方，即对耳轮 13 区	颈椎病等相应部位疾病

6.3.4 三角窝部位

三角窝部总计分为5区，共有5穴。（图2-6-5，表2-6-4）

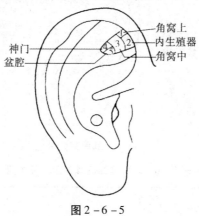

图2-6-5

表2-6-4 三角窝部位耳穴定位及主治

穴名	定位	主治
角窝上（IF$_1$）	在三角窝前1/3的上部，即三角窝1区	高血压
内生殖器（IF$_2$）	在三角窝前1/3的下部，即三角窝2区	妇科病、男性病
角窝中（IF$_3$）	在三角窝中1/3处，即三角窝3区	哮喘、咳嗽、肝病等
神门（IF$_4$）	在三角窝后1/3的上部，即三角窝4区	失眠、多梦、各种痛证、咳嗽、哮喘、眩晕、高血压、过敏性疾病、戒断综合征
盆腔（IF$_5$）	在三角窝前1/3的下部，即三角窝5区	盆腔炎、附件炎等盆腔内病证

6.3.5 耳屏部位

耳屏部总计分为4区，共有9穴。

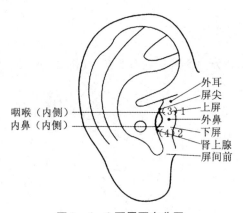

外耳
屏尖
上屏
外鼻
下屏
肾上腺
屏间前

咽喉（内侧）
内鼻（内侧）

图 2 - 6 - 6 耳屏耳穴分区

表 2 - 6 - 5 耳屏部位耳穴定位及主治

穴名	定位	主治
上屏（TG_1）	在耳屏外侧面上 1/2 处，即耳屏 1 区	咽炎，单纯性肥胖
下屏（TG_2）	在耳屏外侧面下 1/2 处，即耳屏 2 区	鼻炎，单纯性肥胖
外耳（TG_{1u}）	在屏上切迹前方近耳轮部，即耳屏 1 区上缘处	各类耳病，如耳鸣、眩晕等
屏尖（TG_{1p}）	在耳屏游离缘上部尖端，即耳屏 1 区后缘处	五官炎症、痛证
外鼻（$TG_{1,2i}$）	在耳屏外侧面中部，即耳屏 1、2 区之间	各类鼻病，如鼻渊等
肾上腺（TG_{2p}）	在耳屏游离缘下部尖端，即耳屏 2 区后缘处	低血压、昏厥、休克、炎症、哮喘、过敏性疾病、无脉症等
咽喉（TG_3）	在耳屏内侧面上 1/2 处，即耳屏（3）区	咽喉肿痛、声音嘶哑、咽炎等
内鼻（TG_4）	在耳屏内侧面下 1/2 处，即耳屏（4）区	各类鼻病，如鼻渊、鼻塞流涕等
屏间前（TG_{zi}）	在屏间切迹前方耳屏最下部，即耳屏 2 区下缘处	眼病

注：（3）和（4）这在 1、2 区的内侧面，从外面看不到。

6.3.6 对耳屏部位

对耳屏部总计分为4区共有8穴。

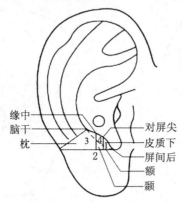

图2-6-7 对耳屏部位分区

表2-6-6 对耳屏部位耳穴及主治

穴名	定位	主治
额（AT_1）	在对耳屏外侧面的前部，即对耳屏1区	额窦炎、头痛、头晕、失眠、多梦
屏间后（AT_{11}）	在屏间切迹后方对耳屏前下部，即对耳屏1区下缘处	眼病
颞（AT_2）	在对耳屏外侧面的中部，即对耳屏2区	偏头痛
枕（AT_3）	在对耳屏外侧面的后部，即对耳屏3区	头痛、眩晕、哮喘、癫痫、神经衰弱
皮质下（AT_4）	在对耳屏内侧面，即对耳屏4区	痛证、间日疟、神经衰弱、假性近视、胃溃疡、腹泻、高血压、冠心病、心律失常、失眠
对屏尖（$AT_{1,2,4i}$）	在对耳屏游离缘的尖端，即对耳屏1、2、4区交点处	哮喘、腮腺炎、皮肤瘙痒、睾丸炎、附睾炎
缘中（$AT_{2,3,4i}$）	在对耳屏游离缘上，对屏尖与轮屏切迹之中点处，即对耳屏2、3、4区交点处	遗尿、内耳眩晕、功能性子宫出血
脑干（$AT_{3,4i}$）	在轮屏切迹处，即对耳屏3、4区之间	头痛、眩晕、假性近视

6.3.7 耳甲部位

耳甲部总计分为 18 区，共有 21 穴。（图 2-6-8，表 2-6-7）

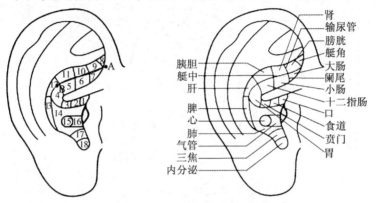

图 2-6-8 耳甲部位耳穴分区

表 2-6-7 耳甲部位耳穴定位及主治

穴名	定位	主治
口（CO_1）	在耳轮脚下方前 1/3 处，即耳甲 1 区	面瘫、口腔炎、胆囊炎同、胆结石、戒断综合征、牙周炎、舌炎
食道（CO_2）	在耳轮脚下方中 1/3 处，即耳甲 2 区	食道炎、食道痉挛
贲门（CO_3）	在耳轮脚下方后 1/3 处，即耳甲 3 区	贲门痉挛、神经性呕吐
胃（CO_4）	在耳轮脚消失处，即耳甲 4 区	胃炎、胃溃疡、失眠、牙痛、消化不良、恶心呕吐
十二指肠（CO_5）	在耳轮脚及部分与 AB 线之间的后 1/3 处，即耳甲 5 区	十二指肠球部溃疡、胆囊炎、胆结石、幽门痉挛、腹胀、腹泻、腹痛
小肠（CO_6）	在耳轮脚及耳轮部分与 AB 线之间的中 1/3 处，即耳甲 6 区	消化不良、腹痛、心动过速、心律不齐
大肠（CO_7）	在耳轮脚及部分耳轮与 AB 线之间的前 1/3 处，即耳甲 7 区	腹泻、便秘、痢疾、咳嗽、痤疮

（续表）

穴名	定位	主治
阑尾（$CO_{6,7i}$）	在小肠区与大肠区之间，即耳甲 6、7 区交界处	单纯性阑尾炎、腹泻、腹痛
艇角（CO_8）	在对耳轮脚下方前部，即耳甲8 区	前列腺炎、尿道炎
膀胱（CO_9）	在对耳轮下脚下方中部，即耳甲 9 区	膀胱炎、遗尿、尿潴留、腰痛、坐骨神经痛、后头痛
肾（CO_{10}）	在对耳轮下脚下方后部，即耳甲 10 区	腰痛、耳鸣、神经衰弱、水肿、哮喘、遗尿症、月经不调、遗精、阳痿、早泄、眼病、五更泻
输尿管（$CO_{9,10i}$）	在肾区与膀胱区之间，即耳甲 9、10 区交界处	输尿管结石绞痛
胰胆（CO_{11}）	在耳甲艇的后上部，即耳甲11 区	胆囊炎，胆结石、胆道蛔虫症、偏头痛、带状疱疹、中耳炎、耳鸣、听力减退、胰腺炎、口苦、胁痛
肝（CO_{12}）	在耳甲艇的后下部，即耳甲12 区	胁痛、眩晕、经前期紧张症、月经不调、更年期综合征、高血压、假性近视、单纯性青光眼、目赤肿痛
艇中（$CO_{6,10i}$）	在小肠区与肾区之间，即耳间 6、10 区交界处	腹痛、腹胀、腮腺炎
脾（CO_{13}）	耳腔的后上部，即耳甲 13 区	腹胀、腹泻、便秘、食欲不振、功能性子宫出血、白带过多、内耳眩晕、水肿、痿证、内脏下垂
心（CO_{15}）	在耳腔正中凹陷处，即耳甲15 区	心动过速、心律不齐、心绞痛、无脉证、自汗、盗汗、癔证、口舌生疮、心悸怔忡、失眠、健忘

（续表）

穴名	定位	主治
气管（CO_{16}）	在心区与外耳门之间，即耳甲16区	咳嗽、气喘、急慢性咽炎
肺（CO_{14}）	在心、气管区周围处，即耳甲14区	咳喘、胸闷、声音嘶哑、痤疮、皮肤瘙痒、荨麻疹、扁平疣、便秘、戒断综合征、自汗、盗汗、鼻炎
三焦（CO_{17}）	在外耳门后下，肺与内分泌区之间，即耳甲17区	便秘、腹胀、水肿、耳鸣、耳聋、糖尿病
内分泌（CO_{18}）	在屏间切迹内，耳甲腔的底部，即耳甲18区	痛经、月经不调、更年期综合征、痤疮、间日疟、糖尿病

6.3.8 耳垂部位

耳垂部总计分为9区共有8穴。

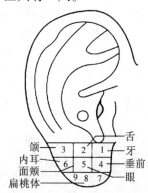

图 2-6-9 耳垂部位耳穴分区

表 2-6-8 耳垂部位耳穴定位及主治

穴名	定位	主治
牙（LO_1）	在耳垂正面前上部，即耳垂1区	牙痛、牙周炎、低血压
舌（LO_2）	在耳垂正面中上部，即耳垂2区	舌炎、口腔炎

（续表）

穴名	定位	主治
颌（LO_3）	在耳垂正面后上部，即耳垂3区	牙齿痛、颞颌关节功能紊乱症
垂前（LO_4）	在耳垂正面前中部，即耳垂4区	神经衰弱、牙痛
眼（LO_5）	在耳垂正面中央部，即耳垂5区	假性近视、目赤肿痛、迎风流泪
内耳（LO_6）	在耳垂正面后中部，即耳垂6区	内耳眩晕、耳鸣、听力减退
面颊（LO_{5,6i}）	在耳垂正面，眼区与内耳区之间，即耳垂5、6区交界处	周围性面瘫、三叉神经痛、痤疮、扁平疣
扁桃体（LO_{7,8,9}）	在耳垂正面下部，即垂7、8、9区	扁桃体炎、咽炎

6.3.9 耳根及耳背部位

耳背及耳根部总计分为5区共有9穴。（图2-6-10，表2-6-9）

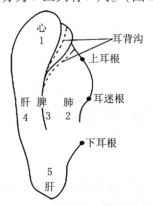

图2-6-10 耳背及耳根部位耳穴分区

表2-6-9 耳背及耳根部位耳穴定位及主治

穴名	定位	主治
耳背心（P_1）	在耳背上部，即耳背1区	心悸、失眠、多梦
耳背肺（P_2）	在耳背中内部，即耳背2区	咳喘、皮肤瘙痒

穴名	定位	主治
耳背脾（P₃）	在耳背中央部，即耳背3区	胃痛、消化不良、食欲不振、腹胀、腹泻
耳背肝（P₄）	在耳背中外部，即耳背4区	胆囊炎、胆结石、胁痛
耳背肾（P₅）	在耳背下部，即耳背5区	头痛、眩晕、神经衰弱
耳背沟（P₆）	在对耳轮沟和对耳轮上、下脚沟处	高血压、皮肤瘙痒
上耳根（R₁）	在耳郭与头部相连的最上处	鼻衄、哮喘
耳迷根（R₂）	在耳轮脚沟的耳根处	胆囊炎、胆结石、胆道蛔虫症、鼻炎、心动过速、腹痛、腹泻
下耳根（R₃）	在耳郭与头部相连的最下处	低血压、下肢瘫痪

6.4 耳穴的临床应用

6.4.1 辅助诊断

人体疾病的发生，往往会在耳郭的相应部位出现不同的病理反应（阳性反应），如皮肤色泽、形态改变（变形、变色、脱屑、丘疹），局部痛阈降低，耳穴电阻下降等。以上改变可以借助下列检查法加以判定，结合临床症状、体征，从而起到辅助诊断的作用。

6.4.2 疾病治疗

（1）各种疼痛性病证：如偏头痛、三叉神经痛、肋间神经痛等神经性疼痛；扭伤、挫伤、落枕等外伤性疼痛；各种外科手术所产生的伤口痛；胆绞痛、肾绞痛、心绞痛、胃痛等内脏痛证。

（2）各种炎性病证：如急性结膜炎、牙周炎、咽喉炎、扁桃体炎、胆囊炎、腮腺炎、支气管炎、风湿性关节炎、面神经炎等。

（3）功能紊乱性病证：如心脏神经官能症、心律不齐、高血压、多汗证、眩晕、胃肠神经官能症、月经不调、遗尿、神经衰弱、癔证等。

（4）过敏与变态反应性疾病：如过敏性鼻炎、支气管哮喘、过敏性结肠炎、荨麻疹、过敏性紫癜等。

（5）内分泌代谢性疾病：如单纯性肥胖、糖尿病、甲状腺功能亢进或低下、绝经期综合征等。

（6）其他：如用于手术麻醉，预防感冒、晕车、晕船，戒烟、戒毒，美容、延缓衰老、防病保健等。

6.5 耳穴的操作

6.5.1 耳穴的选穴原则

（1）辨证取穴：根据中医的脏腑、经络学说辨证选用相关耳穴。如皮肤病，按"肺主皮毛"的理论，选用肺穴；目赤肿痛，按"肝开窍于目"的理论，选用肝穴；骨折的病人，按照"肾主骨"的理论选取肾穴。

（2）对证取穴：即可根据中医理论对证取穴，如耳中与膈肌相应，可以治疗呃逆，又可凉血清热，用于治疗血证和皮肤病；也可根据西医学的生理病理知识对证选用有关耳穴，如月经不调选内分泌；神经衰弱选皮质下等。

（3）对应取穴：直接选取发病脏腑器官对应的耳穴。如眼病选眼穴及屏间前、屏间后穴；胃病取胃穴；妇女经带疾病取内分泌穴。

6.5.2 耳穴的刺激方法

（1）毫针法

针具选择：选用 28～30 号粗细的 0.5～1 寸长的毫针。

操作方法：进针时，押手固定耳郭，刺手持针速刺进针；针刺方向视耳穴所在部位灵活掌握，针刺深度宜 0.1～0.3cm，以不穿透对侧皮肤为度；多用捻转、刮法或震颤法行针，刺激强度视患者病情、体质和敏感性等因素综合决定；得气以热、胀、痛，或局部充血红润多见；一般留针 15~30 分钟，可间歇行针 1~2 次。疼痛性或慢性疾病留针时间可适当延长；出针时，押手托住耳背，刺手持针速出，同时用消毒干棉球压迫针孔片刻。

（2）电针法

针具选择：选用 28~30 号粗细的 0.5~1 寸长的毫针；G6805 型电针仪。

操作方法：押手固定耳郭，刺手持针速刺进针；得气后连接电针仪，多选用疏密波、适宜强度，刺激 15~20 分钟；起针时，先取下导线，押手固定耳郭，刺手持针速出，并用消毒干棉球压迫针孔片刻。

（3）埋针法

针具选择：揿针型皮内针为宜。

操作方法：押手固定耳郭并绷紧欲埋针处皮肤，刺手用镊子夹住皮内针柄，速刺（压）入所选穴位皮内，再用胶布固定并适度按压，可留置 1~3 天，期间可嘱患者每日自行按压 2~3 次；起针时轻轻撕下胶布即可将针一并取出，并再次消毒。两耳穴交替埋针，必要时双耳穴同用。

（4）压子法

压子选择：压子又称压豆或埋豆，以王不留行、磁珠、磁片等为主，或油菜子、小绿豆、莱菔子等表面光滑、硬度适宜、直径为 2mm 左右的球状物为宜，使用前用沸水烫洗后晒干备用。

操作方法：将所选"压豆"贴于 0.5cm×0.5cm 的透气胶布中间，医师用镊子将其夹持，敷贴于所选耳穴并适当按揉，以耳穴发热、胀痛为宜；可留置 2~4 天，期间可嘱患者每日自行按压 2~3 次。

（5）穴位注射法

针具选择：1ml 注射器和 26 号注射针头。

操作方法：在所选耳穴处常规消毒后，押手固定耳郭，刺手持注射器将按照病情所选用的药物缓慢推入耳穴皮内或皮下 0.1~0.3ml，耳郭可有红、热、胀、痛等反应；注射完毕用消毒干棉球压迫局部片刻，一般注射 2~3 穴，3~5 次为 1 个疗程。

6.5.3 耳针法的注意事项

（1）严格消毒，防止感染。因耳郭在外，表面凹凸不平，结构特殊，针刺前必须严格消毒，有创面和炎症部位禁针，针刺后如针孔发红、肿胀应及时涂 2.5% 碘酒，防止化脓性软骨膜炎的发生。

（2）对扭伤和有运动障碍者，进针后宜适当活动，有利于提高疗效。

（3）习惯性流产的孕妇应禁针。

（4）患有严重器质性病变和伴有高度贫血者，不宜针刺，对严重心脏病、高血压患者不宜行强刺激。

（5）耳针治疗时应注意防止发生晕针，如发生应及时处理。

7. 头针

头针法又称头皮针法，是指在头部特定部位针刺的治疗方法。大量实验结果表明，针刺头部穴区对皮层功能有调节作用，可改善脑血流图，有收缩血管、改善血管弹性等作用。大脑皮层的功能在相应的头皮部位存在一定的折射关系，主要表现为采用针刺等方法刺激相应的头皮部位，可影响相应的大脑皮层功能。

7.1 头针法刺激部位

标准化头针线共 14 条，分别位于额区、顶区、颞区、枕区 4 个区域的头皮部。（图 2 - 7 - 1）

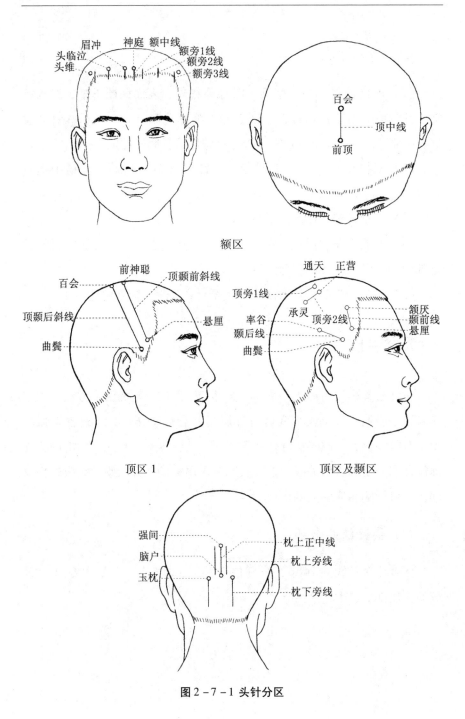

额区

顶区 1

顶区及颞区

图 2 - 7 - 1 头针分区

7.2 头针的主治

中枢神经系统疾患：脑血管疾病所致的偏瘫、失语、假性延髓性麻痹，小儿神经发育不全和脑性瘫痪，颅脑外伤后遗症，脑炎后遗症，以及癫痫、舞蹈病和震颤麻痹等。疼痛和感觉异常：头痛、三叉神经痛、颈项痛、肩痛、腰背痛、坐骨神经痛、胆绞痛、胃痛、痛经等各种急慢性疼痛病证，以及肢体远端麻木、皮肤瘙痒等病证。皮层内脏功能失调所致疾患：高血压、冠心病、溃疡、性功能障碍和月经不调，以及神经性呕吐、神经性腹泻等。

7.3 头针的操作方法

应根据病情和操作部位选择不同型号的毫针。局部选用75%乙醇消毒棉球或棉签在施术部位由中心向外环行擦拭。医师双手用肥皂水清洗干净，再用75%乙醇消毒棉球擦拭。

7.3.1 进针方法

一般宜在针体与皮肤成15°~30°角进针，然后平刺进入穴线内。采用快速进针，将针迅速刺入皮下，当针尖达到帽状腱膜下层时，指下感到阻力减小，然后使针与头皮平行，根据不同穴线刺入不同深度。进针深度宜根据患者具体情况和处方要求决定。一般情况下，针刺入帽状腱膜下层后，使针体平卧，进针0.5~1.5寸为宜。

7.3.2 行针方法

在针体进入帽状腱膜下层后，医师肩、肘、腕关节和拇指固定不动，以保持毫针相对固定。示指第1、2节呈半屈曲状，用示指第1节的桡侧面与拇指第1节的掌侧面持住针柄，然后示指掌指关节做伸屈运动，使针体快速旋转，要求捻转频率在200次/分左右，持续行针2~3分钟。

7.3.3 出针方法

先缓慢出针至皮下，然后迅速拔出，拔针后必须用消毒干棉球按压针孔，以防出血。

7.3.4 一般疗程

每日1次或隔日1次，10次为1个疗程。两个疗程之间间隔5~7天。

7.4 头针注意事项

囟门和骨缝尚未骨化的婴儿、颅骨缺损或开放性脑损患者、孕妇不宜用头皮针治疗。头颅手术部位，头皮严重感染、溃疡和创伤处不宜使用，可在其对侧取相应头皮针治疗线进行。头皮针刺入时要迅速，注意避开发囊、瘢痕。针刺深浅及方向，应根据治疗要求，并结合患者年龄、体质及敏感性决定。留针时不要随意碰撞针柄，以免发生弯针和疼痛。严重心脏病、重度糖尿病、重度贫血、急性炎症和脑血管意外急性期患者或血压、病情不稳定者不宜使用。对精神紧张、过饱、过饥者应慎用。

知识点 6　针灸治疗学知识点概要

针灸治疗疾病是以中医基础理论为指导，依照患者的具体情况进行辨证论治，以明确疾病的病因病机、病位、病性及病情的标本缓急，运用针灸的方法进行治疗。而针灸处方则是在此基础上，选择适当的腧穴、刺灸及补泻方法组合而成，是针灸治病的重要步骤。依方施术，通其经脉，调其气血，阴平阳秘，从而达到防病治病的目的。

1. 针灸治疗作用

古代医家在长期的临床医疗实践中，总结出针灸具有调和阴阳、疏通经络、扶正祛邪的治疗作用。现代临床及实验研究不仅从多学科、多角度证实了针灸的治疗作用，也使人们对针灸治疗作用机制的认识得到深入。

1.1 疏通经络

疏通经络是指运用针灸等方法，通过腧穴和针灸手法的作用，使瘀阻的经络疏通、气血畅达，从而发挥其正常生理功能，是针灸最基本和最直接的治疗作用。

针灸疏通经络主要是根据经络循行、选择相应的腧穴和针灸手法的作用，使经络通畅，促使气血的正常运行，达到治疗疾病的目的。如经络闭阻不通，"不通则痛"而出现的痛证，针灸正是利用其疏通经络的作用，通过刺激经络、腧穴，使经络通畅、气血调和，达到"通则不痛"的治疗效果。

1.2 调和阴阳

调和阴阳是指运用针灸等方法，通过经络、腧穴和针灸手法的作用，使机体从阴阳的失衡状态向平衡状态转化，是针灸治病最终要达到的根本目的。

针灸调和阴阳的作用主要是通过经络、腧穴配伍和针刺手法来实现的。如中风后出现足内翻，经络辨证为阳（经）缓而阴（经）急，治疗时可采用补阳经、泻阴经的刺法。胃火炽盛牙痛，属阳热偏盛，治宜清泻胃火，取足阳明胃经荥穴内庭，针用泻法以泻胃火；肾阴虚牙痛，属肾阴不足，治宜滋补肾阴，取足少阴肾经原穴太溪，针用补法以补肾阴。

1.3 扶正祛邪

扶正是指扶助正气，提高机体的抗病能力；祛邪是指祛除病邪，消除致病因素的影响。扶正与祛邪是针灸治病的根本法则和手段。

针刺要起到扶正祛邪的作用，除了采用相应的补泻手法之外，还与机体所处的功能状态、选用腧穴的相对特异性等因素有关。不少腧穴能鼓舞人体正气，促使功能旺盛，具有扶正补虚作用，如关元、气海、命门、膏肓等；一些腧穴能疏泻病邪，具有祛邪泻实作用，如人中、委中、十二井穴、十宣等。但绝大部分腧穴则具有良性的双向调节作用，如中脘、内关、三阴交、合谷、太冲、足三里等，既可用于扶正，又可用于祛邪。

2. 针灸治疗原则

针灸治疗原则是针灸治疗疾病必须遵循的准绳，整个治疗过程中，均应以治疗原则为指导。根据中医治疗疾病的基本思想，结合针灸治疗疾病的具体实践，常将针灸治疗原则归纳为补虚与泻实、清热与温阳、局部与整体、治标与治本、同病异治与异同治、三因制宜等几个方面。

2.1 补虚泻实

"虚"是指人体的正气虚弱；"实"是指邪气偏盛。补虚就是扶助人体的正气，增强脏腑器官的功能，补益人体的阴阳气血以抗御疾病。泻实就是祛除邪气，以利于正气的恢复。针灸的"补虚"与"泻实"，是通过针和灸的方法激发机体本身的调节机能，从而产生补泻的作用，达到扶正祛邪的目的。

所谓"虚则补之"，就是虚证采用补法治疗。"虚则实之"意同"虚则补之"。针刺治疗虚证用补法，主要是通过针刺手法的补法以及穴位的选择和配伍等实现的。如在有关脏腑经脉的背俞穴、原穴施行补法，可改善脏腑功能，补益阴阳、气血等的不足；此外，应用偏补性能的腧穴如关元、气海、命门、肾俞等穴，也可起到补益正气的作用。

所谓"陷下则灸之"，属于"虚则补之"范畴，也就是说气虚下陷的治疗原则是以灸治为主。针灸临床对于因脏腑经络之气虚弱，中气不足，对气血和内脏失其升提固摄能力而出现的一系列病证，如久泻、久痢、遗尿、脱肛等，常灸百会、神阙、气海、关元等穴补中益气、升阳举陷。

所谓"实则泻之"，就是实证采用泻法治疗。"盛则泻之""满则泻之""邪盛则虚之"都是泻损邪气的意思，可统称为"实则泻之"。针刺治疗实证用泻法，主要是通过针刺手法的泻法以及穴位的选择和配伍等实现的。如在穴位上施行捻转、提插、开阖等毫针泻法，或用三棱针放血，或用梅花针重叩出血，可以起到祛除人体病邪的作用；此外，应用偏泻性能的腧穴如十宣、水沟、素髎、丰隆、血海等，也可达到祛邪的目的。

所谓"宛陈则除之"，是实证用泻法的一种。"宛"同"瘀"，有瘀结、瘀滞之义。"陈"即"陈旧"，引申为时间长久。"宛陈"泛指体表络脉瘀阻之类的病证。"除"即"清除"，指清除瘀血的刺血疗法。《素问·针解》篇说："宛陈则除之，是出恶血也。"由体表络脉瘀阻而引起的病证，应以三棱针点刺出血为治法，属于实者泻之的范畴。如外伤扭挫，或气滞血瘀形成的肿痛，或邪入营血，郁结不解和久病入络、青紫肿胀，可选用局部络脉或瘀血部位施行三棱针点刺出血术，以活血化瘀，消肿止痛。如病情较重者，可从患处局部以三棱针点刺后加拔火罐

（血罐），这样可以排出更多的恶血，促进病愈。又如腱鞘囊肿、小儿疳积的点刺放液也属此类。

所谓"不盛不虚以经取之"是指本经自病采用本经循经取穴治疗。"不盛不虚"，并非病证本身无虚实可言，而是脏腑经络的虚实表现不明显或虚实兼而有之。主要是由于脏腑经络本身一时性的气血紊乱，而不涉及其他脏腑、经脉，属于本经自病。《灵枢·禁服》："不盛不虚，以经取之，名曰经刺。"《难经·六十九难》："不盛不虚以经取之者，是正经自病也。"治疗应按本经循经取穴，以原穴和五输穴最为适宜。针下得气后，多采用平补平泻的针刺手法，使本经的气血调和，脏腑功能恢复正常。此原则最能体现针灸的调整作用，故在临床应用甚为广泛。

2.2 清热温寒

清热是指热证用"清"法，温寒是指寒证用"温"法。这与治寒以热、治热以寒的意义是一致的。《灵枢·经脉》："热则疾之，寒则留之。"这是针对热性病证和寒性病证制定的治疗原则。

"热则疾之"，"热"指邪热亢盛，或为外感风寒，风热引起的表热证；或为五脏六腑有热的里热证；或为气血壅盛于经络局部的局部热证。"疾"是快速的意思。这里是指治疗方法，即疾刺快出针。在针灸临床中，如表热证，常取大椎、曲池、合谷等穴，浅刺疾出，以宣散热邪；五脏热者，选相应背俞穴而刺之，以泻其热；热在经络、皮部者，可毫针散刺，或三棱针点刺，或皮肤针叩刺局部出血，以疏散其热。此外，热证还可用"透天凉"针法。

"寒则留之"，"寒"指疾病的性质属寒，或为外感寒邪引起的表寒证；或为寒湿痹阻经脉的寒痹证；或为阳气不足引起的脏寒证。在针灸临床中，寒性病证的治疗原则是针灸并用，深刺而久留针，以达温经散寒的目的。因寒性凝滞而主收引，针刺时不易得气，故应留针候气；加艾灸更能助阳散寒，使阳气得复，寒邪乃散。如寒邪在表，留于经络者，艾灸施治最为适宜；若寒邪在里，凝滞脏腑，则针刺应深而久留，或配合"烧山火"针法，或加用艾灸、温针灸法最为适宜。

2.3 治病求本

治病求本是指治疗疾病时要抓住疾病的本质，针对疾病的本质进行治疗。"标"和"本"是相对的概念。在中医学中有丰富的内涵，可以说明病变过程中各种矛盾的主次关系。如从正邪关系上看，正气是本，邪气是标；从疾病的发生上看，病因是本，症状是标；从病变的部位上看，内脏是本，体表是标；从发病的先后上看，先病是本，后病是标。治病求本是一个基本法则。临床上常会遇到疾病的标本缓急等特殊情况，这时要灵活掌握，处理好治标和治本的关系。若标病急于本病，如不及时处理，可能危及生命或影响本病的治疗，应"急则治标"。"缓则治本"是指在标病不急时，针对病证本质进行治疗的一种治疗原则。这个原则对于指导慢性病和急性病的恢复期的治疗更有意义。"标本同治"是指在标病和本病并重情况下，应当采取标本同治的方法。

2.4 三因制宜

"三因制宜"是指因时、因地、因人制宜，即根据患者所处的季节（包括时辰）、地理环境和治疗对象的不同情况而采取适宜的治疗方法。

2.4.1 因人制宜

因人制宜是指在疾病治疗过程中，应考虑到人的年龄、性别、体质不同的特点，因人而异，区别对待，制定适宜的治疗原则。

2.4.2 因地制宜

因地制宜是指在疾病治疗过程中，应考虑到不同地域、不同生活环境、不同生活习惯与方式的背景特点，根据这些差异制定适宜的治疗原则。

2.4.3 因时制宜

因时制宜是指在疾病的治疗过程中，根据不同时间、不同季节气候的特点，制定适宜的治法，选方用药，选经用穴。

3. 选穴和配穴

3.1 选穴原则

选穴原则就是临证选穴应该遵循的基本法则，包括近部选穴、远部选穴、辨证选穴和对证选穴。近部选穴和远部选穴是主要针对病变部位而确定腧穴的选穴原则；辨证、对证选穴是针对疾病表现出的证候或症状而选取穴位的原则。

3.1.1 近部选穴

近部选穴是指选取病变局部或邻近部位的腧穴的选穴方法，是腧穴普遍具有近治作用的体现，常用于治疗部位较局限或体表反应较为明显的病证。如肩痛取肩髃，眼病取睛明，耳病取耳门、听宫，胃痛取中脘、梁门等。

3.1.2 远部选穴

远部选穴是指在病变部位所属和相关的经络上，距病位较远的部位选取腧穴的方法，是腧穴普遍具有远治作用的体现，是"经络所过，主治所及"治疗规律的体现。

3.1.3 辨证选穴

辨证选穴是指针对某些全身症状或疾病的病因病机而辨证选取腧穴的方法，是中医理论和腧穴主治功能的体现。

3.1.4 对证选穴

对证选穴，亦称随证选穴，是指针对疾病的特殊症状而选取腧穴的原则。临床常选用一些具有特殊功效或在临床中有较好疗效的腧穴来治疗，亦称经验取穴，是腧穴特殊治疗作用及临床经验在针灸处方中的具体运用。如昏厥选人中、十宣、十二井穴，高热选大椎、曲池，不寐选内关、神门，哮喘选定喘，虫积选百虫窝等。此外，阿是穴的选取在临床上治疗仆击、扭伤、痹证等可收到较好的疗效。

3.2 配穴方法

配穴方法是指在腧穴主治特性和选穴原则基础上，根据不同病证选择具有协同作用的两个或两个以上的腧穴进行配伍应用的方法，是针灸处方中的重要内容。临床上具体配穴方法多种多样，总体上可归纳为两大类，按经配穴法和按部配穴法。

3.2.1 按经配穴法

按经配穴法是指按照经络理论和经络之间的联系配穴的方法，主要包括本经配穴法、表里经配穴法、同名经配穴法、子母经配穴法。

（1）本经配穴法

本经配穴法是指某一脏腑、经脉发生病变时，即选用该脏腑、经脉的腧穴配成处方的方法。如少阳头痛可取胆经率谷、风池、侠溪；胃火牙痛可取胃经颊车、内庭；肺病咳嗽可取中府、尺泽、太渊等。

（2）表里经配穴法

表里经配穴法是以脏腑、经脉的阴阳表里配合关系为依据的配穴方法。当某一脏腑经脉发生疾病时，取本经和其相表里的经脉腧穴配合成方。如风热袭肺导致的感冒咳嗽，可取肺经的尺泽穴和大肠经的曲池、合谷；胃脘痛可取胃经梁门、足三里和脾经公孙；心绞痛可取心包经内关和三焦经外关。特定穴应用中的原络配穴法也是本法在临床上的具体运用。

（3）同名经配穴法

同名经配穴法 是将手足同名经的腧穴相互配合的方法，是基于同名经"同气相通"的理论。如牙痛、面瘫、阳明头痛取手阳明经的合谷配足阳明经的内庭；落枕、急性腰扭伤、太阳头痛取手太阳经的后溪配足太阳经的昆仑等。

3.2.2 按部配穴法

按部配穴法是结合人体腧穴分布的部位进行腧穴配伍的方法，主要包括远近配穴法、上下配穴法、前后配穴法、左右配穴法。

（1）上下配穴法

上下配穴法是指将腰部以上腧穴和腰部以下腧穴配合应用的方法，在临床上应用较为广泛。《灵枢·终始》篇："病在上者下取之，病在下者高取之，病在头者取之足，病在腰者取之腘。"如头项强痛，上取大椎，下配昆仑；胃脘痛取内关、足三里；胸腹满闷取内关、公孙；子宫脱垂取百会、气海等。

（2）前后配穴法

前后配穴法 是指将人体前部和后部的腧穴配合应用的方法，主要指将胸腹部和背腰部的腧穴配合应用，又称"腹背阴阳配穴法"，在《内经》中称之为"偶刺"。此法多用于治疗脏腑病证，在临床上应用广泛。如咳嗽、气喘，取天突、膻中、肺俞、定喘；胃脘疼痛，取中脘、梁门、胃俞、脊中等。

（3）左右配穴法

左右配穴法是指将人体左侧和右侧的腧穴配合应用的方法。本法是根据人体十二经脉左右对称分布和部分经脉左右交叉的特点总结而成的配穴组方的方法。此法源于《内经》中的"缪刺"和"巨刺"，左病可以右取，右病可以左取，还可以左右同时并取。如左侧偏头痛，可选同侧的太阳、头维和对侧的外关、足临泣；左侧面瘫可选用同侧的太阳、颊车、地仓和对侧的合谷；如胃痛可选用双侧足三里、胃俞等。

4. 特定穴应用

特定穴是指十四经穴中具有某种特殊治疗作用和特定名称的一类腧穴的总称，包括五输穴、原穴、络穴、背俞穴、募穴、八会穴、八脉交会穴、郄穴、下合穴、交会穴等。因分布、特性和作用的不同，临床应用范围较广，在选穴配伍上也有一定的特点。

4.1 五输穴

五输穴是指十二经穴分布于肘、膝关节以下的井、荥、输、经、合五类腧穴的总称。十二经脉中每条经有 5 个穴位属于五输穴，故人体共有五输穴 60 个。在临床上的应用非常广泛，是远部选穴的主要穴位。

临床上井穴多用于治疗五脏六腑的急症、重症，以及精神异常诸证。有泻热、开窍、醒神等作用；荥穴用于治疗脏腑、经脉的热证。有泻热止痛作用；输穴用于治疗发作性疾病及关节病变。有疏通经气、通络止痛作用；经穴用于治疗喘咳寒热、失音等内脏病。有调整脏腑功能作用；合穴用于治疗脏腑功能紊乱病证、经脉盛满有瘀血者。有调整脏腑功能、疏通经络作用。

此外五输穴具有五行属性，根据其五行生克制化的原理，可采用《难经·六十九难》提出的"虚者补其母，实者泻其子"的原则进行施治。其中可依五输穴之五行属性进行补泻，也可依经脉之五行属性选穴针治。具体运用时可分本经子母补泻法和异经子母补泻法。如肝经属木，肝经实证可泻行间，行间为肝经荥（火）穴，即实则泻其子，而肝经虚证可补曲泉，曲泉为肝经合（水）穴，即虚则补其母，这是本经子母补泻法。又如肝经实证，还可泻心经荥穴少府（子经本穴），肝虚证，补肾经合穴阴谷（母经本穴），这是异经子母补泻法。其他各经，依次类推。

人体气血在经络中的运行，随时间条件的不同，有着相应的周期性盛衰变化的规律。《难经·七十四难》云："春刺井，夏刺荥，季夏刺输，秋刺经，冬刺合。"春夏之季，阳气在上，人体之气行于浅表，故应浅刺井、荥；秋冬之季，阳气在下，人体之气潜伏于里，故宜深刺输、经、合。此外，古代医家总结出以五输穴配合阴阳五行为基础，运用天干地支配合脏腑，按时取穴的方法，即子午流注针法。子午流注针法是根据一日之中十二经脉气血盛衰开阖的时间，择时与五输穴相配的一种针法。它作为一种特殊的择时选穴治疗疾病的方法，具有深厚的中医理论基础和重要的临床应用价值。

4.2 原穴和络穴

原穴是脏腑的原气输注、经过和留止的部位。原穴与三焦有密切关系，三焦为原气之别使，三焦之气源于肾间动气，输布全身，调和内外，宣导上下，关系着脏腑气化功能，而原穴就是其所留止之处。因此，原穴主要用于治疗相关脏腑的疾病，也可协助诊断。

络穴是络脉由经脉别出部位的腧穴，也是表里两经联络之处。络穴除可治疗其络脉的病证，又能"一络通二经"，对表里两经有加强联络的作用，故还可治疗表里两经的病证。

原穴和络穴既可单独应用，也可相互配合应用。临床上常把先病经脉的原穴和后病的相表里的经脉络穴相配合，称为原络配穴法或主客原络配穴法，属表里经配穴法的范畴。它以原发疾病经脉的原穴为主，以相表里经脉的络穴为客。一主一客相互配合，疏通内外，贯穿上下，对相表里脏腑、经脉的病证均有较好的疗效。如肺经先病，先取其经的原穴太渊，大肠后病，再取该经络穴偏历。反之，大肠先病，先取本经原穴合谷，肺经后病，后取该经络穴列缺。

4.3 背俞穴和募穴

背俞穴位于背腰部的膀胱经第1侧线上，是脏腑之气输注于背腰部的腧穴，又称"背俞穴"；募穴均位于胸腹部，是脏腑之气汇聚于胸腹部的腧穴，故又称为"腹募穴"。每一脏腑均有各自的背俞穴和募穴。

背俞穴和募穴都是脏腑之气输注和汇聚之处，在分布上大体按所对应脏腑所在部位的高低而上下排列，临床上主要用于治疗相关脏腑的病变，腑病多选其募穴，脏病多选其俞穴。如肺经虚热咳嗽，可取肺之背俞穴肺俞；寒邪犯胃出现的胃痛，可取胃之募穴中脘。另外，背俞穴和募穴还可用于治疗与对应脏腑经脉相联络的组织器官疾患，如肝开窍于目，主筋，目疾、筋病可选肝俞；肾开窍于耳，耳疾可选肾俞。由于俞、募穴均与脏腑之气密切联系，因此，临床上俞募穴可以单独应用，也可相互配合应用，以发挥其协同作用，此为俞募配穴法，该法属前后配穴法范畴。如胃痛，取胃俞、中脘；咳喘，取肺俞、中府等。

脏腑发生病变时，常在俞、募穴上出现阳性反应物，如压痛、结节、条索状物、敏感点等，因此诊察按压俞、募穴，可结合其他症状判断脏腑疾患。俞募二穴可相互诊察疾病，即审募而察俞，察俞而诊募。

4.4 郄穴

郄穴是脏腑气血深聚的部位。十二经脉各有一个郄穴，加上阴维脉、阳维脉、阴跷脉、阳跷脉也各有一个郄穴，共计十六个郄穴。临床上，郄穴是治疗本经循行部位和相应脏腑病证的重要穴位，尤其在治疗急症方面有独特的疗效。阴经的郄穴多治急性血证，阳经的郄穴多治急性痛证。如急性胃脘痛，取胃经郄穴梁丘；肺病咯血，取肺经郄穴孔最等。脏腑疾患也可在相应的郄穴上出现疼痛或压痛，有助于诊断。郄穴除单独使用外，常与八会穴配合使用，故有"郄会配穴"之称。如孔最配血会膈俞治疗肺病咯血效果尤佳，梁丘配腑会中脘治疗急性胃脘痛疗效更显等。

4.5 八脉交会穴

八脉交会穴是十二正经与奇经八脉脉气相通的八个腧穴，具有主治本经和奇经病证的作用。八脉交会穴的主治范围比较广，不仅主治本经经脉循行所过的四肢躯干、头面五官病变，也主治奇经八脉的有关病证。在临床上，当奇经八脉出现相关病变时，可以用相对应的八脉交会穴来治疗。如腰脊强痛、角弓反张等督脉病证，可取通督脉的后溪；胸腹气逆而拘急的冲脉病证，可取通冲脉的公孙。此外，按一定的原则两穴配伍，可以治疗两脉相合部位的病证。即把公孙和内关、后溪和申脉、足临泣和外关、列缺和照海相配，治疗有关部位的病证，此属于上下配穴法的范畴。

4.6 八会穴

八会穴是指人体气、血、脏、腑、筋、脉、骨、髓等精气聚会处的八个腧穴，即脏会章门，腑会中脘，气会膻中，血会膈俞，筋会阳陵泉，脉会太渊，骨会大杼，髓会绝骨。这八个穴位虽属于不同经脉，但对于各自所会的脏、腑、气、血、筋、脉、骨、髓相关病证有特殊的治疗作用，临床上常把其作为治疗这些病证的主要穴位。如五脏之病，可取章门；六腑之病，可取中脘；血证可取膈俞；气病可取膻中等。

4.7 下合穴

下合穴是指六腑之气下合于下肢三阳经的六个腧穴，又称"六腑下合穴"。它们主要用于治疗六腑病证。《灵枢·邪气脏腑病形》指出："合治内腑"，概括了下合穴的主治功能。六腑胃、大肠、小肠、胆、膀胱、三焦的下合穴依次分别为足三里、上巨虚、下巨虚、阳陵泉、委中、委阳。临床上六腑病证均可选用各自相应的下合穴进行治疗。如胃脘痛取足三里；胁痛、呕吐、黄疸可取阳陵泉；肠痈可取上巨虚；泻痢可取下巨虚。另外，下合穴也可协助诊断。

4.8 交会穴

交会穴是指两经或两经以上经脉交叉、会合部位的腧穴。历代文献对交会穴的记载略有不同，但绝大部分内容出自《针灸甲乙经》。交会穴有治疗本经和所交会经病证的作用，根据"经脉所通，主治所及"的原理，临床上常选用交会穴治疗多经病证。如三阴交本属足太阴脾经腧穴，它又是足三阴经的交会穴，因此，它不仅治疗脾经病证，也可治疗足少阴肾经和足厥阴肝经的病证。

5. 针灸治疗常见病证

5.1 中风后遗症

中风后遗症是指急性脑血管病后遗的肢体瘫痪、口角歪斜、语言不利等证，属于中医的"中风""偏枯"等范畴。本病是由于脏腑功能尚未复常，痰浊、瘀血阻滞经络，经气运行失常所致。

5.1.1 辨证

多为一侧肢体瘫痪，伴有麻木或疼痛，口角歪斜，舌强语謇，吞咽困难。

5.1.2 治疗

主穴：内关（双）、人中、三阴交、极泉、委中、尺泽。

配穴：吞咽困难加风池、翳风、完骨；手指拘挛加合谷；语言謇涩加上廉泉、金津、玉液；足内翻加丘墟、照海。

操作方法：先刺内关穴直刺 0.5～1 寸，采用提插捻转结合泻法；再刺人中穴，向鼻中隔方向斜刺 0.3～0.5 寸，采用重雀啄手法，以流泪或眼球湿润为度；刺三阴交时、沿胫骨内侧面与皮肤呈 45°，用提插补法，下肢抽动三次为度；刺下极泉，直刺 1～1.5 寸，施用提插泻法，以上肢抽动 3 次为度；直刺尺泽 1 寸，用提插泻法，针感从肘关节传到手指或手动外旋，以手外旋抽动 3 次为度；针刺委中穴，仰卧位抬起患侧下肢取穴，术者用左手握住患肢踝关节，以术者肘部顶住患肢膝关节，刺入穴位后，针尖向外 15°，进针 1～1.5 寸，用提插泻法，以下肢抽动 3 次为度。针刺风池、完骨、翳风，三穴均向喉结方向斜刺，进针 2～2.5 寸。施用小幅度，高频率捻转补法，即捻转幅度小于90°，捻转频率为 120～160 转/分钟，行手法 1 分钟。要求双手操作同时捻转，留针 15 分钟；针刺合谷穴，针尖向三间穴方向，透刺 1～1.5 寸，施用提插泻法，以握固的手指自然伸展为度；针刺上廉泉，向舌根部斜刺 2 寸，施用提插泻法，以舌根部麻胀感为度；金津、玉液用三棱针点刺出血 1～3ml 为度；丘墟穴进针向照海部位透刺，透刺应缓慢前进，从踝关节的诸骨缝隙间逐渐透过，进针为 2～2.5 寸，以局部出现胀痛感为度。

5.2 失眠

失眠是指经常不能获得正常睡眠为特征的病证。临床表现为入睡困难，或易醒，或醒后难以入睡，或睡眠不深，严重时彻夜不眠。失眠多由劳倦思虑过度、情志失常、饮食不节、久病体虚等原因，使心、肝、脾、肾功能失调，阴血不足，影响心神而致病。现代医学的神经衰弱、更年期综合征等疾病，出现不寐的临床表现时，可参考本节进行辨证论治。

5.2.1 辨证

（1）肝郁化火

急躁易怒，心烦不寐，多梦，甚至彻夜不眠，伴有头晕头胀，目赤耳鸣，口干而苦，胸闷胁痛，不思饮食，便秘溲赤，舌红苔黄，脉弦数。

（2）心肾不交

心悸不安，心烦不寐，伴头晕耳鸣，腰酸足软，健忘遗精，五心烦热，潮热盗汗，口干津少，舌红少苔，脉细数。

（3）心脾两虚

不易入睡，多梦易醒，心悸健忘，神疲食少，伴头晕目眩，四肢倦怠，腹胀便溏，面色少华，舌淡苔薄，脉细无力。

5.2.2 治疗

（1）体针疗法

主穴：神门、三阴交、百会、四神聪、申脉、照海。

配穴：肝郁化火证：加行间、侠溪；心肾不交证：加心俞、大陵、肾俞、太溪；心脾两虚证：加心俞、脾俞、足三里。

操作方法：毫针刺，泻申脉，补照海。

（2）耳针疗法

选穴：神门、皮质下、心、肝、脾、肾、交感。

操作方法：每次选 3～5 穴，毫针刺，轻刺激，每日 1 次，每次留针 30 分钟，10 次为 1 疗程。或用王不留行子贴压，每 5～7 日更换 1 次，双耳交替使用。

5.3 感冒

感冒是指以鼻塞、流涕、喷嚏、头痛、恶寒、发热、全身不适、脉浮等为主要临床表现的一种外感疾病。一年四季均可发病，以冬、春季节为多，在外感病中最为常见。本病的发生主要由于体虚，抗病能力减弱，当气候剧变时，人体卫外功能不能适应，邪气乘虚由皮毛、口鼻而入，引起一系列肺卫症状。由于发病季节的不同及体质的差异，证候表现分为风寒、风热两大类，并有夹暑夹湿之兼证。若因风寒湿邪，则毛窍闭塞，阳气郁阻，肺气失宣；若因风热暑燥，则腠理疏泄失畅，泻热灼肺，肺失清肃。

5.3.1 辨证

（1）风寒束表

恶寒重，发热轻，头痛无汗，四肢酸楚，鼻塞声重，喷嚏，流清涕，咳嗽，痰稀而白，口不渴或喜热饮，舌苔薄白，脉浮或浮紧。

（2）风热犯表

发热重，恶寒轻，汗出或汗出不畅，口干而渴，鼻塞，流黄涕，咽喉乳蛾红肿疼痛，头痛，咳嗽，痰黄稠黏，舌苔薄黄，脉浮数。

（3）暑湿伤表

发热，微恶风，汗少，肢体酸重，头重胀痛，咳嗽痰黏，鼻流浊涕，心烦口渴，小便短赤，胸闷泛恶，口中黏腻，渴不多饮，舌苔薄黄腻，脉濡数。

5.3.2 治疗

（1）体针疗法

主穴：风池、大椎、合谷、列缺。

配穴：风寒加风门、肺俞；风热加尺泽、曲池；暑湿加中脘、足三里；鼻塞、流涕加上星、迎香；咽喉肿痛加少商点刺出血。

操作方法：毫针刺，用泻法。少商点刺放血，属于风寒大椎和风门可加用灸法，属于风热，大椎可刺络拔罐。

（2）三棱针法

取穴：耳尖、少商、商阳、尺泽等穴，每次选用 1～2 穴，点刺或刺络出血。适用于风热犯表、暑湿伤表证。

（3）拔罐疗法

取大椎、大杼、风门、身柱、肺俞等穴，每次选 2～3 穴，留罐 10 分钟；或在背部督脉、膀胱经走罐。适用于风寒束表证。

5.4 咳嗽

咳嗽为呼吸系统疾病的主要症状，根据其发病原因，概分为外感咳嗽与内伤咳嗽两大类。外感咳嗽是由于外邪侵袭肺卫而引起；内伤咳嗽则为脏腑功能失调所致。本证的发生，其原因有二：一为外感风寒、风热之邪，从口鼻皮毛而入，肺卫受感，于是肺气壅遏不宣，清肃之令失常；二为他脏病变，累及肺脏而致。或脾失健运，聚湿生痰，上犯于肺；或肝郁化火，上逆烁肺，肺失清肃均可导致咳嗽。

5.4.1 辨证

（1）风寒袭肺

咳嗽声重，痰稀色白，伴头身疼痛，鼻塞，流清涕，恶寒发热，无汗，苔薄白，脉浮或浮紧。

（2）风热犯肺

咳嗽痰黄，稠而不爽，口渴咽痛，身热，或头痛，恶风汗出，苔薄黄，脉浮数。

（3）痰湿蕴肺

咳嗽痰多，色白质稀，胸脘满闷，身重倦怠，苔白腻，脉濡滑。

（4）肝火犯肺

气逆呛咳阵作，痰少质黏，每因情绪波动而发，面红咽干，咳时引胁作痛，舌红，苔薄黄少津，脉弦数。

（5）肺肾阴虚

起病缓慢，干咳少痰，或痰中带血，潮热颧红，失眠盗汗，五心烦热，形瘦乏力，舌红少苔，脉细数。

5.4.2 治疗

（1）体针疗法

主穴：肺俞、膻中、天突、列缺。

配穴：风寒配风池、合谷；风热配大椎、曲池；痰湿蕴肺加足三里、丰隆；肝火犯肺加行间、鱼际；肺肾阴虚加肾俞、太溪和膏肓。

操作方法：根据证候虚实选用补泻。对于风寒束肺和痰湿蕴肺者，背俞穴可以用灸法或拔罐。

（2）穴位贴敷疗法

选穴：定喘、肺俞、大椎、风门、膏肓、天突、膻中。

操作方法：用白芥子、甘遂、细辛、延胡索、肉桂、胆南星等量研成细粉过 100 筛，取药粉适量加入基质，调成糊状制成直径 1cm 圆饼，贴在穴位上，每次选取 3～4 个腧穴，胶布固定 2～4 小时，每 3 日交换1 次腧穴，10 次为 1 疗程。

5.5 胃痛

胃痛可见于急、慢性胃炎，消化性溃疡，胃神经官能症，胃癌等疾病中，临床上可出现上腹胃脘部疼痛，食欲减退，或饱胀嗳气、恶心呕吐等主要症状。胃痛急性发作多因感受外邪，饮食不慎等，导致脾胃纳运失常，胃失和降，浊气上逆。慢性胃痛多因寒积于中，胃气不和，脾与胃相表里，虚寒或禀赋不足，中阳素虚，内寒产生，胃失温降；或情志不畅，劳倦过度，久病体虚，导致肝郁气滞、中焦虚寒、胃阴不足等发病。

5.5.1 辨证

（1）寒邪客胃

胃痛暴作，得温痛减，遇寒加重；恶寒喜暖，口淡不渴，或喜热饮，舌淡，苔薄白，脉弦紧。

（2）饮食伤胃

胃脘疼痛，胀满拒按，嗳腐吞酸，或呕吐不消化食物，其味腐臭，吐后痛减，不思饮食，大便不爽，得矢气及便后稍舒，舌苔厚腻，脉滑。

（3）肝气犯胃

胃脘胀痛，连及两胁，攻撑走窜，每因情志不遂而加重，善太息，不思饮食，精神抑郁，夜寐不安，舌苔薄白，脉弦滑。

（4）瘀血停胃

胃脘疼痛，状如针刺或刀割，痛有定处而拒按，入夜尤甚。病程日久，胃痛反复发作而不愈，面色晦暗无华，唇黯；舌质紫暗或有瘀斑，脉涩。

（5）脾胃虚寒

胃脘隐痛，遇寒或饥时痛剧，得温或进食则缓，喜暖喜按。伴面色不华，神疲肢怠，四末不温，食少便溏，或泛吐清水。舌质淡而胖，边有齿痕，苔薄白，脉沉细无力。

（6）胃阴不足

胃脘隐痛或隐隐灼痛。伴嘈杂似饥，饥不欲食，口干不思饮，咽干唇燥，大便干结，舌体瘦，质嫩红，少苔或无苔，脉细而数。

5.5.2 治疗

主穴：内关、中脘、足三里。

配穴：寒邪客胃加神阙、梁丘；肝气犯胃加期门、太冲、阳陵泉；瘀血停胃加膈俞、膻中；饮食伤胃加梁门、天枢；脾胃虚寒加气海、脾俞、胃俞；胃阴不足加胃俞、太溪、三阴交。

操作方法：肝气犯胃和瘀血停胃证可用平补平泻或泻法；脾胃虚寒和胃阴不足证可用补法，虚寒证加灸。神阙穴只用灸法。

5.6 便秘

便秘主要是由于肠功能紊乱而引起的。其临床主要表现是大便秘结不通，排便艰涩难下，排便周期延长；或粪质不硬，虽有便意，而排便不畅为主要临床表现的一种病证。便秘是由于素体阳盛，嗜食辛辣厚味，烟酒过度；或情志不舒；或劳倦内伤、年老体弱，病后或产后气血未复，导致肺、脾胃、肾等脏腑功能失调，津液不足，大肠传导失司所致。

5.6.1 辨证

（1）实秘

便次减少，经常三五日1次或更长时间，临厕努责，燥结难下。如属热邪壅结，则见身热、烦渴、口臭喜冷，脉滑实，苔黄燥；气机郁滞者，每见脘腹胀满或疼痛，噫气频作，纳食减少，脉弦，苔薄腻。

（2）虚秘

便秘如因气血虚者，则见面色唇爪㿠白无华，头晕心悸，神疲气怯，舌淡苔薄，脉虚细等。如阴寒凝结，则见腹中冷痛，喜热畏寒，脉沉迟，舌质淡，苔白等证。

5.6.2 治疗

体针疗法

主穴：大肠俞、天枢、支沟、上巨虚。

配穴：热结加合谷、曲池；气滞加中脘、行间；气血虚弱加足三里、气海；阳虚加灸肾俞、命门。

操作方法：虚证用补法，实证用泻法，阳气虚可用灸法。

耳针疗法

选穴：直肠下段、大肠、皮质下、膈、肝、脾。

操作方法：每次选3～5穴，常规操作，强刺激，留针30分钟。或用王不留行子压耳法。

5.7 头痛

头痛是指以患者自觉头部疼痛为主要临床表现的一种病证。头痛可以单独出现，亦可出现于多种急、慢性疾病中。头痛的病因不外乎外感与内伤两类。外感多因六淫外邪侵袭，上扰清空，壅塞经络，络脉不通；内伤多责之于肝阳上亢、痰瘀阻滞，或气血不能上荣等致肝、脾、肾三脏功能失调，发为头痛。

5.7.1 辨证

（1）风邪袭络

头痛时作，痛势较剧，痛连项背，遇风受寒则发，苔薄白，脉浮紧。

（2）肝阳上亢

头胀痛而眩，心烦易怒，夜寐不宁，或兼胁痛，面红口苦，舌红苔薄黄，脉弦。

（3）气血虚弱

头痛绵绵，头晕目眩，遇劳则甚，神疲乏力，面色不华，舌淡脉细弱。若因瘀血阻络，症见头痛经久不愈，痛处固定不移，痛如锥刺，舌紫或有瘀斑，脉细涩。

（4）痰浊内阻

头痛昏蒙，胸脘满闷，呕恶痰涎，苔白腻，脉滑或弦滑。

（5）气滞血瘀

头痛经久不愈，痛处固定不移，痛如锥刺，或有头部外伤史，舌质紫，苔薄白，脉细或细涩。

5.7.2 治疗

体针疗法

主穴：风池、百会、太阳。

配穴：风邪袭络证，按头痛部位配穴，前头痛加印堂、上星、阳白、合谷；侧头痛加率谷、外关、足临泣；巅顶痛配涌泉、太冲；后头痛配天柱、后溪、昆仑。肝阳上亢加太冲、太溪、行间；气血虚弱加气海、足三里、脾俞；痰浊内阻加阴陵泉、丰隆；气滞血瘀加合谷、三阴交、膈俞。

操作方法：随证每次选 4 ~ 6 穴，气血虚弱用补法并灸，其余诸证用泻法或平补平泻，瘀血者可点刺太阳出血。

耳针疗法

选穴：皮质下、枕、前额、颞、肝、胆和神门。

操作方法：每次选 3 ~ 4 穴，常规操作，强刺激，留针 30 分钟。或用王不留行子压耳法。

5.8 面瘫

本病指茎乳孔内急性非化脓性炎症所致的周围性面神经麻痹，又称之为"口眼歪斜"。临床表现为起病突然，多在睡眠醒来时发现面部肌肉板滞、麻木、瘫痪，不能做蹙额、皱眉、鼓腮等动作，口角歪向健侧，漱口漏水，进餐时食物常常停滞在病侧齿颊之间；病侧额纹鼻唇沟消失，眼睑闭合不全，迎风流泪。少数病人初起有耳后耳下及面部疼痛。本病多由正气不足，经络空虚，卫外不固，风邪乘虚侵袭阳明少阳经络，以致经气阻滞，经筋失养，筋肉纵缓不收而发病。

5.8.1 辨证

辨证要点：起病突然，常在睡眠醒来时发现面部肌肉板滞、麻木、瘫痪，不能做蹙额、皱眉、鼓腮等动作，口角歪向健侧，漱口漏水，进餐时食物常常停滞在病侧齿颊之间病侧额纹鼻唇沟消失，眼睑闭合不全，迎风流泪。少数病人初起有耳后耳下及面部疼痛。部分患者初起时有耳后疼痛，还可出现患侧舌前2/3味觉减退或消失，听觉过敏等证。

（1）风寒阻络

突发口眼歪斜，多有面部受凉史，如迎风睡眠、电风扇或空调对着一侧面部吹风过久等。一般无外感表证。

（2）风热阻络

面往往继发于感冒发热、中耳炎、牙龈肿痛之后，伴有耳内、乳突轻微作痛。

5.8.2 治疗

（1）体针疗法

主穴：攒竹、阳白、四白、颊车、地仓、颧髎、合谷。

配穴：风寒阻络加风池、风门；风热阻络加大椎、曲池；气血虚弱加脾俞、胃俞、足三里、三阴交；乳突后疼痛加翳风；鼻唇沟变浅加迎香透睛明；人中沟歪斜加水沟或口禾髎；颏唇沟歪斜加承浆或夹承浆。抬眉困难：加眉冲、头临泣、头维。诸穴针用平补平泻法。

操作方法：颊车、地仓采用透刺法，阳白向下平刺；面部诸穴用平补平泻法，四肢部腧穴用泻法；病初期针刺手法宜轻，后期可加艾灸。

（2）皮肤针疗法：叩刺阳白、颧髎、地仓、颊车，以局部潮红为度，隔日1次。适用于发病初期或恢复期。

5.9 腰痛

腰痛是指腰部疼痛，为临床常见的一种症状。其疼痛部位或在脊中，或在一侧、或两侧俱痛。腰痛多因感受风、寒、湿邪，邪入经脉，痹阻不通；或因闪挫跌仆，气滞血瘀，经脉不通而致腰痛；也有因体虚精亏，房劳伤肾，腰府失养所致腰痛。

5.9.1 辨证

（1）寒湿痹阻

腰部重痛、酸麻，或拘急强直不可俯仰，或痛连骶、臀、股、腘，疼痛时轻时重，每遇天寒阴雨发作或加剧，苔白腻，脉沉迟缓。

（2）气血瘀滞

多有腰部外伤史，腰痛如刺，痛有定处，痛处拒按，日轻夜重，轻者俯仰不便,重则不能转侧。舌质暗紫,或有瘀斑,脉涩。

（3）肾气虚损

起病缓慢,隐隐作痛,或酸多痛少,绵绵不已,腰腿酸软无力,劳则更甚。如兼神倦,腰冷,滑精,四肢不温,舌淡,脉沉细者为肾阳虚。如伴有虚烦咽干、手足心热,溲黄,舌红,脉细者为肾阴虚。

5.9.2 治疗

（1）体针疗法

主穴：肾俞、大肠俞、腰夹脊穴、委中、阿是穴。

配穴：寒湿加风府、腰阳关；血瘀加膈俞、次髎；肾虚加命门、太溪、大钟。

操作方法：肾虚者用补法,寒湿和血瘀治者用泻法,血瘀可在委中点刺放血。

（2）耳针疗法

选穴：腰骶椎、肾、神门、皮质下。

操作方法：每次选2~3穴,常规操作,中重刺激,留针30分钟。或用王不留行子压耳法。

5.10 坐骨神经痛

坐骨神经痛是指在坐骨神经通路及其分布区域的疼痛。临床表现为疼痛有腰部经臀部、大腿、小腿后外侧向足部放射,多为一侧疼痛,弯腰或活动下肢时加重。可由多种原因引起。临床分为原发性和继发性两类,否则按受损部位又分为根性和干性两种。本证属于中意的"痹证""腰痛"和"腰腿痛"范畴主要由感受风寒湿邪,经络痹阻；或肾气虚损,经络失养；或外伤闪挫,经络气血瘀滞而致腰腿疼痛。

5.10.1 辨证

（1）寒湿痹阻

多发于感受寒湿之后,腰腿疼痛重着,屈伸不利自觉患部寒冷,每遇阴雨寒冷病势加重。苔白或白腻，脉沉。

（2）肾气虚弱

起病缓慢，隐隐作痛，日久不愈，腰腿酸软无力，劳则更甚。舌淡，脉沉细。

（3）气血瘀滞

多有腰部外伤史，腰腿疼痛如刺，痛有定处，痛处拒按，日轻夜重，轻者俯仰不便，重则不能转侧。舌质暗紫，或有瘀斑，脉涩。

5.10.2 治疗

体针疗法

主穴：3~5 腰夹脊穴、大肠俞、环跳、委中、阳陵泉、悬钟、丘墟。

配穴：寒湿痹阻加腰阳关、秩边、承扶、飞扬、昆仑；肾气虚弱加肾俞、大钟；气滞血瘀加水沟、后溪。

操作方法：根据病情每次选 4~5 个穴。寒湿者，针用泻法，温针灸或艾条灸并可加拔火罐；肾虚者，针刺用补法，温针灸或艾条灸；有瘀滞者，针刺用泻法，委中穴及其附近的瘀阻络脉点刺放血。

5.11 落枕

落枕是以颈部强痛，活动受限为主要特征的一种病证，多见于成人。多由劳后体乏，睡卧不当；或枕头不适，风寒乘虚而入；或颈部扭伤，均可导致气血痹阻，不通则痛。

5.11.1 辨证

晨起始觉颈部不适，或头歪向一侧，左右转动不便。患侧颈项酸痛，可影响及肩。局部肌肉痉挛，压痛明显，轻者一般 3~5 日即可缓解，也有反复发作者。

5.11.2 治疗

（1）体针疗法

主穴：外劳宫、肩井、后溪、阿是穴。

操作方法：针刺用泻法，向针刺远端穴，并让患者活动颈部，后刺局部穴，起针后，可在局部拔火罐。

（2）耳针疗法

选穴：颈、颈椎和压痛点。

操作方法：强刺激，同时让患者活动颈部，留针 15～20 分钟。

5.12 颈椎病

颈椎病是指由于颈椎与颈部软组织，如椎间盘、黄韧带、脊髓鞘膜等发生病理改变，刺激或压迫颈神经根、脊髓、血管、交感神经和其周围组织而引起的综合证候群。临床上可分为软组织型、神经根型、脊髓型、椎动脉型、交感神经型等。本病为中老年人最常见，以 40～50 岁发病率最高。颈部软组织劳损和椎间盘退行性病变是引起本病的主要原因，外伤、劳累、风寒外感、枕头及卧姿不当常为诱发因素。中医认为，年高体弱，肝肾不足，正气亏虚，筋骨失养，为本病内因，外感风寒、湿、热，或扭挫损伤为本病的外因，二者相互作用，致使太阳经经气不利，气血运行不畅，或筋脉失其所濡，或日久气滞血瘀，经脉闭阻不通而发为本病。

5.12.1 辨证

（1）外感风寒

颈项强痛，或痛连肩臂，肢冷手麻，或觉沉重，受风遇寒加重，伴周身酸痛，苔薄白，脉浮紧。

（2）气滞血瘀

颈项肩臂酸胀疼痛或刺痛，或肿胀，或向手臂放射，伴有头晕头痛，精神抑郁、紧张时加重，舌苔白，脉弦涩。

（3）肝肾不足

起病缓慢，颈项肩臂麻木隐痛，日久不愈，劳累后加重，伴眩晕、视物模糊、耳鸣耳聋、腰膝酸软、舌淡，苔白，脉沉细无力。

5.12.2 治疗

（1）体针疗法

主穴：3～5 颈夹脊穴风池、完骨、大椎、天柱、合谷、中渚。

配穴：感风寒加外关、风门、肩井；气血瘀滞加曲池、肩髃、膈俞、阳陵泉；肝肾不足加肝俞、肾俞、悬钟。

治疗方法：虚证用补法，实证用泻法，可以用灸法和拔罐。

（2）耳针疗法

选穴：颈、颈椎、肩、神门。

操作方法：每次选 2～3 穴，常规操作，中重度刺激，留针 30 分钟。或用王不留行子压耳法。

5.13 肩关节周围炎

肩关节周围炎是由于肩关节退行性病变，加之长期劳损、感寒，或外伤等原因，而导致的关节囊和关节周围软组织慢性炎症病变。临床以肩部疼痛和肩关节运动功能障碍为主要症状，早期以疼痛为主，后期以肩部功能障碍为主，好发年龄在 50 岁左右。本病属于中医的"痹证"范畴。多由风寒湿邪乘虚而入，或年老体弱，筋脉失养，或气血凝滞使经络痹阻，气血不行，经筋失用，发生本病。

5.13.1 辨证

早期为阵发性疼痛，常因天气变化及劳累而诱发，其疼痛可向颈部和上臂放散，或呈弥散性疼痛。以后逐渐发展至持续性疼痛，并逐渐加重，昼轻夜重，严重者不能睡眠，不能向患侧侧卧；病延日久，肩关节的上举、外展、内旋活动明显受限，影响梳头、摸背、穿衣等动作。严重者，肘关节功能亦受限，屈肘时不能抬肩。

5.13.2 治疗

（1）体针疗法

主穴：肩髃、肩髎、肩贞、臂臑、阿是穴、条口透承山。

配穴：肩前疼痛加合谷、曲池、足三里；肩外侧和肩胛疼痛加后溪、外关、天宗、阳陵泉；肩背部疼痛加曲垣、天宗。

操作方法：针刺用泻法。先针刺远端腧穴，条口透承山，并让患者活动肩关节，后刺局部腧穴，可以配合运用艾灸和拔罐。

（2）电针疗法

选穴：肩髃、肩髎、肩贞、曲池、阿是穴。

操作方法：每次选用 1~2 穴，针刺得气后。通以脉冲电流 10 分钟。每日 1 次。

5.14 带状疱疹

带状疱疹是以沿周围神经分布区域皮肤出现簇状水疱群，成带状排列，局部有烧灼样刺痛为主证的一种急性疱疹性皮肤病。好发于一侧的胸部、头面部、眼、腹部、股部等处。中医认为本病多因肝经郁火和脾经湿热内蕴，复又感受风湿热毒，以致引动肝火，湿热蕴蒸，浸淫肌肤而发。当邪阻经络日久，气血运行不畅，血瘀阻络，则局部疼痛迁延不愈。

5.14.1 辨证

发疹前患部皮肤灼热，呈束带状刺痛，伴有轻度发热、倦怠乏力、食欲不振等症状。继之皮肤潮红，出现不规则红斑，随之在红斑上生有集簇样粟状丘疹，1 日内迅速变为绿豆至黄豆大小的簇集成群的水疱，中间夹以血疱或脓疱，疱疹中心凹陷，如脐窝状，聚集一处或数处，呈带状排列。2~3 周后，疱疹逐渐干燥结痂，最后痂退而愈。愈后不留瘢痕，少数患者遗留有不定时疼痛感。

5.14.2 治疗

（1）体针疗法

主穴：阿是穴、相应的夹脊穴。

配穴：肝经火毒加太冲、行间、侠溪；脾经湿热加阴陵泉、内庭、血海；发热者加大椎；发于胸胁部位的加支沟、期门、膈俞、肝俞。

操作方法：针刺用泻法。在病变部位多针围刺，也可用灸法。或用三棱针点刺疱疹及周围，拔火罐，令每罐出血3~5ml。

（2）皮肤针法

用皮肤针叩刺疱疹周围皮肤，中强度刺激，可加拔火罐，每日1~2次。

5.15 四肢软组织扭伤

四肢软组织扭伤是指肩、肘、腕、髋、膝、踝关节周围软组织损伤，但无骨折、脱臼和皮肤破损，以局部肿胀、疼痛和关节活动受限为主证的外科病证。本病多因用力不当或闪挫跌仆，伤及筋肉脉络，气滞血瘀而成。

5.15.1 辨证

扭伤部位因瘀阻而肿胀疼痛，伤处皮肤青紫，患肢关节有不同程度的功能障碍，常伴有局部热痛。如红色多系皮肉受伤，青色多系筋伤，紫色多系瘀血留滞。新伤局部微肿，肌肉压痛，表示伤势较轻；如红肿高耸，关节屈伸不利，表示伤势较重。

5.15.2 治疗

（1）体针疗法

主穴：局部阿是穴。

配穴：肩部加肩髃、肩髎、肩井；肘部加曲池、小海、天井；腕部加阳池、阳溪、阳谷、外关；髋部加环跳、秩边、承扶；膝部加梁丘、膝阳关、阳陵泉；踝部加解溪、昆仑、丘墟。

操作方法：针刺用泻法，可用灸法和火罐。

（2）耳针疗法

取穴：反应点、神门。

操作方法：中强刺激，留针 20～30 分钟，每日 1 次。陈旧伤可用王不留行子压耳法。

5.16 痛经

痛经是指妇女凡在经期或经行前后，出现周期性小腹疼痛，或痛引腰骶，以致影响工作和正常生活者。生殖器官无明显异常者称原发性痛经，因生殖器官的自行病变而致的称为继发性痛经。本病多因经期受寒饮冷，寒邪客于冲任；或情志抑郁，郁怒伤肝，致肝郁气滞，经血滞于胞宫；或素体虚弱，或大病久病，气血亏虚，或禀赋素弱，肝肾不足，以致冲任气虚血少，胞脉失养，而发痛经。

5.16.1 辨证

（1）寒湿凝滞

少腹冷痛，拒按，得热痛减。经血量少，畏寒肢冷，苔白，脉沉紧者为寒凝。

（2）气滞血瘀

经期或经前小腹胀痛，经行不畅，量少，色紫黑夹有血块，伴有胸胁乳房胀痛，舌质紫或有瘀点，脉弦。

（3）气血不足

经期或经后小腹隐痛，痛势绵绵不休，喜揉喜按，量少，伴有神疲乏力，腰骶酸痛，头晕心悸，舌淡，脉细弱。

（4）肝肾两虚

经后小腹隐痛，月经先后不定期，经量或多或少，舌淡红无血块，伴，腰膝酸软，夜卧不宁，头晕耳鸣，舌红少苔，脉细。

5.16.2 治疗

（1）体针疗法

主穴：中极、次髎、三阴交。

配穴：寒湿凝滞加归来、关元、水道；气滞血瘀加太冲、血海；气血不足加脾俞、足三里；肝肾两虚加肝俞、肾俞、太溪。

操作方法：经前 3~5 天开始治疗。实证用泻法，可加灸；虚证用补法，也可用灸法。

（2）耳针疗法

选穴：内生殖器、皮质下、交感、内分泌、肝、肾。

操作方法：每次取 2~4 穴，毫针中强刺激，亦可用王不留行子压耳。为防止复发，每于月经来潮前 3 天开始治疗。

5.17 乳少

乳少是指产后乳汁分泌甚少或全无的病证。本病的主要发病机理一为化源不足，二为瘀滞不行。如素体气血虚弱，又因分娩失血过多，气血耗损，致气血生化之源不足，而不能化生乳汁，或因素性抑郁，或产后情志不遂致肝郁气滞，乳汁运行不畅而致缺乳。

5.17.1 辨证

（1）气血不足

产后乳少，甚或全无，乳汁清稀，乳房柔软，无胀痛，食少神倦，面色无华，舌淡少苔，脉细弱。

（2）肝郁气滞

产后乳少，乳房胀硬疼痛，情志抑郁，胸胁胀满，食欲不振，苔薄，脉弦细。

5.17.2 治疗

主穴：乳根、膻中、少泽。

配穴：气血不足加脾俞、足三里、三阴交；肝郁气滞加期门、太冲。

操作方法：少泽穴点刺放血。虚证用补法，实证用泻法。

5.18 胎位不正

正常胎位中，绝大多数为枕前位。如果妊娠 30 周后，经产前检查发现胎位呈枕后位、臀位、横位等称胎位不正。常见于多产或产妇腹壁松弛孕妇。本病多因孕妇素体虚弱，中气不足，无力促胎调转，或孕后肝郁不舒，气机失畅，胎儿不得回转，以致胎位不正。

5.18.1 辨证

胎位不正可通过妊娠后期腹壁成肛门检查而发现。在临产时常表现为宫颈扩张缓慢、宫缩不强、胎儿窘迫成死亡，有的可发生产道损伤。

5.18.2 治疗

主穴：至阴。

操作方法：灸至阴矫正胎位，操作时嘱孕妇放松裤带，平卧床上，或坐在靠背椅上，采用艾条灸双侧至阴穴 15～20min，每日 1～2 次，灸至胎位正常。

5.19 小儿遗尿

小儿遗尿是指 3 周岁以上儿童在睡眠中小便自遗，醒后方觉，并反复出现的一种儿科常见病证。轻者数日遗尿 1 次，重者每夜自遗。中医认为本病多因肾气不足，下元虚寒，封藏失职，膀胱气化失职，固摄无权而致；或因肺脾气虚，上虚不能制下，膀胱约束无力，致使小便自遗。

5.19.1 辨证

（1）肾阳不足

睡中遗尿，甚者一夜数次，尿清而长，神疲乏力，面色苍白，畏寒肢冷，腰膝酸软，小便频数，舌淡，脉沉迟无力。

（2）肺脾气虚

睡中遗尿，劳累后尿床加重，尿频量少，常自汗出，精神不振，少气懒言，四肢乏力，纳呆便溏，舌淡，脉细。

5.19.2 治疗

主穴：中极、关元、膀胱俞、百会、三阴交。

配穴：肾阳不足加肾俞、命门；肺脾气虚配肺俞、脾俞、气海、足三里。

操作方法：毫针刺用补法或温针灸或灸法。

5.20 目赤肿痛

目赤肿痛为多种眼疾中的一个急性症状，以目赤、睑肿、疼痛为主证。本病多因外感风热时邪，侵袭目窍，郁而不宣；或因肝胆火盛，循经上扰，血壅气滞于目，致使目赤肿痛。

5.20.1 辨证

（1）风热外袭

起病较急，目睛红赤，沙涩灼热，羞明流泪，眵多清稀，伴头痛，苔薄黄，脉浮数。

（2）肝胆火盛

起病较缓，病初眼有异物感，视物不清，继而白睛红赤肿痛，畏光羞明，眵多胶结，伴口苦咽干，烦热不寐，溲赤便结，舌红，苔黄，脉弦数。

5.20.2 治疗

（1）体针疗法

主穴：太阳、睛明、风池、太冲、合谷。

配穴：风热外袭加上星、曲池；肝胆火盛加行间、侠溪。

操作方法：针刺用泻法，不能用灸法。太阳、上星可点刺出血。

（2）挑刺

选穴：肩胛区寻找敏感点或大椎旁 0.5 寸处。

操作方法：所选穴位常规消毒，用 6 号注射针头挑断皮下白色纤维2～3 根，用干棉球按压伤口。

5.21 耳鸣耳聋

耳鸣、耳聋是指听觉异常。耳鸣以自觉耳中鸣响，耳聋以听力减退或听觉丧失。两者虽有不同，但往往同时存在，后者多由前者发展而来。两者由于在病因病机及针灸治疗方面大致相同。本病多因风邪侵袭，壅遏耳窍；或因情志不畅，肝胆火旺，循经上犯闭阻；或因肾虚气弱，精气不能上达于耳所致。

5.21.1 辨证

（1）实证

起病迅速，耳聋，或耳中流脓，鸣声隆隆不断，按之不减。兼头痛、眩晕、目红面赤、口苦咽干、烦躁善怒，舌红，苔黄，脉弦者，为肝胆火旺；可见畏寒、发热，苔薄白或苔黄，脉浮者，为外感风邪。

（2）虚证

起病缓慢，耳聋，耳中如蝉鸣，时作时止。劳累加剧，按之鸣声减弱。兼见头晕，腰膝酸软乏力，舌红，苔少，脉细数。

5.21.2 治疗

主穴：翳风、听会、听宫、中渚。

配穴：肝胆火旺加太冲、侠溪；风邪侵袭加外关、合谷；肾气虚弱加肾俞、太溪。

操作方法：实证用泻法，虚证用补法。

5.22 咽喉肿痛

咽喉肿痛是口咽部和咽喉部位病变的一个主要病证，以咽喉部红肿疼痛、吞咽不适为特征。本病多因风热犯肺，热邪熏灼肺系；或因过食辛辣煎炒，引动胃火上蒸，津液受灼，煎炼成痰，痰火蕴结；或肺肾阴虚，虚火上炎，灼于咽喉而致咽喉肿痛。

5.22.1 辨证

（1）风热侵袭

咽喉红肿疼痛，吞咽困难，伴有发热、恶寒、头痛，苔薄白，脉浮数。

（2）肺胃热盛

咽喉疼痛逐渐加剧，吞咽困难，痰多黏稠，伴有口干渴、便秘、溲黄，舌红，苔黄厚，脉洪大。

（3）肺肾阴虚

咽喉不适，口干，疼痛较轻，或吞咽时觉疼痛，入夜症状加重，伴口干咽燥、五心烦热，舌红，苔少，脉细数。

5.22.2 治疗

（1）实证

主穴：少商、廉泉。

配穴：风热侵袭加合谷、关冲；肺胃热盛加内庭、鱼际。

操作方法：少商点刺放血，其余腧穴用泻法。

（2）虚证

主穴：廉泉、鱼际、太溪、列缺、照海。

配穴：潮热盗汗加阴郄、三阴交、复溜。

操作方法：主穴用平补平泻，配穴用补法，不用灸法。

5.23 单纯性肥胖

肥胖系机体生化或生理功能改变，致使体内膏脂堆积过多引起的病证。临床上一般以体重超过标准体重的20%，且常伴有食欲异常、睡眠异常、口干、排便异常等症状。本病多因脾胃功能失常，气血阴阳失调，导致肥胖发生。如胃肠腑热，则食欲旺盛，纳食过多，脂膏积存；脾胃虚弱，则使痰湿内生，流于肌腠；或真元不足，气化失常，水湿滞留而发生肥胖。

5.23.1 辨证

（1）胃肠腑热

食欲旺盛，消谷善饥，口干喜饮，怕热多汗，急躁易怒，大便闭结，小便黄赤，舌质红，苔黄腻，脉滑数。

（2）脾胃气虚

食欲不振，食后腹胀，神疲乏力，嗜睡懒言，大便稀溏，舌淡边有齿印，苔薄白，脉细缓。

（3）脾肾阳虚

面色㿠白，气短而喘，动则汗出，头晕腰酸，口渴饮少，或怕冷肢肿，女性多伴月经不调，男子或见阳痿，舌质淡嫩，苔少，脉沉细无力。

5.23.2 治疗

（1）体针疗法

主穴：中脘、曲池、天枢、丰隆、阴陵泉、支沟、内庭、太冲。

配穴：胃肠腑热加合谷、足三里；脾胃气虚加脾俞、胃俞、足三里、太白；脾肾阳虚加气海、关元、肾俞、命门；便秘加天枢、支沟、阳陵泉；腹型肥胖加归来、下脘、中极。

操作方法：胃肠腑热用泻法，脾胃气虚和脾肾阳虚用补法或平补平泻。

（2）耳针疗法

选穴：饥点、胃、内分泌、口、食道、肺、胃、胰胆。

操作方法：毫针刺，或用王不留行子贴压，每天在餐前、睡前自行按压3次，每次2~3分钟，双耳交替，10次为1疗程。

图书在版编目（CIP）数据

中国针灸：英、汉／张卫东，王丕敏主编．—太原：山西科学技术出版社，2020.7

ISBN 978 - 7 - 5377 - 5853 - 6

Ⅰ.①中… Ⅱ.①张… ②王… Ⅲ.①针灸学—英、汉 Ⅳ.①R245

中国版本图书馆 CIP 数据核字（2019）第 071094 号

中国针灸

ZHONGGUOZHENJIU

出　版　人：赵建伟

主　　　编：张卫东　　王丕敏

责 任 编 辑：王　璇

封 面 设 计：吕雁军

出 版 发 行：山西出版传媒集团·山西科学技术出版社

地　　　址：太原市建设南路 21 号　邮编：030012

编辑部电话：0351 - 4922135　　　邮箱：shanxikeji@ qq. com

发 行 电 话：0351 - 4922121

经　　　销：全国新华书店

印　　　刷：山西基因包装印刷科技股份有限公司

网　　　址：www. sxkxjscbs. com

微　　　信：sxkjcbs

开　　　本：720mm×1010mm　　1/16　　印张：34. 75

字　　　数：690 千字

版　　　次：2020 年 7 月第 1 版　2020 年 7 月山西第 1 次印刷

书　　　号：ISBN 978 - 7 - 5377 - 5853 - 6

定　　　价：148 元

本社常年法律顾问：王葆柯

如发现印、装质量问题，影响阅读，请与编辑部联系调换。